Body Sculpting with Silicone Implants

Nikolas V. Chugay • Paul N. Chugay
Melvin A. Shiffman

Body Sculpting with Silicone Implants

With contribution of Dr. Barry Friedberg
and Allen Andrews

Springer

Nikolas V. Chugay
Long Beach
CA
USA

Melvin A. Shiffman
Tustin
CA
USA

Paul N. Chugay
Long Beach
CA
USA

ISBN 978-3-319-04956-4 ISBN 978-3-319-04957-1 (eBook)
DOI 10.1007/978-3-319-04957-1
Springer Heidelberg Dordrecht London New York

Library of Congress Control Number: 2014936601

Printed on acid-free paper

Springer is part of Springer Science+Business Media (www.springer.com)

Preface

The Road Less Traveled

Body sculpting with implants is something that surgeons have been doing for over 50 years, since the advent of breast augmentation implant procedures in the early 1960s. I personally have been performing body implant surgery, outside of breast augmentation, for over 20 years and have seen all manner of patients and conditions requiring or wanting muscle sculpting. The first body implant procedure that I became familiar with was, of course, breast augmentation surgery. I think most of us that do body implants begin with breast enlargement procedures and grow into doing other muscle augmentation procedures. Breast augmentation is a relatively facile procedure with immediate results for both patient and surgeon. It is for that reason that muscle augmentation procedures are equally gratifying—immediate gratification.

My experience with body implants began just over 20 years ago when there was a patient that wanted to have a calf enlargement procedure. It was a procedure that I had not performed to that point but was willing to learn. I went to Dr. Bircoll in Beverly Hills and watched him perform several calf enlargement procedures. The procedure appeared to be technically easy to perform with results that were good. Since beginning calf augmentation in the early 1990s, I have performed calf augmentation procedures on body builders, on patients that had difficulties with clubfoot deformity and congenital defects of the legs, and on patients with acquired asymmetries from trauma. Calf implants have really served well in helping these patients to achieve symmetry and improved self-esteem.

The early work with calf implants made me wonder about augmenting other muscle groups. It was around that same time period that another patient approached me about doing buttock augmentation. I was aware of the work done by Gonzalez Ulloa in Mexico City. He had used silicone gel prostheses placed on top of the gluteus muscle to augment the buttock region. Some of his early works were done with patients that had suffered deformities in the gluteal region as a result of trauma or injections of various filler materials with subsequent infection and necessity to reconstruct the gluteal area. After reading about some of his early cases, I was intrigued and began studying the anatomy of the region and considered the possibility of placing the gluteal implant under the gluteus maximus muscle and on top of the gluteus medius muscle. Robles had published about a procedure where he had placed the silicone prosthesis under both the maximus and medius muscles but saw that sciatic irritation was produced because of the proximity of the implant to the sciatic nerve due to deep implant placement. After reading about his work, I spoke with my professor and mentor, Ivo Pitanguy, about the possibility of placing the implant above the medius muscle. He encouraged me to proceed with the idea. Similarly, my discussions with Richard Webster resulted in words of encouragement for placement of the implants below the gluteus maximus but above the medius muscle. I then proceeded to design an anatomic solid silicone implant as the implants at that time were very hard and difficult to position under the gluteus muscle. Our initial results on 20 patients was published in the *American Journal of Cosmetic Surgery* in 1997. All of the patients in the series had a good cosmetic improvement without evidence of sagging as the prosthesis was well supported by the overlying gluteus maximus, which acted as a hammock for the prosthesis. In the original buttock augmentation procedures, it was my custom to place the incision in the superior portion of the buttock; however, this left noticeable scars. I then adapted the technique of Gonzalez Ulloa and placed the implants through an intergluteal incision. The original implant that I had designed was manufactured for me by ABT Corp. and measured 4.1 cm in length by 12.5 cm in width by 2.8 cm in height.

After my work in buttock augmentation, I began to explore pectoral augmentation. In evaluating the work of existing surgeons, I noted that the implants were not well supported in the lateral aspect. In order to correct this matter, the pectoral augmentation procedure was modified through the axillary approach to include reinforcement in the lateral aspect. The pectoralis was well visualized during the operative procedure and was then reapproximated to the lateral chest wall/rib periosteum to prevent lateral migration of the implant and palpability of the lateral portion of the implant.

As the popularity of the pectoral augmentation procedure grew, there were more and more patients asking for augmentation of their arms as well. It so happened that I was attending a course in New York City hosted by Sherrell Aston when a publicist asked if I was doing any other sculpting procedures with implants. My office manager at the time was with me in New York and said to the publicist that "Dr. Chugay is considering doing biceps augmentation in the near future." The publicist was all excited and then called me for more information. Hating to make my office manager out to be a liar, I had to come up with a biceps augmentation procedure. In my initial work, the implant was placed in the submuscular plane. This, however, caused significant postoperative pain and involved more risk in the process of dissection. Later, I began to place the implants in a subfascial plane that improved the safety of the procedure. The procedure was initially designed to help patients that had suffered trauma to the biceps muscle and had a depression or deformity in the area of the biceps. It was also quite useful in reconstruction of the arm when large tumors had been excised and created asymmetry between the two extremities. I found it equally useful in giving patients more volume in the area of the biceps when they were unable to achieve that added volume through exercise on their own. Later, as the procedure became more popular, I had body builders wanting the procedure done as the incision was well hidden in the axilla and amplified their already large arms. Our work in biceps augmentation has been published in the *American Journal of Cosmetic Surgery*, and it continues to be a popular surgery with excellent results in over 200 patients.

Triceps augmentation came as a natural add-on to the existing list of muscle augmentation procedures. Quite a number of patients wanted to have their triceps enlarged, and I developed an implant to position in the triceps region along the long head of the triceps muscle, beneath the fascia.

Next, in the list of muscle augmentation procedures came the development of the deltoid augmentation procedure. At the time that I had developed the triceps implant, I had a patient that presented with marked hypoplasia of the right deltoid. He was a principal of a high school and had been bothered for some time by his students about the asymmetry of his arms. He had undergone multiple procedures to improve the deformity but without significant results. So, he asked me whether I could design an implant that can be placed in the area of his rudimentary deltoid muscle, perhaps submuscularly, that would give him the bulk and the volume that he wanted. So, I had an implant developed for me by Aesthetic and Reconstructive Technologies, Inc. (AART, Reno, Nevada). Since they had helped me in enhancing my gluteal implant and biceps implants and developed my triceps implant, I knew that I could trust them with this new adventure. Within a few weeks, we had the deltoid implant ready. The surgery was then scheduled. Plans were made for an incision right over the deltoid muscle. Dissection would then be carried through the rudimentary deltoid muscle to a submuscular plane. Postoperatively, the patient was ecstatic with the result even though the improvement was not dramatic and he was not perfectly symmetric. To him, the change was huge and it gave him more self-confidence, thereby achieving our goal with the procedure.

So the saga continued. Next, in our list of muscle augmentation procedures came hip augmentation. I had a transgender patient that approached me about the possibility of building out her hips. The patient had a masculine and very narrow hip area which she wanted to have made into a more feminine hip. We designed an implant that was very similar to some of the smaller buttock implants, made of a soft silicone material. In this patient, we placed our custom-made implant on top of the fascia lata, in a very superficial position. The patient was ecstatic with the result; but, I was not entirely pleased as you could still see the well-delineated edges of the implant. The capsule that formed around the implant was also visible when the patient was examined months after the procedure. I proceeded to develop a procedure where the implant would be placed right along the lateral aspect of the femur. The implant was placed under the fascia lata, over the top of the femoral shaft. My early experience with this procedure was similarly published in the *American Journal of Cosmetic Surgery*. Since that time, I have had quite a few patients, particularly Asians with poor development of the hip area and transgender patients, benefit from the procedure. We have also seen females with developed hip regions, wanting more of a Kardashian or J Lo figure, benefit from the implant in the lateral hip/thigh region to create a more accentuated hourglass figure.

Now, after all these procedures, you will naturally ask what comes next. Well, we are looking at various options. There are some implants available for six-pack abdominal augmentation. However, these implants can shift and produce very unnatural results if complications occur. Also, the implants do not move fluidly with the patient. We have looked at possibly developing six small prostheses that would be placed under the rectus abdominis fascia in the area bounded by the inscriptions of the rectus abdominis. This would then accentuate a patient's already defined abdominal musculature and create a more natural-appearing six-pack abs.

Over the years, I have had a great deal of fun developing and perfecting these procedures. They literally added an extra zest to my practice. I hope that you will enjoy reading about the various procedures that I have developed/ improved upon.

The next generation of muscle augmentation procedures will rest with my son, Paul Chugay. He has recently joined me in practice and continues to be the coauthor on our works in the field of muscle augmentation. We are performing many of these procedures together, allowing me to pass on my knowledge and experience to him. It has been a great deal of fun teaching him how to perform these procedures, and together we are constantly improving upon what I have already been able to design/improve upon.

I hope this book will be of use to you and help you in taking care of your patients. Should you ever have any questions/concerns, I am at your service.

Nikolas V. Chugay, DO

Contents

1 Body Implants: Overview

Allen Andrews

Introduction

Biomaterials, as a category, have exploded over the past decade with new materials being developed and qualified for use in medical applications. Along with all of the new materials, silicone has maintained its position as arguably the best known and positioned as the gold standard. Silicone is a generic, extremely broad term for materials that contain a backbone consisting of repeating silicon-oxygen atoms where each silicon atom also has two organic groups (Fig. 1.1). These organic groups (-R) are most commonly methyl but may also be vinyl, trifluoropropyl, phenyl, or a myriad of other organic groups. By varying these groups, different physical and chemical properties may be conferred on the resultant polymer. Most silicone polymers can be placed into three general categories based on their methodology of curing or polymerization: addition cure (most common), condensation cure, and peroxide cure.

Curing or Polymerization

Addition cure utilizes the addition of a silylhydride to a site of unsaturation, normally a vinyl group. This reaction is catalyzed by a metallic compound, usually platinum. The catalyst may be present in a concentration range of 5–20 ppm, but most commonly is present at the lower end such as 7–8 ppm. Should multiple silylhydrides be preset in the same molecule, they will react with vinyl groups in the prepolymer creating a crosslinked network. Most silicone polymers used in medical devices are manufactured using the addition cure system. This system is routinely a two-part system where one part contains the platinum catalyst, vinyl functionality, and sometimes an inhibitor. The other part contains the silylhydride crosslinker as well as the presence of vinyl functionality on the silicone backbone. These two parts when mixed thoroughly can be pumped, poured, or injected into containers (molds) which are configured in the shape desired. There is a finite time during which this can occur. This is called the working time. Beyond this time, the mixture becomes too thick to work with and is unusable. Once in the container (mold), heat is then used to activate the mixture initiating the cure or vulcanization process resulting in an elastomer. These same basic sequences are used for easily flowable materials such as liquid silicone rubber (LSR) or thick, non-pumpable polymers such as high consistency rubber (HCR).

Condensation cure may be one- or two-part systems and utilizes hydrolyzable groups on both the crosslinker and polymer components. The one-part system is more common. When removed from their storage containers, they react with moisture from the atmosphere which diffuses through the polymer. This results in the hydrolysis of the reactive group on the crosslinker molecule. The silanol species

N.V. Chugay et al., *Body Sculpting with Silicone Implants*,
DOI 10.1007/978-3-319-04957-1_1, © Springer International Publishing Switzerland 2014

Fig. 1.1 Molecular formula for silicone

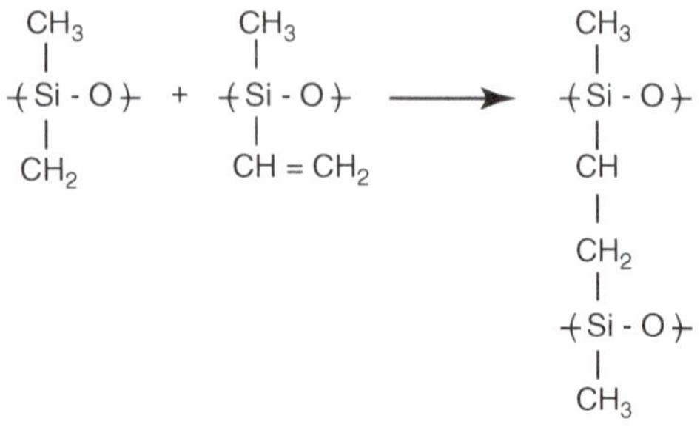

As these reactions are repeated, the crosslink network results.

formed can then react with a hydrolyzable group attached to the polymer end. When repeated on the same crosslinker molecule, the crosslink network results. These one-part systems are referred to as room temperature vulcanization (RTV). Though not used routinely in the primary fabrication of medical components, RTVs are commonly used as an adhesive to bond other silicone materials together. Two-part RTVs are occasionally used in the fabrication of medical parts where part thickness exceeds 0.2 in. (5 mm).

Peroxide cure utilizes the decomposition of an organic peroxide to form a free radical that produces polymerization with the backbone polymer. Peroxide cure systems are currently not commonly used in medical device applications due to issues with residual peroxides and their decomposition products such as PCBs. Historically, post-curing (elevated heat and/or vacuum) treatments have been used to volatilize or remove the offending materials. These days most manufacturers simply use another curing (vulcanization or polymerization) system such as the addition cure system.

From a practical standpoint, the overwhelming majority of medical products on the market today utilize addition cure vulcanization during the fabrication of silicone elastomers including gels. The most common of these use the methyl functional organic group (-R) and when cured are called polydimethylsiloxane or abbreviated as PDMS. The molecular weight and physical properties of these polymers can vary dramatically from low molecular weights (silicone oils) to high molecular weights and/or with high degrees of crosslinking (Sh-D molded parts).

Design and Manufacture

The design and manufacture of silicone implants for cosmetic, plastic, and reconstructive therapies requires knowledge of and insight into the physiological and mechanical interactions that take place between the implant, tissues that surround the implant, and where on the body the implant is located. This understanding must also contemplate the normal daily activities and forces envisioned for the individual. As an example, implants designed for the breast are expected to perform their function in a very different physiological environment from an implant designed for the buttock or gluteus. Both at their essence are simple void fillers; however, forces exerted on the gluteal area are far greater and more demanding than those exerted on the chest area. Similarly, there are different requirements for bone on-lay products such as a chin implant versus a nasal implant. The former is used to augment or replace bone while the latter is used to augment or replace cartilage. It is a core design belief for AART, Inc. (AART), to closely match or mimic the physical properties of the native tissues that they are augmenting or replacing.

Implants provided by AART (Aesthetic and Reconstructive Technologies, Inc., Reno, NV) are divided into two major groups: body contouring implants such as calf, gluteal, pectoral, etc. and facial implants such as chin, malar (cheek), nasal, etc. All of the implants are manufactured utilizing state-of-the-art Implant Grade raw materials. Other manufacturers such as PIP in France, which used food grade silicone instead of Implant Grade for its gel breast implant, have created controversy casting negative impressions over all in the industry, physicians and manufacturers alike.

Body contouring implants are larger in volume and designed to augment or replace muscle, fat, or a combination. The physical properties (e.g., hardness) of implants vary depending on application area. Generically, the softest normally is associated with the buttock or gluteal area. Chest implants for males generically are harder and calf implants are somewhere in the middle depending on the desires of the patient and/or surgeon. Implants for other muscle groups such as biceps, triceps, or quadriceps follow suit.

Facial implants by their nature are substantially smaller in volume and are designed to augment or replace bone or cartilage. These implants are substantially harder and can be more complex. In keeping with its philosophy, AART varies the physical properties dependent on the needs of the application site, for example, chin (harder) or nasal (softer). As the nasal is replacing cartilage, it should be softer to minimize skin erosion (wearing its way through the skin). Everyone remembers Michael Jackson. Consideration of implant edges and edge location is paramount in facial implants.

Due to patient's unique aesthetic considerations, custom implants are a third major grouping. AART has three approaches to custom implants. They are presented below in order of increasing cost.

1. The first is a simple description by the surgeon sometimes with a hand drawing providing the appropriate dimensions.
2. The second is the production of a moulage or visual sample using materials available to the surgeon or AART's Moulage Kit, a two-part self-reacting silicone.
3. The third option is to utilize digital data to design an implant with high precision and that is unique to the individual. Generally, a CAT scan or MRI is taken of the patient and the implant is designed to present the aesthetic result desired. The implant can be visualized separately as well as within the framework of the scan (Figs. 1.2 and 1.3).

   While the cost is more for a custom implant, many consider the personalization and additional adjustments for their unique needs well worth the additional cost.

AART manufactures all of its implants in an appropriate controlled atmosphere room (Nominal Class 10,000 (ISO 7)) and specific tasks such as curing in Class 100 ovens or trimming and washing under a Class 1,000 laminar flow hood (Figs. 1.4, 1.5, 1.6, and 1.7). Utilization of these technologically advanced workstations to perform specific tasks is not required by the regulatory agencies but ensures enhanced cleanliness and minimizes contamination potential.

The following are the most commonly used body implant styles and sizes as employed by Dr. Nikolas Chugay and Dr. Paul Chugay (Figs. 1.8, 1.9, 1.10, 1.11, 1.12, 1.13, 1.14, 1.15, 1.16, 1.17, 1.18, 1.19, 1.20, and 1.21).

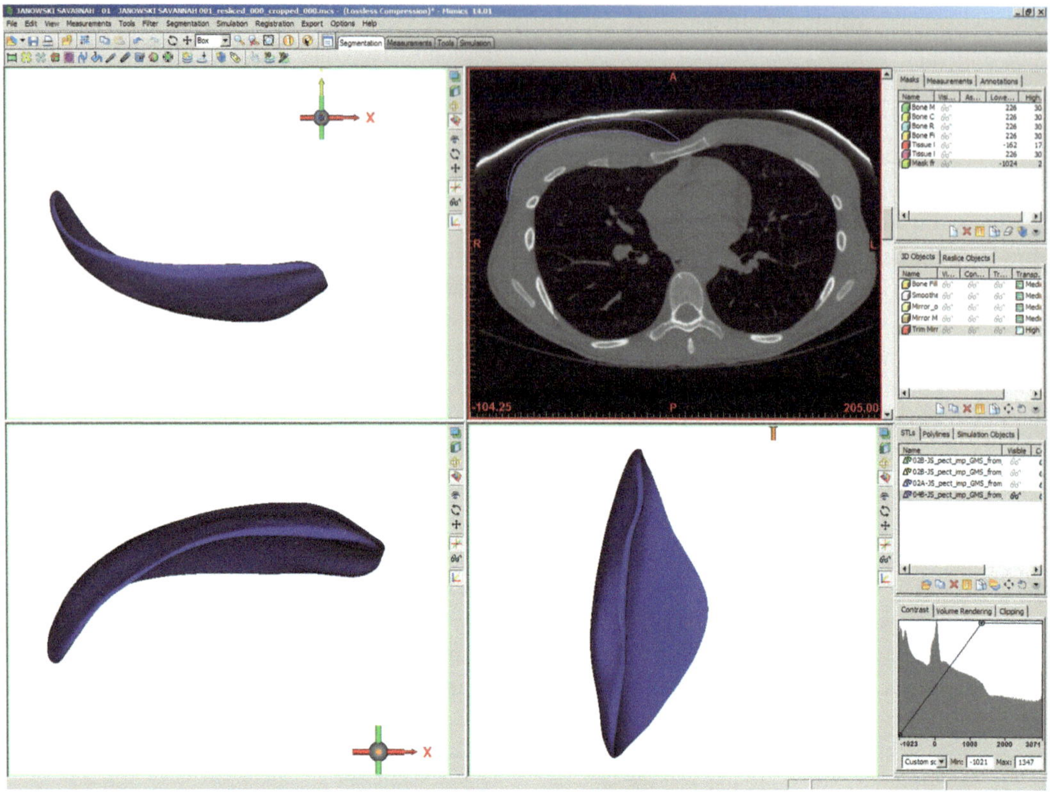

Fig. 1.2 Rendering of implant based on CT of patient presenting for pectoral augmentation

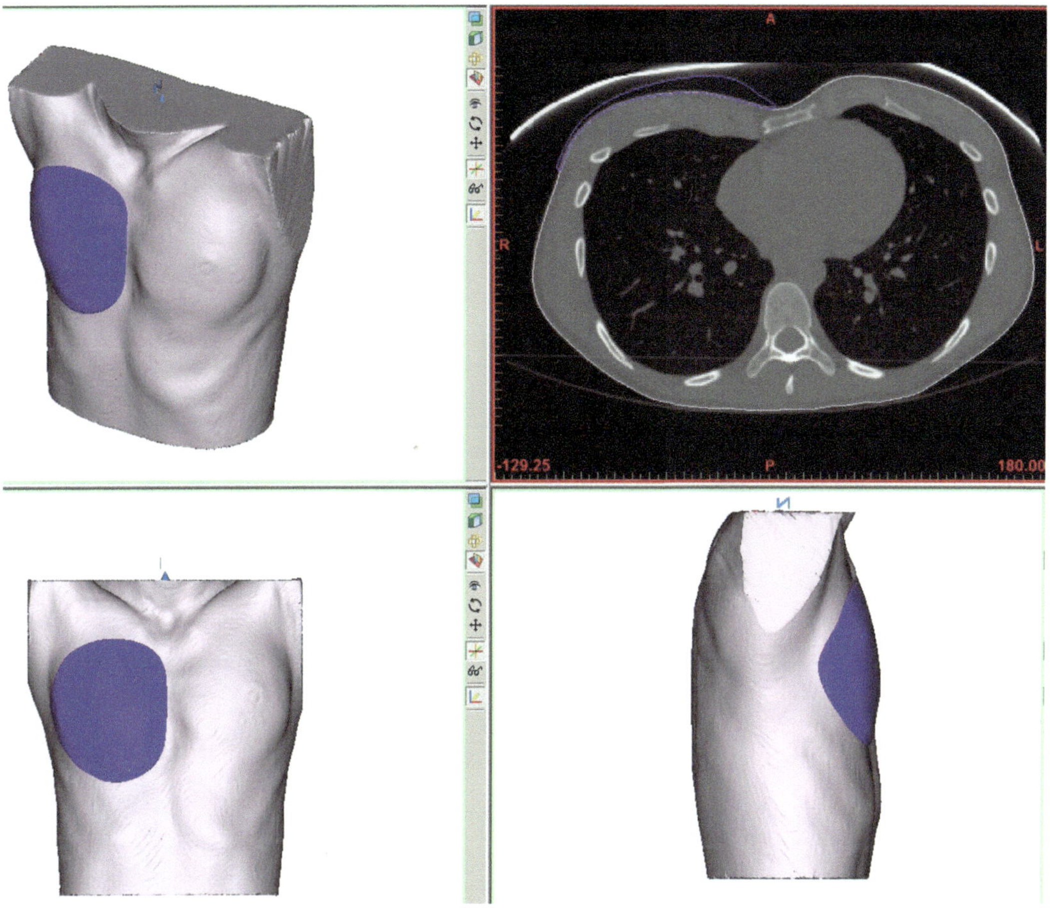

Fig. 1.3 Another view of rendering of implant based on CT of patient presenting for pectoral augmentation

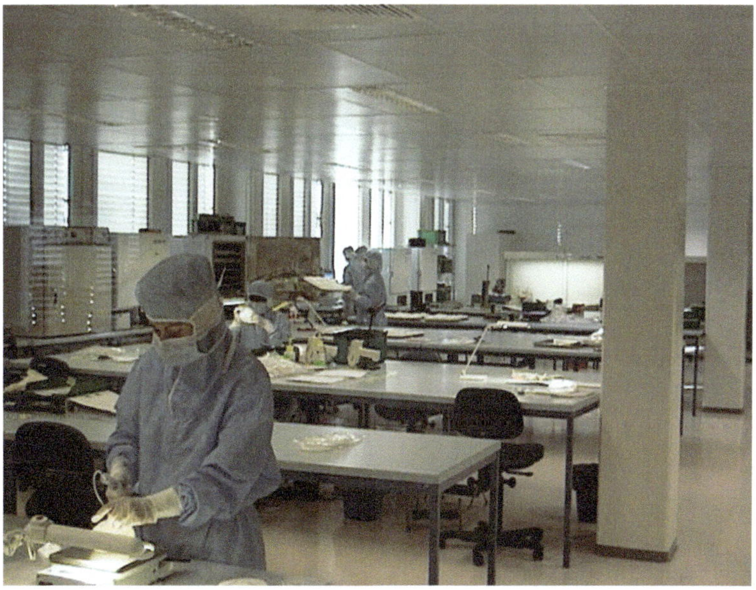

Fig. 1.4 Clean room assembly

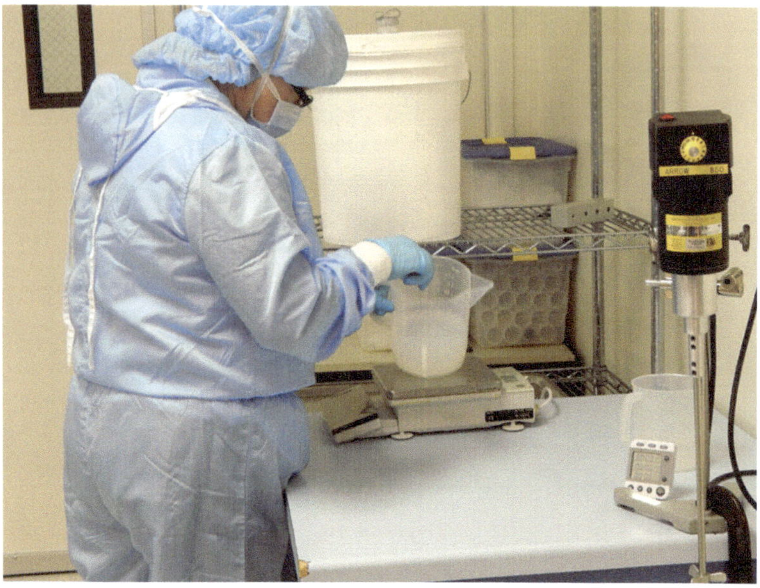

Fig. 1.5 Clean room mixing

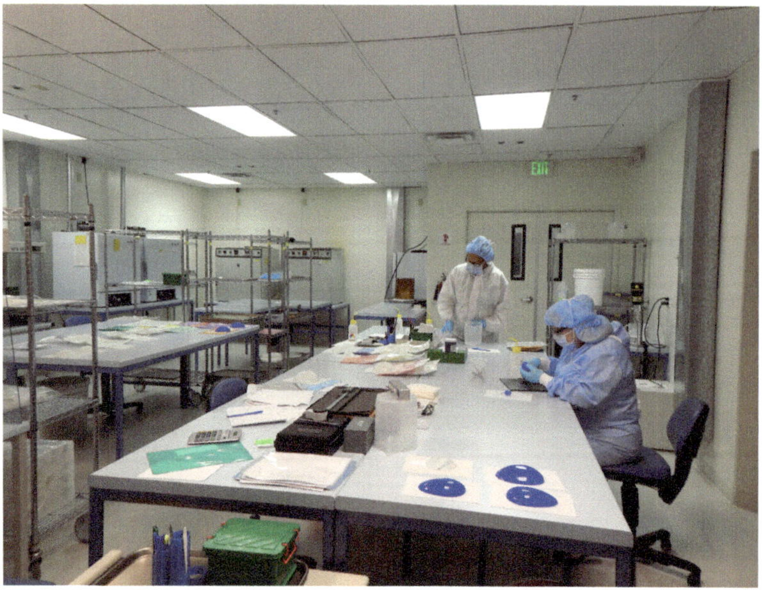

Fig. 1.6 Clean room demolding and trimming

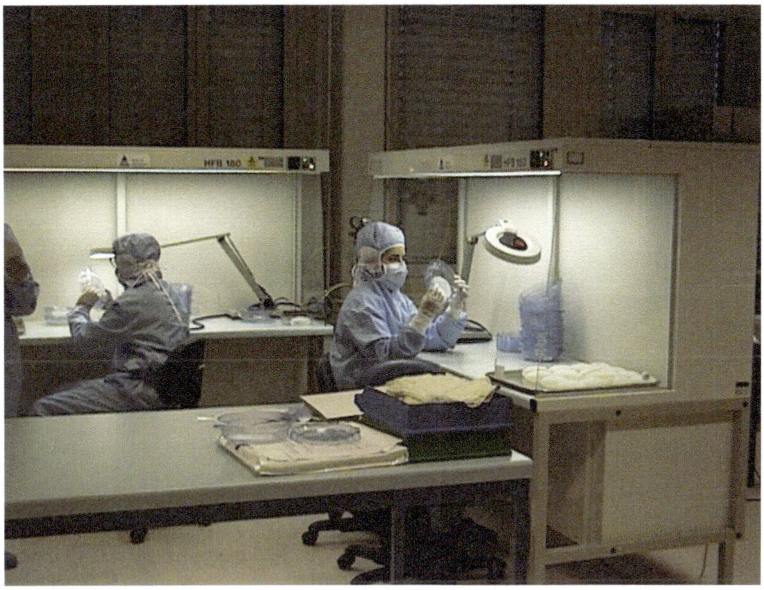

Fig. 1.7 Clean room packaging

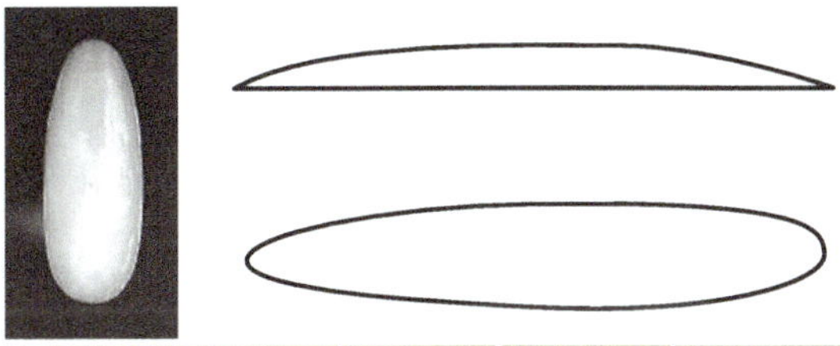

Size	Catalog#	Width	Length	Projection	Volume (cc)
1	600–801	6.2	16.3	2.3	151
2	600–802	5.8	13.3	2.0	60
3	600–803	5.9	13.3	2.4	86

Fig. 1.8 Biceps implants

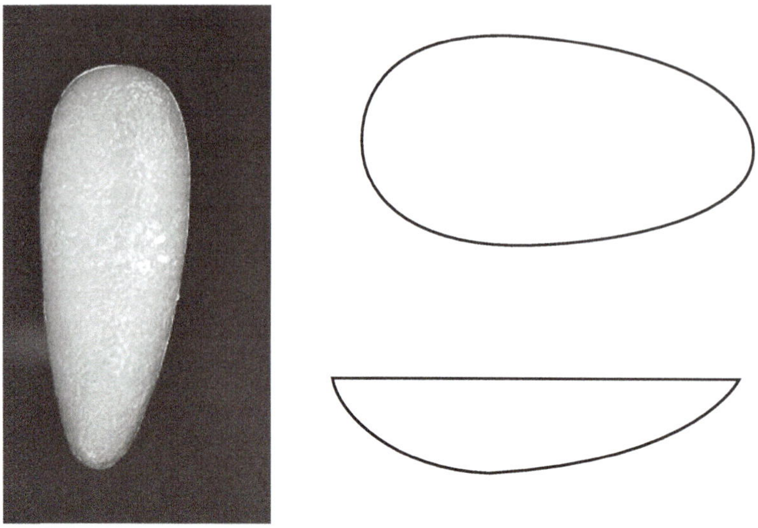

Size	Catalog#	Width	Length	Projection	Volume (cc)
1	600–820	10.0	5.0	2.2	
2	600–825	15.0	6.0	2.2	

Fig. 1.9 Triceps implants

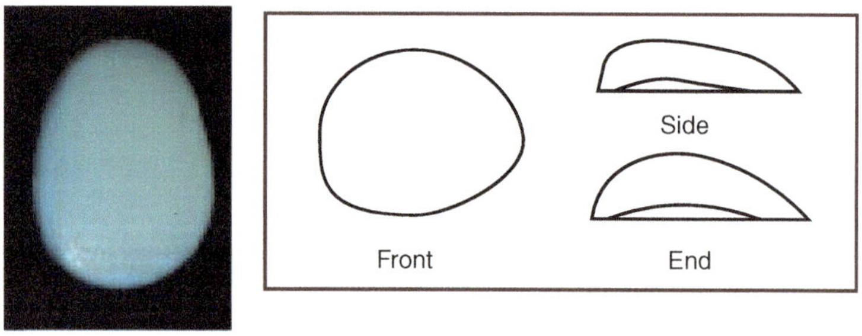

Style 1

	Catalog#	Width	Length	Projection	Volume (cc)
Size 1	500–101	14.7	11.4	2.7	234
Size 2	500–102	15.4	12.0	3.0	273
Size 3	500–103	16.1	13.7	3.1	349
Size 4	500–104	15.5	12.0	2.1	189
Size 5	500–105	16.1	12.5	2.3	222
Size 6	500–106	17.0	14.6	2.5	289

Fig. 1.10 Pectoral implants: style 1

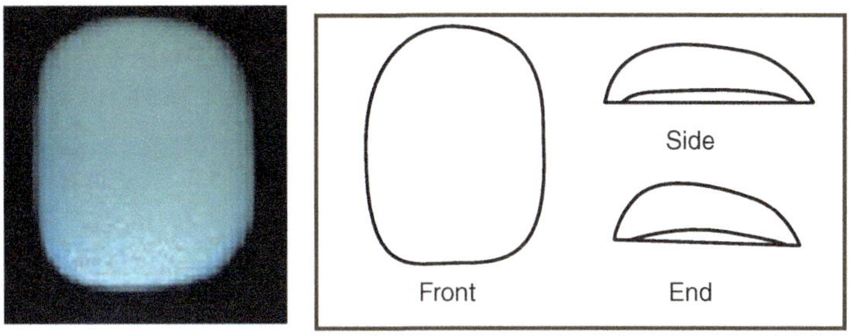

Fig. 1.11 Pectoral implants: style 2

Style 2	Catalog#	Width	Length	Projection	Volume (cc)
Size 0	500–200	13.3	14.8	1.9	230
Size 1	500–201	13.0	15.4	2.2	294
Size 2	500–202	13.8	16.1	2.7	367
Size 3	500–203	13.9	16.6	2.9	409

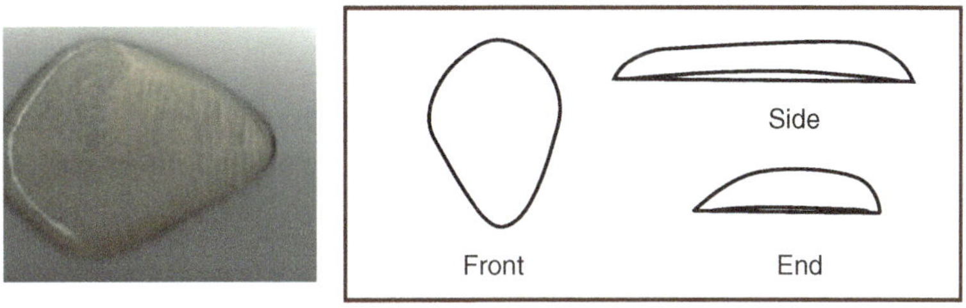

Fig. 1.12 Pectoral implants: style 3

Style 3 Catalog#		Width	Length	Projection	Volume (cc)
Size 1	500–301	13.8	18.5	2.5	300
Size 2	500–302	14.9	18.9	2.7	328

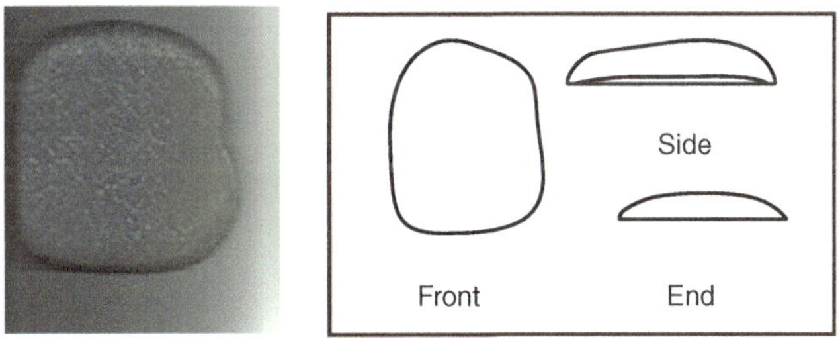

Style 4	Catalog#	Width	Length	Projection	Volume (cc)
Size 1	500–401	11.4	16.8	2.3	231
Size 2	500–401	13.4	16.0	2.3	349
Size 3	500–403	14.5	17.0	2.5	449
Size 4	500–404	15.5	18.0	2.5	490

Fig. 1.13 Pectoral implants: style 4

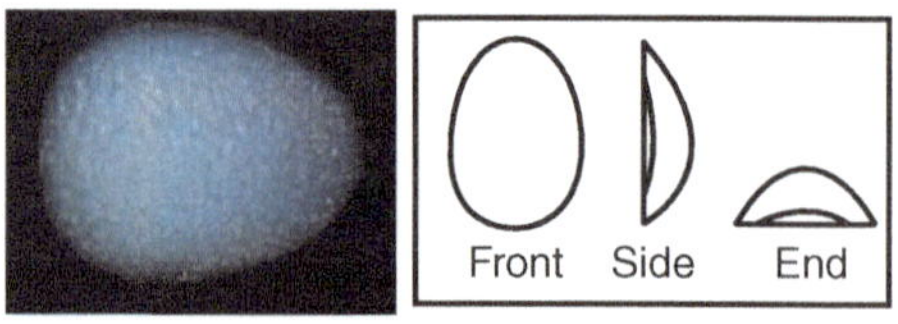

Fig. 1.14 Buttock implants: style 1

Size	Catalog#	Width	Length	Projection	Volume (cc)
1	501–101	10.4	15.0	2.5	207
2	501–102	11.0	15.6	3.1	250
3	501–103	13.5	18.0	4.6	545
4	501–104	11.1	16.2	3.2	303
5	501–105	11.5	16.6	3.6	328
6	501–106	12.9	18.0	4.2	435

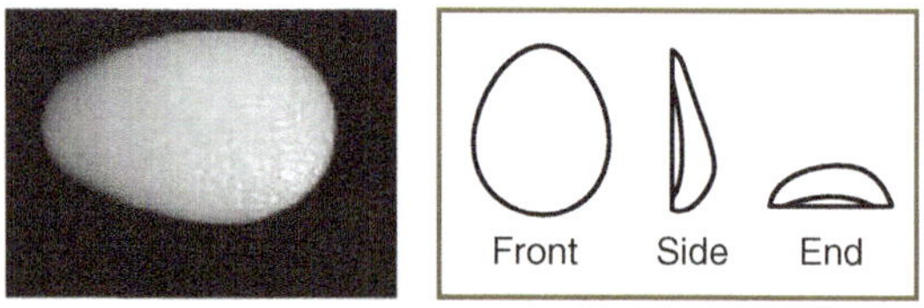

Fig. 1.15 Buttock implants: style 2

Size	Catalog#	Width	Length	Projection	Volume (cc)
1	501–201	12.4	14.5	2.5	194
2	501–202	12.7	15.4	2.9	234
3	501–203	12.8	16.5	3.3	292
4	501–204	13.4	18.0	3.8	375
5	501–205	14.6	19.3	4.8	575
6	501–206	12.5	16.4	4.6	430

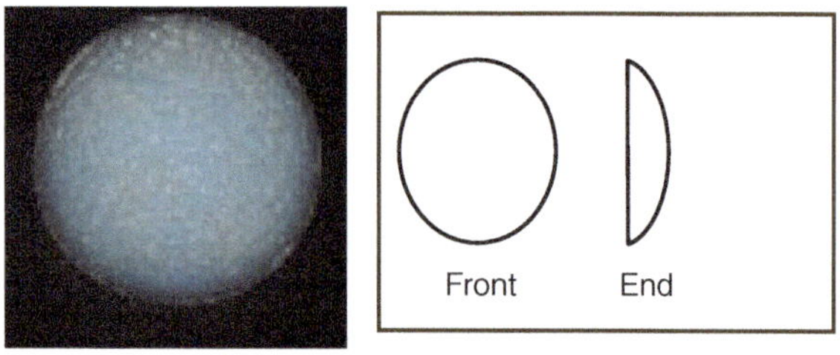

Size	Catalog#	Diameter	Projection	Volume (cc)
0	501–300	10.5	2.5	117
1	501–301	12.5	2.8	189
2	501–302	13.4	3.6	276
3	501–303	14.5	3.8	379
4	501–304	13.4	4.9	434
5	501–305	13.5	3.7	301
6	501–306	15.0	5.5	713
7	501–307	12.5	4.0	296
8	501–308	12.0	3.5	215
9	501–309	15.0	4.5	485
10	501–310	15.0	5.0	550

Fig. 1.16 Buttock implants: style 3

Fig. 1.17 Hip implants

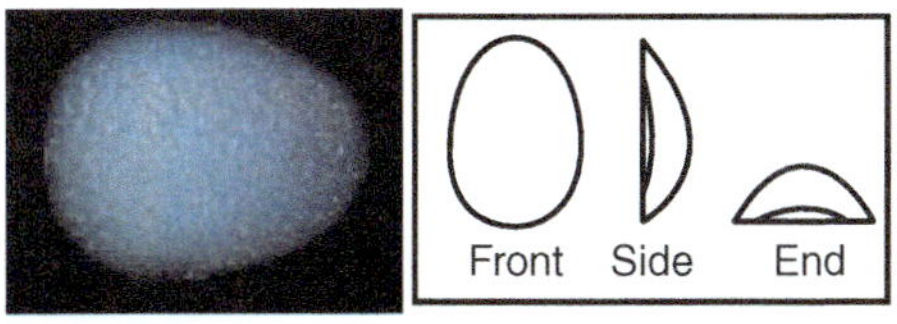

Size	Catalog#	Width	Length	Projection	Volume (cc)
1	501–101	10.4	15.0	2.5	207
2	501–102	11.0	15.6	3.1	250
3	501–103	13.5	18.0	4.6	545
4	501–104	11.1	16.2	3.2	303
5	501–105	11.5	16.6	3.6	328
6	501–106	12.9	18.0	4.2	435

Fig. 1.18 Calf implants: style 1

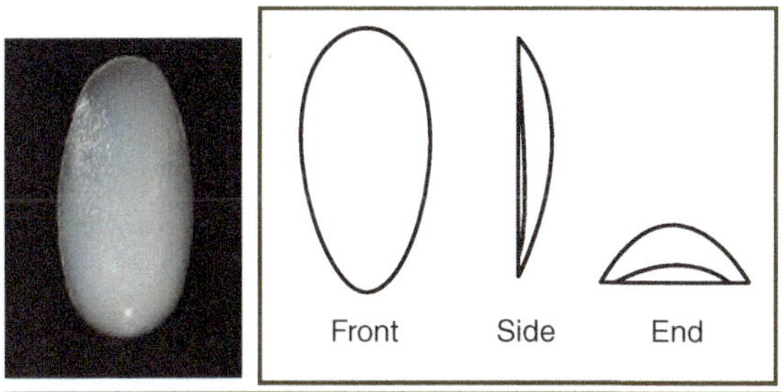

Size	Catalog#	Width	Length	Projection	Volume (cc)
1	501–101	6.2	12.7	1.6	53
2	501–102	6.9	13.9	1.7	68
3	501–103	7.8	14.2	1.9	91
4	501–104	9.5	16.3	2.0	131
5	501–105	11.3	17.3	2.7	275
6	501–106	9.5	16.3	2.5	147
7	501–107	9.7	17.2	2.3	192

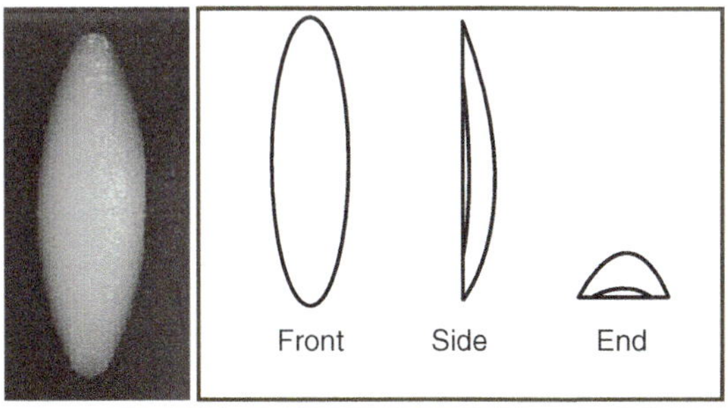

Size	Catalog#	Width	Length	Projection	Volume (cc)
1	502–201	6.1	17.4	2.1	94
2	502–202	6.5	20.7	2.3	126

Fig. 1.19 Calf implants: style 2

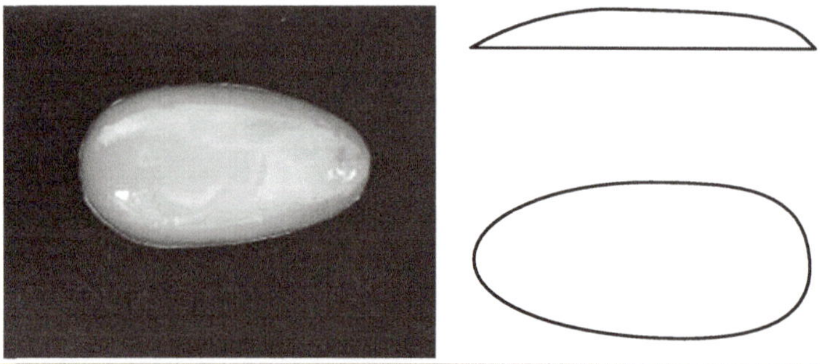

Fig. 1.20 Calf implants: style 3

Size	Catalog#	Width	Length	Projection	Volume (cc)
0	502–300	5.2	12.5	1.5	49
1	502–301	6.5	14.0	1.7	72
2	502–302	6.7	14.3	1.8	80
3	502–303	8.0	14.6	2.0	133
4	502–304	9.5	16.5	2.2	163
5	502–305	6.2	13.5	1.6	68
6	502–306	6.5	14.5	1.8	81
7	502–307	7.9	14.7	2.0	110
8	502–308	9.1	17.1	2.0	144
9	502–309	5.7	12.4	1.5	47

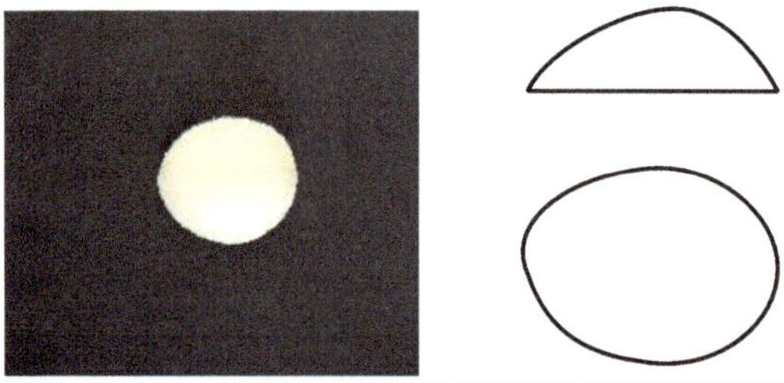

Size	Catalog#	Width	Length	Projection	Volume (cc)
1	1100–01DEL	8.0	10.0	2.0	116
2	1100–01DEL	8.0	10.0	3.0	115
3	1100–01DEL	8.0	10.0	4.0	161

Fig. 1.21 Deltoid implants

Propofol-Ketamine (PK) Anesthesia in Body Implant Surgery

2

Barry Friedberg

Poetry in Motion

All cosmetic surgery, including body implant surgery, can be performed under local anesthesia alone. When awake patients have pain during the case, they may move, but they also communicate verbally of their inadequate analgesia, i.e., "Ouch!" (Fig. 2.1).

More often than not, general inhalation anesthesia (GA) or propofol-opioid (i.e., alfentanil or remifentanil) total intravenous anesthesia (TIVA) is used for greater control of patient movement. Greater patient movement control obscures vital information about inadequate local analgesia to the (postoperative) detriment of the patient. No postoperative patient benefit could be determined when preemptive local analgesia was injected after induction of GA and prior to incision as seen in a meta-analysis of 80 studies [1].

Figure 2.2 clearly illustrates brain function is not necessary to produce movement. Movement in a sedated patient may also occur with or without brain involvement. Without the ability to discern brain-generated movement from that generated from the spinal cord, one remains stuck in the twentieth century mode of anesthesia wherein all patient movement had to be treated as if it might be a sign of patient awareness or recall.

Patient movement under sedation is almost always the patient's request for more local analgesia (Fig. 2.3). Brain-monitored propofol permits the differentiation between the need for more local analgesia (spinal cord-generated movement) and the need for more propofol (brain-generated movement). The ability to differentiate, and subsequently more appropriately treat, the two distinctly different types of patient movement results in less inappropriate types (and amounts) of adjuvant drugs being given to sedated patients.

Some surgeons direct their own diazepam (or midazolam)-ketamine anesthesia [2] with an impressive safety record. However, benzodiazepine sedation has no reliable, reproducible clinical signs for adequacy of brain protection from negative ketamine side effects. Currently available cerebral cortical monitors do not reliably measure benzodiazepine effect.

Direct measurement of anesthetic effect on the cerebral cortex has only been available since the 1996 FDA approval of the Bispectral Index® (BIS) (Aspect Medical Systems, Inc.) monitor. While

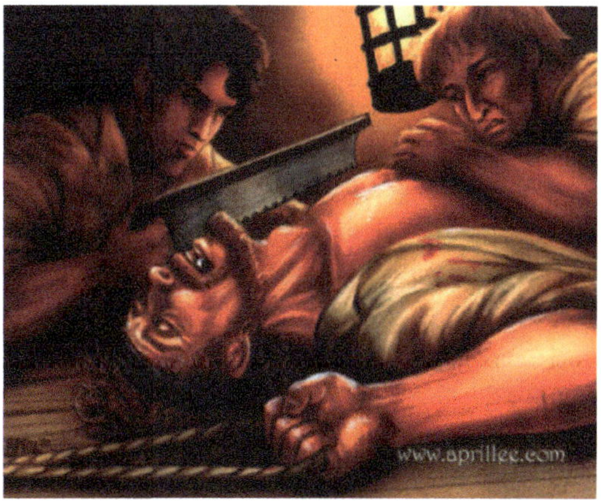

Fig. 2.1 Surgery without pain: an achievable PK goal

N.V. Chugay et al., *Body Sculpting with Silicone Implants*,
DOI 10.1007/978-3-319-04957-1_2,

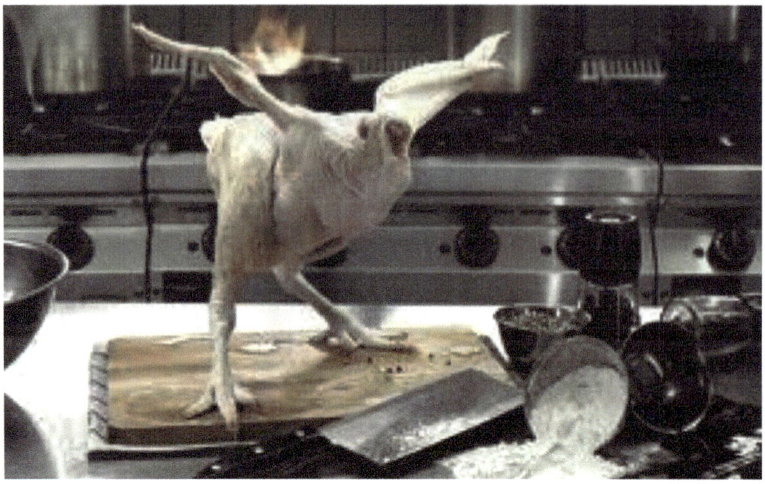

Fig. 2.2 Headless chicken generating movement

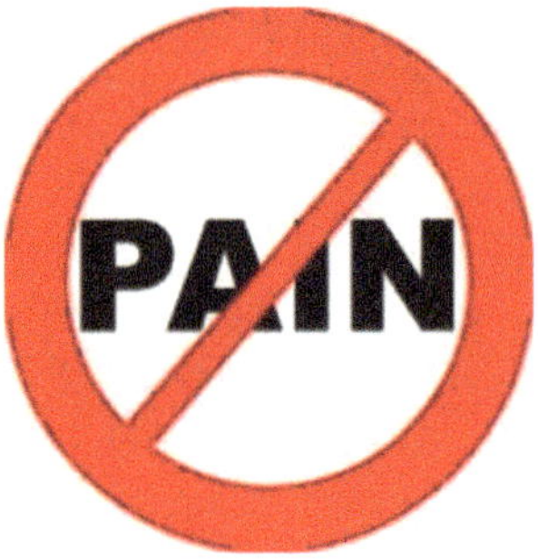

Fig. 2.3 Adequate local analgesia is a critical element of PK anesthesia

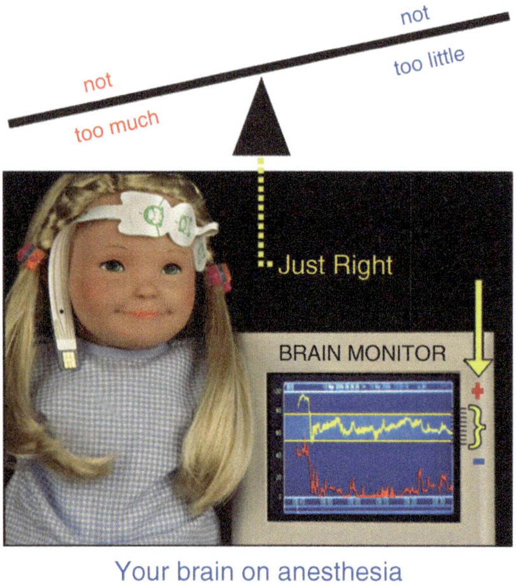

Fig. 2.4 BIS/EMG monitored PK MAC (aka "Goldilocks" anesthesia)

cerebral cortical monitoring does not replace vital signs, like heart rate and blood pressure, vital signs only reflect brain stem activity (Fig. 2.4).

Brain stem activity (i.e., vital signs) simply cannot reliably guide the cerebral cortical effect, as was standard anesthetic practice prior to 1996. The net result of this void of cortical effect information was routine over-medication to prevent under-medication (anesthesia awareness). Complex activities like processing hearing, feeling, and recall occur in the cerebral cortex. Clearly, then direct cerebral cortical monitoring should be part of the twenty-first century anesthetic practice.

Over the past 21 years, propofol-ketamine (PK) monitored anesthesia care (MAC) has appeared as an alternative to both GA and propofol-opioid TIVA. From March 26, 1992 through December 25, 1997, PK anesthesia was more art than science. With the addition of BIS/EMG monitoring on December 26, 1997, numerical reproducibility was achieved [3].

Propofol-Ketamine TIVA [4] or "Ketofol"

There is no precise definition of what ketofol is. Generally ketofol refers to the 50:50 mixture of ketamine and propofol, 0.5 mg/kg of each

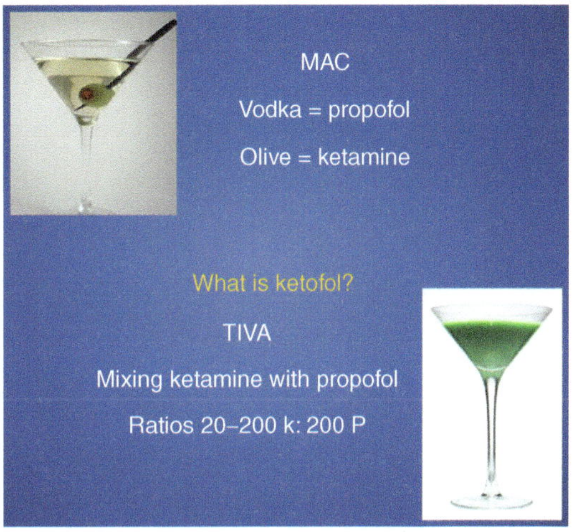

Fig. 2.5 Vodka martinis illustrating the difference between PK MAC and PK TIVA (aka ketofol)

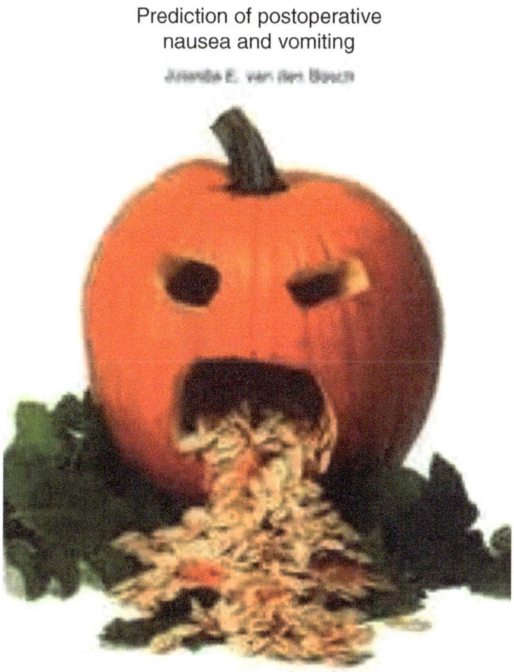

Fig. 2.6 Emesis is our nemesis

(Fig. 2.5). However, a broader definition considered that ketofol is the combination of ketamine and propofol, regardless of the ratio to each other (the initial dose of each can be scaled up to 3 mg/kg). When they are used in infusion, the dose is 100 μg/kg/min.

The principle objection to ketofol is the inability to ascertain the amount of hypnosis (propofol effect) and the degree of NMDA block (ketamine effect) with induction and prior to the initial local anesthetic injection. The secondary objection is the potential for exceeding 200 mg ketamine during the case, potentially prolonging emergence. Conversely, PK MAC clearly defines hypnosis (BIS <75, baseline EMG) prior to dissociation (immobility with injection).

Anesthesia considerations for body implant cosmetic surgery revolve around the three parties' concerns – the patient, surgeon, and anesthesiologist. The key consideration is that the patient is the first priority! The patient wants (1) not to hear, feel, or remember their surgery, a cerebral cortical effect, and (2) to awaken promptly without pain, prolonged emergence, or postoperative nausea and vomiting (PONV) (Fig. 2.6), a function of anesthetic technique.

The surgeon wants a motionless patient during the surgery and the fewest possible postoperative concerns. Numb patients rarely move under sedation. Without a brain monitor to assure adequate propofol sedation levels (i.e., BIS <75, EMG baseline vide infra), it is nearly impossible to encourage the surgeon to re-inject a vasoconstricted field.

The anesthesiologist wants reproducibility along with control of the patient's airway and movement during surgery. However, this is confounded by variations in patients' cerebral tolerance to medication effect in addition to their varying ability to metabolize and eliminate the anesthetic agents.

Friedberg's Triad answers the patients' desires, the surgeon's needs, and the anesthesiologist's quandary over what drug or intervention is most appropriate when facing patient movement under sedation.

1. Measure the brain
2. Preempt the pain
3. Emetic drugs abstain

"Measure the brain" means incrementally titrating propofol to BIS <75 with baseline electromyogram (EMG) (Fig. 2.7). Brain measurement provides numerically reproducible propofol levels to protect the brain from negative ketamine side effects.

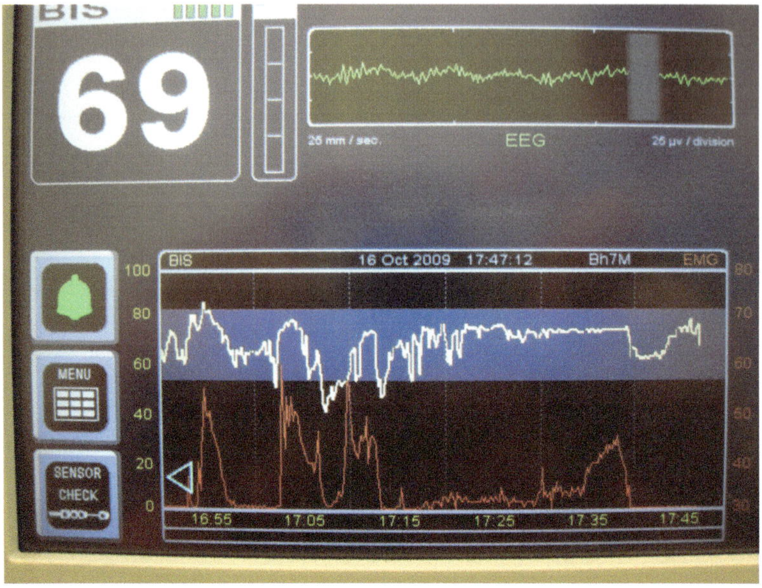

Fig. 2.7 EMG is the lower (*red*) trace

"Preempt the pain" means using a 50 mg dissociative dose of ketamine, independent of adult body weight, to completely saturate midbrain NMDA receptors 3 min prior to skin stimulation (i.e., injection of local analgesia).

"Emetic drugs abstain" simply means scrupulous avoidance of opioids (narcotics) like morphine, meperidine, fentanyl, alfentanil, or remifentanil as well as inhalational agents like forane, sevoflurane, or desflurane (Fig. 2.8). Assurance of adequate local analgesia obviates the need for these troublesome agents. Abstaining from emetic agents also eliminates the need for antiemetic drugs.

Propofol's advantages over inhalational agents include the following:

1. Not a malignant hyperthermia (MH) trigger.
2. Not needing to stock dantrolene, an MH antidote.
3. Antiemetic qualities.
4. Antioxidant qualities: halogenated inhalational agents like forane, desflurane, or sevoflurane are oxidizing agents.
5. Rapid, pleasant emergence likely due to rapid metabolism.
6. Preserved REM sleep patterns.

Unlike benzodiazepines, propofol clinical signs (i.e., loss of lid reflex and loss of verbal response) are reliable and clinically reproducible, and cerebral cortical effect can be measured and, therefore, is numerically reproducible.

Bispectral Index (BIS) Monitor

With the 1983 introduction of pulse oximetry (SpO_2) monitoring, anesthetic mortality declined from 1 in 10,000 in the 1950s to about 1 in 250,000 patients. Additional vital signs of blood pressure, EKG and $EtCO_2$, while important, still only provide a reflection of brain stem activity. However, the part of the brain that processes hearing, feeling, and memory is the cerebral cortex.

For anesthesiologists practicing prior to 1996, there was no direct measure of patient cerebral anesthetic response. To compensate for this lack of information about cortical effect, the anesthesiologist was obliged to over-medicate for fear of not giving enough anesthetic. In 1996, the Food and Drug Administration (FDA) approved Aspect Medical Systems' Bispectral Index (BIS) monitor to directly measure the patients' cerebral drug response.

While the BIS technology has been validated in over 3,500 published scientific studies and found in over 75 % of US hospitals, BIS utilization remains at only about 25 %. There are sev-

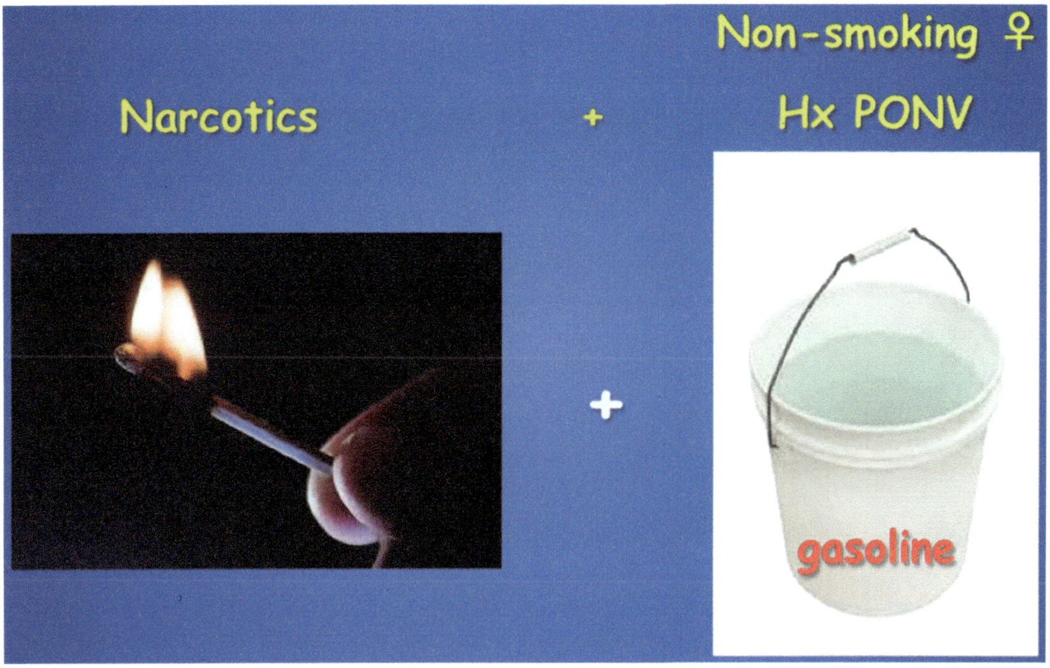

Fig. 2.8 "As long as emetogenic agents are part of the anesthetic regimen, the use of anti-emetics is of limited utility" – Christian Apfel MD, PhD

eral reasons for the underutilization of BIS monitoring. First, the BIS value is a unit-less, derived value that is 15–30 s behind real time (vital signs, like heart rate and blood pressure, are measured in real time). Titrating anesthetics with only the BIS value is akin to trying to drive an automobile with only the rearview mirror information. The factory default setting displays only the BIS value and tracing. A tool that does not provide useful, real-time information is not often used. BIS values delayed from real time are not especially helpful to titrate anesthetics.

The optimal use of BIS is by trending the frontalis muscle electromyogram (EMG) as the secondary trace [5] and responding to EMG spikes as if they were heart rate or blood pressure changes. EMG is to the frontalis muscle what the EKG is to the myocardial muscle, i.e., a real-time, physiologic parameter (Fig. 2.9). While some allege the use of ketamine invalidates the ability to titrate propofol with BIS, there is evidence to the contrary [6], along with 15 years of reproducible clinical practice.

Premedication

Between March 1992 and June 1997, the addition of midazolam premedication was undertaken in the hope of reducing the cost of the average 3–20 ml bottles of propofol (Diprivan® Zeneca). Three groups of patients were informally studied – 0, 2, and 4 mg midazolam premedication, with the 4 mg group selected for cases of 4+ h. Review of the comparative propofol rates revealed no cost-effective reduction with either 2 or 4 mg midazolam premedication [7].

Midazolam premedication was subsequently abandoned in favor of no pharmacologic agents from June 1997 through December 1998. In September 1997, Oxorn published a double-blind Level I RCT showing no propofol-sparing effect from 2 mg midazolam versus none, but a 3× increase in postoperative pain medication was required in the midazolam patient group [8].

In December 1998, oral clonidine premedication was added to the PK regimen. The therapeutic level is 2.5–5.0 mcg/kg [9]. Patients weighing

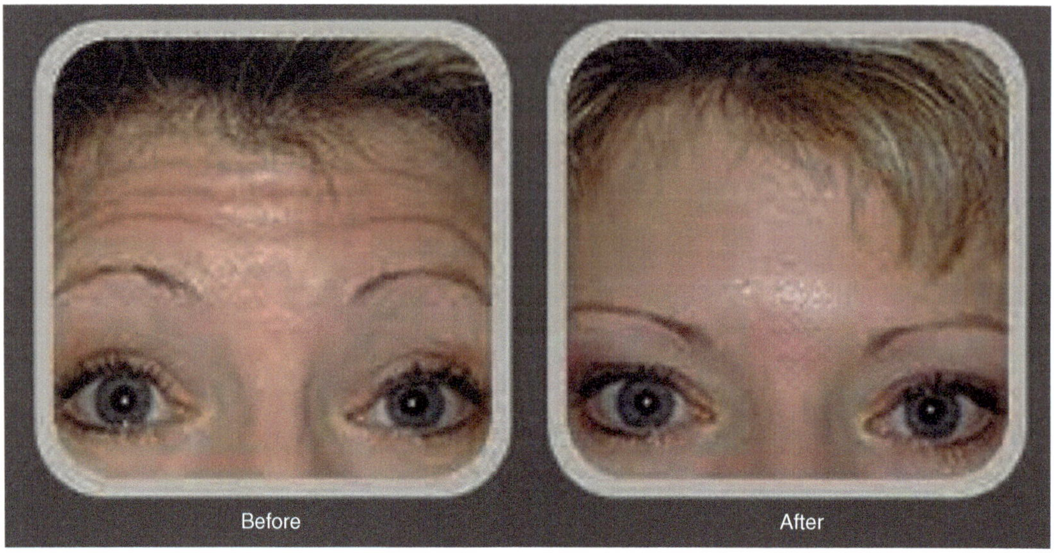

Fig. 2.9 Botox does not eliminate EMG spikes

between 95 and 175 lb require 0.2 mg clonidine to achieve the therapeutic level. For patients with systolic blood pressure <100 mmHg, clonidine should be avoided. An explanation for the salutary postoperative effect on patients' pain has been suggested recently [10].

Two clonidine caveats:

1. Never give clonidine for patients to take at home prior to surgery. In the event of postural hypotension, one is unlikely to have someone to either start an intravenous or place the patient in Trendelenburg. Also, patients are not likely to have their scheduled surgery.
2. Clonidine is available in 0.1, 0.2, and 0.3 mg doses. Only stock 0.1 mg formulation of clonidine to avoid medication dose errors.

Lastly, clonidine premedication is not critical to the success of PK anesthesia. If one has recurrent hypotension with the clonidine, eliminating it from the regimen will not negatively affect the reproducible success of PK anesthesia. While propofol is generic and dramatically less expensive than in the 1990s, given the recent problems sourcing propofol, it may still be worth including propofol-sparing clonidine premedication.

Induction

All patients receive 0.2 mg glycopyrrolate (Robinul®) in the same syringe as 1.5 mL 1 % lidocaine prior to starting the propofol infusion. Glycopyrrolate counteracts the tendency of ketamine to produce excessive salivation. Saliva touching the vocal cords frequently results in laryngospasm and oxygen desaturation. Lidocaine often eliminates the discomfort patients report from the propofol infusion.

Hypnosis first, then dissociation follows Vinnik's concept using propofol instead of diazepam [2] Most anesthesia providers emulate the speedy hare in their approach (i.e., 1,000–2,000 mcg/kg bolus) to starting a case. However, the winning example of the slow and steady tortoise (i.e., sequential 50 mcg/kg doses) (Fig. 2.10) is demonstrated in this YouTube clip at http://www.youtube.com/watch?v=GlQ3Do3b3_I.

Three distinct benefits derive from the incremental type of induction:

1. Patient's airway and drive to breathe are infrequently disturbed, simplifying airway management.

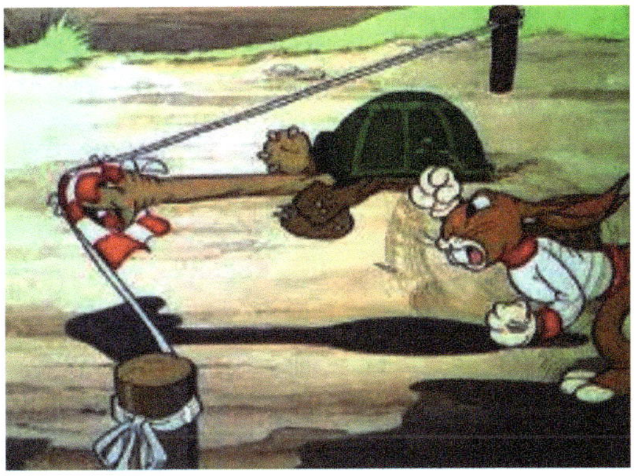

Fig. 2.10 Slow and steady wins the race: airway, breathing, and blood pressure preserved

Table 2.1 PK anesthesia progressive airway algorithm (assumes incremental propofol induction): errors to avoid [13]

1.	Ketamine before propofol: NO
2.	Ketamine at BIS >75: NO
3.	Bolus propofol induction: NO
4.	Inadequate local analgesia: NO
	BIS as fianchetto for adequate propofol and lidocaine
5.	Opioids instead of more lidocaine: NO
6.	Ketamine instead of more lidocaine: NO
7.	>200 mg total ketamine or any in last 20 min. of case: NO
8.	Tracheostomize patient for laryngospasm instead of IV lidocaine: NO
9.	SCH instead of lidocaine for laryngospasm: NO

2. Blood pressure is maintained, unlike that observed with propofol bolus induction that often necessitates ephedrine treatment.
3. Stable brain level of propofol provides protection from the historically reported ketamine side effects of hallucinations [11], dysphorias, and flashbacks.

The induction time of 2.5 min shown in the YouTube clip approximates the more traditional preoxygenation, bolus propofol induction, muscle relaxation, laryngoscopy, endotracheal tube placement, and tube position confirmation times for GA.

Airway Management

Three muscles, the temporalis, orbicularis oris, and genioglossus, are responsible for maintaining the tongue from retrograde airway occlusion. Snoring is one sign of partial airway obstruction while pre-tracheal, sternal notch retraction is more often associated with total airway obstruction.

BIS 60–75 is not a measure of airway patency or brain oxygenation. Only the SpO_2 will measure oxygenation. When incremental propofol induction is administered, the $EtCO_2$ most commonly remains between 38 and 42. If one is not able to observe ventilation, $EtCO_2$ monitoring can display a waveform of the patient's breathing. This author has not used $EtCO_2$ monitoring for BIS/EMG monitored PK MAC and does not mandate its use for others.

Bolus propofol induction produces rapid decreases in all three airway muscles, frequently leading to the need to support the airway with chin lift and positive pressure ventilation. Incremental propofol induction frequently, but not always, tends to maintain tongue muscle support. Propofol, incrementally titrated to BIS 60–75, may still produce airway obstruction. However, obstruction occurs far more infrequently than with bolus induction. Observationally, the mouth, more often than not, tends to remain closed with incremental propofol, while the so-called "O" sign is more characteristic of bolus propofol.

Patient safety with sedation absolutely demands scrupulous attention to airway patency. Management of the airway follows a progressive algorithm (Table 2.1) that depends on what is required to keep the tongue from occluding the airway.

1. Head position: extend and laterally rotate ~30 %, rhytidectomy or facelift position (Fig. 2.11).
2. Shoulder pillow (or 1,000 mL IV bag) (Fig. 2.12): ~30 % increased extension force on genioglossus muscle.
3. Nasal airway #28 FR (Fig. 2.13) ~30 %.
4. LMA #4 (Fig. 2.14): ~5–10 %. No intubation required 21 years, >5,000 patients.
5. Oxygen, supplemental: ~10–20 %.

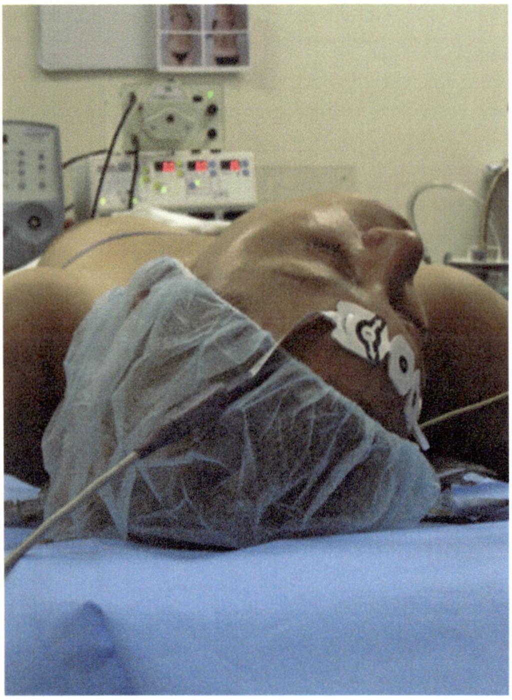

Fig. 2.11 Head position

Dissociation (NMDA Receptor Block)

Although Vinnik's initial ketamine dose is 75 mg [2], this has been reduced to 50 mg independent of adult body weight [5]. The 50 mg ketamine dose will provide complete *N*-methyl-D-aspartate (NMDA) block in ~98 % of adults (Fig. 2.15). A 25 mg dose will produce NMDA block in ~80 % of patients. However, there are no negative consequences to using the 50 mg dose once the brain has been protected with a stable propofol level. Stable propofol brain level will not be produced with a bolus propofol induction. The practical upper aggregate ketamine dose has been found to be 200 mg for day surgery cases. It is useful, therefore, to inject as many of the surgical fields with the initial dissociating 50 mg ketamine dose. Ketamine dissociation is only used to render the patient unresponsive to the local anesthetic injection of a virgin field.

When patient movement (without EMG spike) occurs, necessitating additional local anesthetic

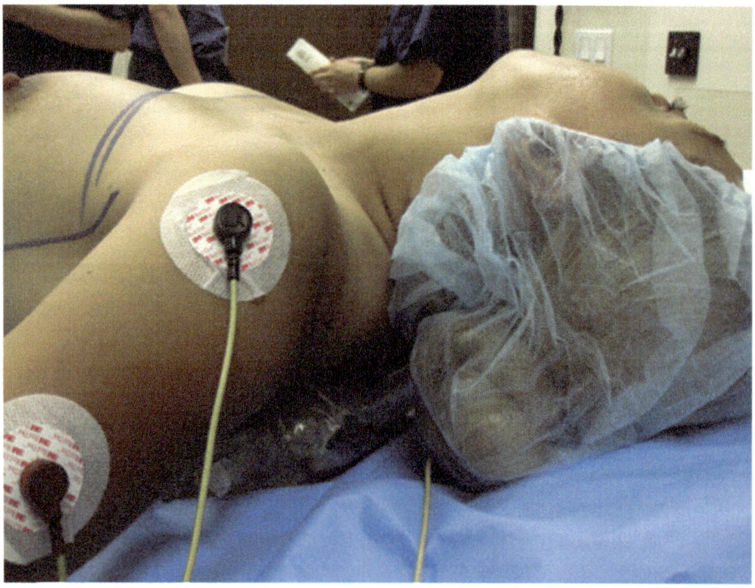

Fig. 2.12 Shoulder pillow (or 1,000 mL IV bag)

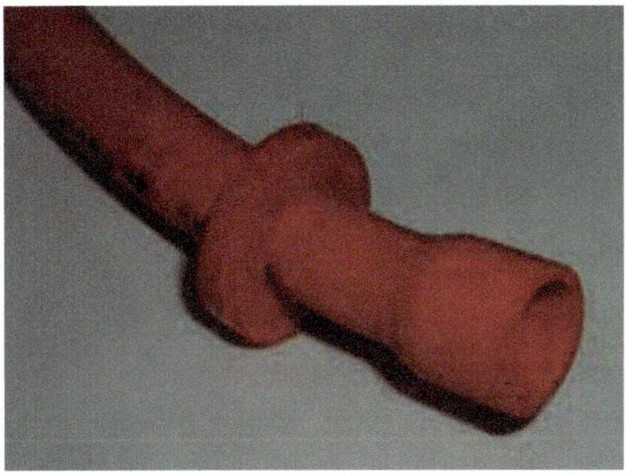

Fig. 2.13 Nasal airway #28 FR

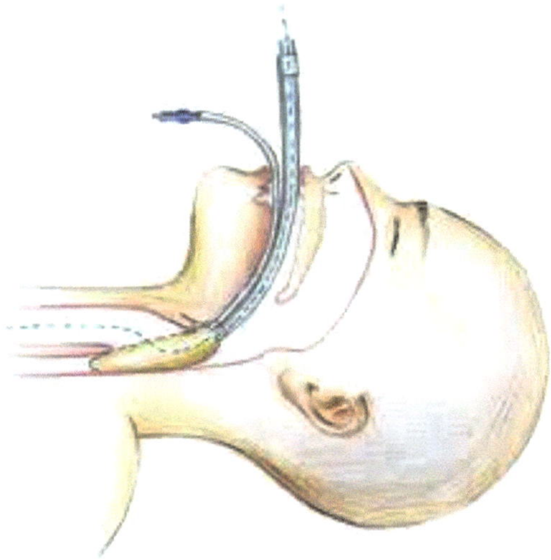

Fig. 2.14 LMA #4

injection, additional ketamine dissociation is rarely required. Paradoxically, there is usually sufficient residual analgesia to block the noxious signal from follow-up local analgesia injection but not enough to continue surgery without that supplementation. Also, once the surgical field has been injected, continuing to administer more ketamine will more often produce an aggregate ketamine dose in excess of 200 mg and a somnolent emerging patient.

Additional ketamine dissociation may be required once the surgical field has been injected a total of three times (i.e., the initial and two subsequent injections to eliminate patient movement). However, cognizance of the aggregate dose must be taken to preserve the rapid emergence and ability to efficiently discharge the patient from the surgical facility. Brain measurement of propofol levels assures continued brain protection for subsequent ketamine doses, should they be necessary.

Ketamine increases the laryngeal or so-called life-preserving reflexes (Fig. 2.16) mentioned in CA AB595 requiring office certification whenever anxiolytics or analgesics are administered in doses likely to depress those reflexes. Recognition of the prodrome of laryngospasm, along with prompt therapy, is essential to the best conduct of the case.

Ketamine-Associated Laryngospasm

The "crowing" sound of laryngospasm is created by the partial vocal cord closure. However, ketamine-associated laryngospasm produces complete vocal cord closure. Hence, no readily recognizable sound occurs with ketamine-associated laryngospasm. The prodrome is a cough or sneeze. Therapy consists of the prompt intravenous bolus injection of lidocaine 1 mg/lb. Like benzodiazepines, propofol hypnosis elevates the seizure threshold of lidocaine. Seizures have not been seen over the 21 years of administering lidocaine 1 mg/lb for ketamine-associated laryngospasm.

Maintenance

The art of the technique lies in defining the basal infusion rate necessary (i.e., "surfing" the level of consciousness) to maintain BIS 60–75 (with

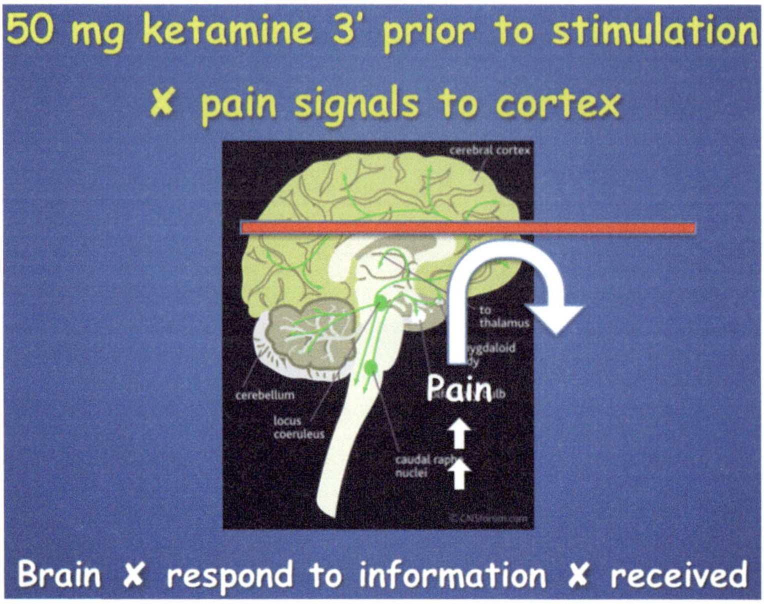

Fig. 2.15 Windup phenomenon eliminated with NMDA block prior to injection

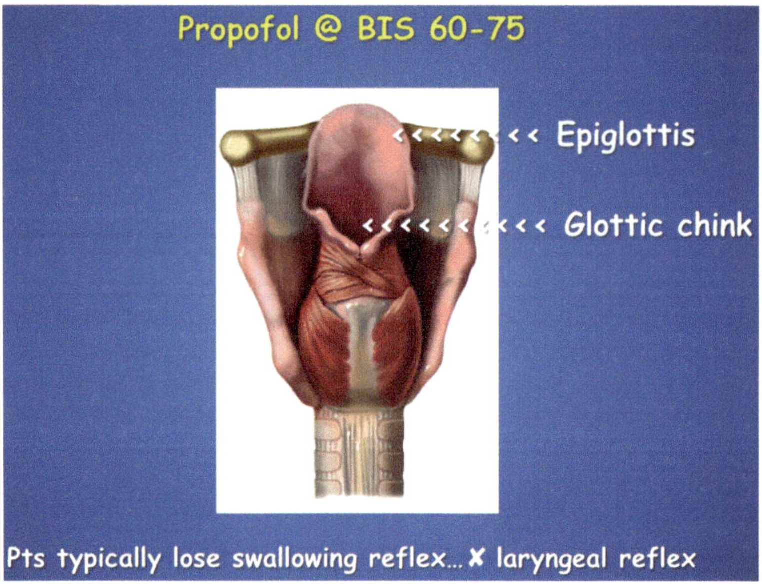

Fig. 2.16 Laryngeal reflexes protect the lungs from aspiration and are life preserving. Ketamine increases laryngeal reflexes, while opioids (narcotics) decrease them

baseline EMG) as well as defining the optimal bolus rate required to return the patient to BIS 60–75 when EMG spike activity is observed. Recall is not dependent on the absolute BIS value observed, but rather on the area under the BIS curve >3–5 min.

The empirically derived initial bolus of 50 mcg/kg^{-1} and basal rate of 25 mcg/kg^{1}/min^{-1} are not "set in stone" but have been found to produce the least trespass to patient airway, breathing, and blood pressure. For instance, when preparing to anesthetize a very elderly or frail patient, one might consider decreasing the bolus and basal rate in half and taking 3–4 min, instead of the customary 2 min, to induce propofol to BIS <75, EMG baseline.

Adjusting Expectations

One cannot provide BIS/EMG PK MAC without prior discussion to secure the surgeon's understanding for the need to supplement local analgesia during the case. Some surgeons appear to perceive the need to supplement local during the case as an affront to their ability to inject local analgesia. Other surgeons mistakenly believe the presence of vasoconstriction guarantees adequate local analgesia. While these are untrue presumptions, care needs to be taken to not insult the surgeon's ego or intellect when the need for additional local analgesia becomes manifest.

BIS/EMG monitoring can explain the differentiation of spinal – versus brain-driven patient movement to the surgeon (Fig. 2.17). Vasoconstriction observed in the surgical field does not guarantee adequate analgesia, especially when there is no EMG activity and propofol BIS levels are 60–75!

"Perfect" local analgesia with the initial injection is not required, but subsequent persistence with local analgesia when required during the case is an absolute requirement for PK success. One then sets the stage for poetry in motion. The anesthesiologist measures the level of hypnosis while the surgeon controls surgical analgesia. The patient benefits enormously by not being hurt during the procedure.

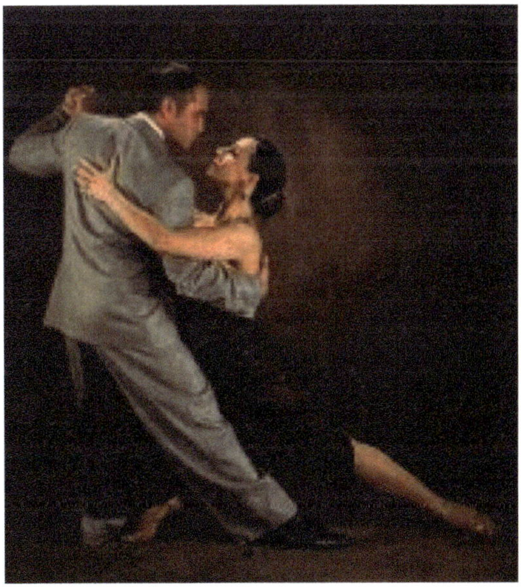

Fig. 2.17 The tango: poetry in motion

Postoperative Pain Management

Patients do not typically exhibit the traumatized "look" of surgery. The dissociative effect precludes intraoperative pain. The major pain signal of violating the skin is never sent to the brain (i.e., dissociation or NMDA block). Hence, patients typically have little or no postoperative discomfort after body implant surgery. The brain cannot wind up from information it never receives. Over the past 15 years of BIS/EMG monitored PK MAC, a minority of >3,000 patients have required postoperative opioids prior to discharge from the office facility.

Much of the postoperative discomfort is a function of muscle spasm secondary to increasing muscle fiber length by the implant placement. This issue can readily be dealt with by prescribing 5–10 mg oral diazepam every 4–6 h. Patients recover quickly and are able to swallow oral medications after BIS/EMG monitored PK MAC. Midazolam (Versed®) 1–2 mg intravenously has infrequently been given for the rare patient. Postoperative opioids like hydrocodone carry the (avoidable) risks of PONV and constipation. Sometimes, patients can avoid postoperative opioids by taking not more than 1,000 mg acetaminophen (Tylenol®) every 8 h to supplement the diazepam relaxation.

Patients will benefit with prolonged postoperative analgesia by placing bupivacaine (Marcaine®) in the implant pockets prior to closing or injecting retrograde in the drains. Since bupivacaine rapidly binds to tissues, it is not necessary to inject the agent with a needle. Depending on the pocket size, 10–25 mL of bupivacaine per pocket is deposited. To avoid cardiotoxicity, never exceed a total of 125 mg or 50 mL 0.25 % bupivacaine. If greater than 50 mL is required, simply dilute 0.25–0.125 % with normal saline (NSS) to have 100 mL to distribute among multiple pockets.

On occasion, there are patients who have been predominantly immobile during surgery but complain bitterly of pain after surgery. These patients are given two "Big Blue" pain pills (i.e., Tylenol® PM) for relief of nonphysical pain. Unless specifically asked for the name of this drug, staff does not customarily mention the proprietary name as the therapeutic efficacy is greatly diminished by doing so.

Postoperative Nausea and Vomiting (PONV)

Avoidance of both opioids and inhalational vapors (i.e., emetogenic agents) has allowed the lowest published rate of PONV (0.6 %) in a high-risk patient population without the need of anti-emetic use [7].

Discussion

Inasmuch as GA and TIVA remain the most commonly performed anesthetics for body implant surgery, the question remains, "Why are more anesthesiologists not offering BIS/EMG PK MAC?"

Because the academic centers rarely expose their trainees to BIS/EMG PK MAC, many anesthesiologists are reluctant to try a technique they have not become familiar with in their residency training. Without being exposed to the real-time use of BIS with EMG as the secondary trace, many anesthesiologists have discarded the idea of using this device. Also, BIS monitors are not always physically available in cosmetic surgery practices. For too many anesthesiologists, the idea of buying their own BIS monitor remains a totally foreign concept they need to shed.

Academic anesthesia centers are still not routinely having residents titrate anesthetics with BIS/EMG. Without being able to differentiate spinal-cord-generated movement (i.e., movement without EMG spike) from cortically generated movement (i.e., movement with EMG spike), it is difficult to convince the surgeon for the need of additional local analgesia as well as spinal cord movement not being a sign of awareness and recall. BIS/EMG PK MAC without dealing with the need for adequate local analgesia will not provide dramatically better outcomes.

Lectures in anesthesia training programs continue to emphasize hallucinations, hypertension, and tachycardia as ketamine's side effects when the drug is administered as a solo agent. Rarely is cognizance taken of the satisfactory elimination of those troublesome side effects when pretreatment with either benzodiazepines [2] or propofol [11] is provided.

BIS monitoring has been FDA approved since 1996. Advocacy of universal BIS monitoring could reduce anesthetic use by 30 % [3], potentially jeopardizing the American Society of Anesthesiologists (ASA) of millions of various forms of drug company (Big Pharma) support dollars. From 1983 to 1990, the ASA also resisted advocacy of pulse oximetry as a standard of care until Medicare mandated the additional SpO_2 fee being bundled as a base charge.

Surgeons who appreciate the value of good local analgesia tend to be more receptive to PK MAC for their patients. They also understand the difference between intraoperating room process and postsurgical *outcomes*. Why should more anesthesiologists seek to offer BIS/EMG PK MAC for elective cosmetic surgery like body implants? Patient safety is improved with a minimally invasive anesthetic regimen. Preservation of native airway, reduced need for supplemental oxygen, and blood pressure stability self-evidently minimize the potential for needing to perform CPR or call 911.

Ketamine does not depress respiration. Respiratory embarrassment is far less likely when only a single respiratory depressant (i.e., propofol) is titrated against both brain stem and cortical response. Patients who experience desaturation with PK MAC frequently recover normal SpO_2 without the need for bag-mask ventilation. Often a simple, transient chin lift will suffice.

Patient satisfaction is dramatically improved for several reasons. Patients emerge from propofol feeling refreshed as opposed to "hung over." Propofol permits REM sleep patterns as well as providing an anti-inflammatory effect. The absence of emetic drugs also provides a nearly zero PONV rate [7], especially important in patients with a previous history of PONV. Ketamine's anti-inflammatory effect supplements that of propofol [12].

Cost-effectiveness is improved when drugs are administered in the optimal fashion. Propofol usage is reduced by 30 % with BIS/EMG monitoring and clonidine premedication [3]. Ketamine usage is most often only one or two 50 mg doses. However, most importantly is that local analgesia instead of excessive propofol, ketamine, or even opioids is employed to accurately deal with the patient's need for intraoperative pain relief. Providing a lack of information to the patient's brain (i.e., dissociation or complete NMDA block) for both the initial local analgesia injection and during the case for supplemental analgesia has led to >3,000 BIS/EMG PK MAC patients not needing opioid relief upon emergence since December 26, 1987.

Outliers are eliminated using BIS/EMG monitoring with an incremental approach to anesthetic induction. Clonidine premedicated patients, on average, require 25–50 mcg/kg/min^{-1} to maintain BIS 60–75. Patients have been observed to require as low as 2.5 mcg/kg/min^{-1} and as high as 185 mcg/kg/ min^{-1} to maintain BIS 60–75 with the same excellent recovery times. Responding to EMG spikes as if they were heart rate or blood pressure changes is the key to avoiding over – and under-medication [5].

Conclusions

Patients are universally happy with BIS/EMG PK MAC anesthesia. Happy patients tend not to file medical liability lawsuits. According to a leading medical liability insurer, anesthesiologists get sued every 8 years on average. For the past 21 years of PK MAC, no patients have filed such an action. Happy patients are also more often likely to return for additional procedures and are more likely to have friends who observe their positive anesthesia outcome and seek out that surgeon for their surgeries. PK MAC anesthesia patients are a positive advertisement and an asset to the cosmetic surgeon.

References

1. Moiniche S, Kehlet H, Berg J. A qualitative and quantitative systemic review of preemptive analgesia for postoperative pain relief. Anesthesiology. 2002;96(3): 725–41.
2. Vinnik CA. An intravenous dissociation technique for outpatient plastic surgery: tranquility in the office surgical facility. Plast Reconstr Surg. 1981;67(6): 799–805.
3. Friedberg BL, Sigl JC. Clonidine premedication decreases propofol consumption during bispectral (BIS) index monitored propofol-ketamine technique for office based surgery. Dermatol Surg. 2000;26(9): 848–52.
4. Guit JB, Koning HM, Coster ML, Niemeijer RP, Mackie DP. Ketamine as analgesic with propofol for total intravenous anesthetic (TIVA). Anaesthesia. 1991; 46(1):24–7.
5. Mathews DM, Clark L, Johansen J, Matute E, Seshagiri CV. Increases in electroencephalogram and electromyogram variability are associated with increased incidence of intraoperative somatic response. Anesth Analg. 2012;114(4):759–70.
6. Friedberg BL. The effect of a dissociative dose of ketamine on the bispectral (BIS) index during propofol hypnosis. J Clin Anesth. 1999;11(1):4–7.
7. Friedberg BL. Propofol-ketamine technique, dissociative anesthesia for office surgery: a five-year review of 1,264 cases. Aesthetic Plast Surg. 1999;23(1):70–4.
8. Oxorn DC, Ferris LE, Harrington E, Orser BA. The effects of midazolam on propofol-induced anesthesia: propofol dose requirements, mood profiles and perioperative dreams. Anesth Analg. 1997;85(3): 553–9.
9. Goyagi T, Tanaka M, Nishikawa T. Oral clonidine premedication reduces awakening concentrations of isoflurane. Anesth Analg. 1998;86(2):410–3.
10. Blaudszun G, Lysakowski C, Elia N, Tramèr MR. Effect of perioperative systemic α2 agonists on postoperative morphine consumption and pain Intensity: systematic review and meta-analysis of randomized controlled trials. Anesthesiology. 2012;116(6): 1312–22.
11. Friedberg BL. Hypnotic doses of propofol block ketamine induced hallucinations. Plast Reconstr Surg. 1993;91(1):196–7.
12. Liu FL, Chen TL, Chen RM. Mechanisms of ketamine-induced immunosuppression. Acta Anesthesiol Taiwan. 2012;50(4):172–7.
13. Friedberg B. PK with BIS monitoring. In: Friedberg B, editor. Anesthesia in cosmetic surgery. New York: Cambridge University Press; 2007.

3 Biceps Augmentation

Introduction

Over the years, there has been an increase in the number of males seeking out cosmetic surgery. Recent statistics by the American Society of Plastic Surgeons show an increase of 5 % in men seeking out cosmetic surgery procedures when comparing 2011–2012 [1]. Despite attempts at betterment through physical activity and weight training, some men are unable to achieve their desired outward appearance. For that reason, they present to a cosmetic surgeon for a host of procedures aimed at improving body contour. Liposuction has ranked in the top five procedures performed by men for the past several years [1, 2]. While being fat is definitely something that men wish to avoid, it seems that more males are concerned with having a muscular physique which is believed to be associated with attractiveness to the female sex and a sign of masculinity [3]. The advent of body implants for augmentation of various muscle groups has brought patients to surgeons' offices seeking augmentation when other measures have failed to give them a more "sculpted" physique [4].

Fascination with the muscular male dates back to antiquity. Stars of the silver screen such as Arnold Schwarzenegger, Sylvester Stallone, and Jason Statham have popularized the muscular and well-built man. Male action figures and Playgirl centerfolds have further demonstrated the obsession with a muscular physique, causing many males to critique themselves and become dissatisfied with their outward appearance [5, 6]. Augmentation of the biceps is one of the muscle groups that lends itself to immediate results with significant improvement in the contour of the male form, with a potential to improve a male's overall impression of himself. Herein, we will discuss the background of the procedure, the operative technique, and common complications seen in bicipital augmentation.

Body Dissatisfaction in Males

Researchers commonly use the concept of an "Adonis Complex" to explain the wide array of secret body image concerns experienced by males. These concerns include everything from body dissatisfaction to muscle dysmorphia (MD), a subtype of body dysmorphic disorder (BDD) found mostly in males, that causes males with either normal or muscular physiques to believe their body is too small or inadequately muscular [5, 7, 8]. Body dissatisfaction has received a lot of attention in male body image research, partly due to its prevalence in Western society. Pope et al. [8] estimated there to be over 50 million males in the United States who were dissatisfied with their muscularity at the beginning of the twenty-first century. This number has most likely risen with various media outlets creating even more unrealistic images of the ideal male body, including the modern and hyper-muscular GI Joe [5] and the lean and muscular Playgirl centerfold model [7]. Pope even went so far as to extrapolate the muscularity of action figures to human size and determined

N.V. Chugay et al., *Body Sculpting with Silicone Implants*,
DOI 10.1007/978-3-319-04957-1_3, © Springer International Publishing Switzerland 2014

that today's GI Joe figure would be just as unattainable to boys as the Barbie doll is for girls [3]. In its most extreme case, muscularity concerns can lead to muscle dysmorphia, which is commonly viewed as the equivalent of anorexia nervosa in females [9]. While females with anorexia perceive themselves to be too big, males with MD perceive themselves to be too small. Ironically, many males with MD are more muscular than their normal counterparts. Males with MD are ashamed and embarrassed of their perceived inadequate muscularity and think about it constantly. Many males with MD also report mood disorders, anxiety disorders, and substance abuse.

Muscle dissatisfaction is associated with numerous psychological problems including depression, low self-esteem, and overall low life satisfaction [9]. The desire for a muscular body has led patients down the road of behavioral problems, disordered eating, use of prohormones, and anabolic steroid use. Although not without its complications, biceps augmentation stands to be an alternative for males who seek to have a more muscular physique and avoids the use of drugs and extreme dieting that are well documented to have deleterious physical and psychological side effects [3, 5, 9].

History of the Procedure

Biceps augmentation was initially used by surgeons to help in the reconstruction of soft tissue defects of the upper extremity left by significant trauma or post-oncologic surgery [10]. While it does not add to the patient's use of the arm, the use of a silastic implant does provide "gratifying cosmetic results" that are durable, leaving surgeons an option for maintaining symmetry of the body. Hodgkinson [11] further added to the literature on the use of solid silicone implants for restoration of symmetry and addition of volume to traumatized extremities. In his article from 2006, he discusses the use of silicone implants to add volume to the upper extremity after ruptures of triceps and biceps muscles and in cases of axillary nerve injury that showed degeneration of the deltoid muscle.

From its initial introduction for reconstructive purposes, the primary author produced research in the area of biceps augmentation for cosmetic purposes in early 2006 [12]. The actual use of biceps implants for cosmetic reasons was begun in 2004, by the primary author, when a 32-year-old recreational body builder presented with a complaint of an underdeveloped biceps region. By the time of publication in 2006, the author had completed a total of 12 augmentations in the submuscular plane, below the biceps brachii muscle. This was followed by a retrospective review of 94 cases in 2009, which further evaluated the procedure and its potential risks and complications [13]. All procedures were performed via an incision in the axilla and placement of the implant in the submuscular plane. In the primary author's experience, greater risks for complications were possible with placement of the implant under the muscle. With placement solely beneath the fascia, the improved contour was similarly noted but without the increased risk of damage to vital neurovascular structures. For that reason, the primary author's standard practice at this time is use of a subfascial approach for implant placement, rather than the submuscular plane. In 2010, Dini and Ferreria [14] evaluated the size of the short head of the biceps muscle and devised an implant based on these dimensions, measuring 20 cm in length, 3 cm in width, and 1.7 cm in height made out of silicone envelope filled with silicone gel. The implant is introduced via an incision in the axilla and placed in a subfascial plane. In 2012, Abadesso and Serra [15] published their work on 32 cases of biceps augmentation for improving the cosmetic appearance of the arms. Their report includes augmentation brachioplasty performed for increase in brachial volume in 16 patients (50 %), to correct sagging skin in 9 (28.1 %), and to improve the appearance of the arm after bariatric surgery in 5 (15.6 %). While the primary author prefers the use of an axillary incision for bicipital augmentation, Abadesso and Serra use a 4 cm long S-shaped incision in the middle of the arm. They then place calf implants into the submuscular plane to achieve the desired augmentation. In patients that require more volume, they combine solid silicone elastomer implants with cohesive gel silicone implants using a 3-0 nylon suture to stack the implants on top of one another.

Indications

Initially, biceps augmentation was introduced as a means to treating asymmetries in the arm region left due to congenital anomalies, trauma producing atrophy of muscles in the upper extremity, and in those patients who suffered volume deficits secondary to trauma or post-oncologic surgery. Biceps augmentation, for purely aesthetic reasons, is indicated for the patient who has hypoplasia in the area of the biceps muscle. It can be used in the patient who has a condition from birth resulting in hypoplasia or may be applied to a patient who is unsuccessful in achieving the desired volume in the region of the biceps, despite aggressive weight training (e.g., body builders).

Contraindications

While not every male presenting for biceps augmentation suffers from muscle dysmorphia, the surgeon must be aware of this and take it into consideration when considering a patient for muscle augmentation surgery. A patient who seems unrealistic in the goals of his surgery should be turned away.

Limitations

In any initial biceps augmentation, patients are instructed on the fact that they can achieve an augmentation of approximately 1 inch in added circumference of the arm. Larger augmentations may require a second operation with larger, custom implants. Also, patients are instructed that while biceps and triceps augmentations can be performed, it is safer to separate this into two separate surgeries to avoid the risk of compartment syndrome in the upper extremity.

Relevant Anatomy

The technique described herein is ideal in that it avoids major neurovascular structures in the upper extremity. However, for completeness sake some of the basic anatomy that is pertinent to the discussion of biceps augmentation will be reviewed.

An axial section through the mid arm shows much of the relevant anatomy for biceps augmentation (Fig. 3.1). Two distinct muscular compartments (anterior and posterior) exist in the upper arm and are separated by the medial and lateral intermuscular septa and humerus [16, 17]. The medial and lateral intermuscular septa arise from the humerus and insert into the brachial fascia, which covers the superficial muscles of the anterior compartment. The anterior compartment is composed of the biceps brachii, brachialis, and coracobrachialis. The posterior compartment is composed of the triceps muscle. The biceps brachii is a long muscle consisting of two heads and functions to flex the elbow and supinate the forearm (Fig. 3.2). The short head arises by a thick flattened tendon from the apex of the coracoid process. The long head arises from the supraglenoid tuberosity at the upper margin of the glenoid cavity. Each tendon is then succeeded by an elongated muscular belly. The two bellies are closely adherent but then unite into a single flattened tendon about 7.5 cm proximal to the elbow joint. This tendon then inserts onto the radius. The fascia overlying the biceps is often referred to as the deep fascia of the arm and is a continuation of the fascia covering the deltoid and pectoralis major. As mentioned previously, it gives off the strong intermuscular septa to the medial and lateral aspects that form the distinction between anterior and posterior compartments of the arm [16].

One of the structures most at risk for injury is the lateral antebrachial cutaneous nerve (Fig. 3.3). This nerve is a continuation of the musculocutaneous nerve and serves as one of the primary sources of sensory innervation to the skin of the forearm in the lateral aspect (Fig. 3.4). It runs along the undersurface of the biceps and can be injured with submuscular placement of the biceps implant. The nerve continues on the undersurface of the biceps brachii muscle until it emerges just lateral to the biceps tendon, 2–4 cm above the elbow crease. For this reason, it is possible to have a compression injury along the course of the nerve when the implant is placed in the submuscular plane and exerts direct pressure on the nerve [18, 19]. The medial antebrachial cutaneous

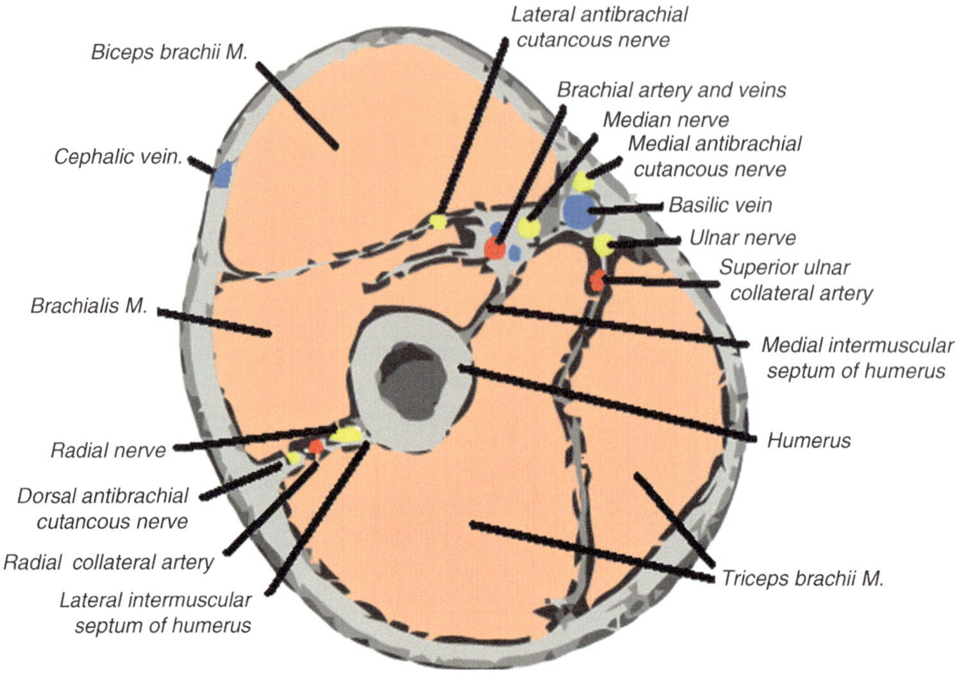

Fig. 3.1 Axial cross section of arm showing humerus with medial and lateral intermuscular septa that separate anterior from posterior compartments of the arm. The anterior compartment is composed of the biceps brachii, brachialis, and coracobrachialis. The posterior compartment is composed of the triceps muscle. Major neurovascular structures are primarily localized to the medial aspect of the arm

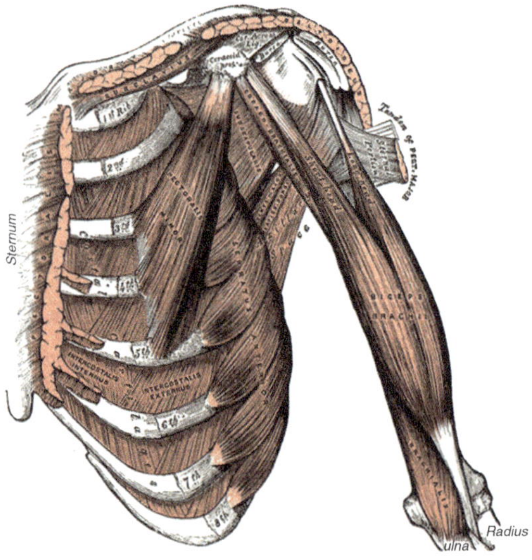

Fig. 3.2 Biceps brachii with long and short heads

nerve is derived from the medial cord of the brachial plexus and serves as a major contributor of sensory nerves of the medial aspect of the forearm (Fig. 3.5). It is more medial in the dissection of the upper arm and is spared in the typical dissection for biceps augmentation, both subfascial and submuscular [18].

The cephalic vein is a major superficial vein of the upper extremity along with the basilic vein. The cephalic vein crosses superficial to the musculocutaneous nerve and ascends in the groove along the lateral border of the biceps brachii, leaving it open to injury with aggressive dissection of the subfascial pocket in the lateral aspect. The basilic vein also plays a major role in the superficial venous drainage of the upper extremity. It runs upward along the medial border of the biceps brachii, perforates the deep

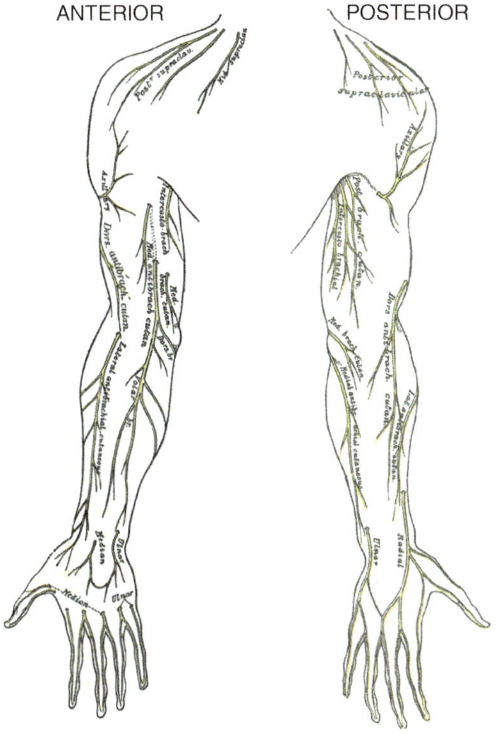

Fig. 3.3 Nerve distribution in the upper extremities (dorsal and ventral views)

fascia slightly below the middle of the arm, and, ascending on the medial side of the brachial artery to the lower border of the teres major, continues onward as the axillary vein. This vessel is spared in a typical subfascial biceps augmentation but may be injured with aggressive medial dissection in the submuscular approach to biceps augmentation.

The brachial artery (a continuation of the axillary artery) commences at the lower margin of the tendon of the teres major, and, passing down the arm, ends about 1 cm below the bend of the elbow, where it divides into the radial and ulnar arteries. At first, the brachial artery lies medial to the humerus; however, it gradually moves in front of the bone as it runs down the arm, and at the bend of the elbow, it lies midway between its two epicondyles. The brachial artery is the major supplier of blood flow to the upper extremities. Because this artery is superficial throughout its entire extent, being covered in front by the integument and the superficial and deep fascia, great care should be taken to preserve its integrity. Risk of injury comes with submuscular approaches to biceps augmentation as very medial dissection can injure the neurovascular bundle.

Consultation/Implant Selection

The consultation begins with a thorough medical history on the patient. Special attention is taken to ask specifically about trauma to the extremity, history of vascular insufficiency which may put blood flow at risk, history of venous insufficiency or arm swelling, and any history of nerve damage or sensory deficits as may be seen in patients with diabetes mellitus. Also, patients with histories of nerve entrapment disorders should be asked about the current state of those nerves and any long-term sequelae. At the time of consultation, the patient is asked what specifically about their arm bothers them as it may be necessary to combine muscle augmentation surgery with adjunct procedures such as liposculpture or brachioplasty to achieve the patient's goals. Preoperative goals are assessed at this point. A patient who has unrealistic expectations and is unable to comply with the strict postoperative instructions is deemed a poor candidate for augmentation. Patients who have congenital anomalies, significant size disparities between the two arms, or bilateral hypoplasia are informed that several surgeries may be required to attain symmetry and achieve the augmentation they desire. Patients are also asked about their current level of activity and muscle building history, taking care to inform the patient of the need to take at least 1 month of time to recover before resuming any vigorous arm building regimens.

After completion of the history, the patient's arms are evaluated. First, symmetry of the two sides is assessed and any disparity is brought to

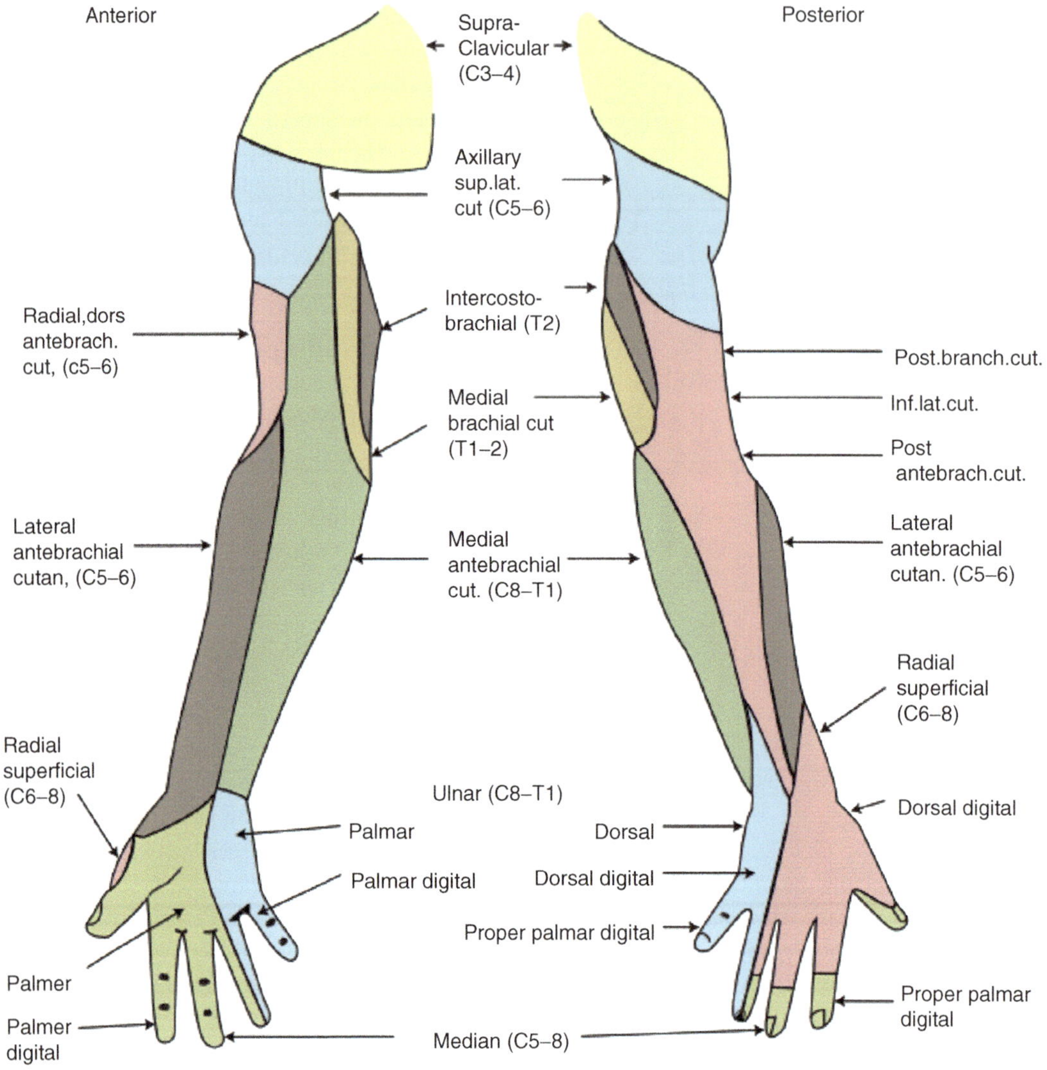

Fig. 3.4 Sensory dermatomes of the nerves of the upper extremity

the attention of the patient. Although the majority of patients present with a preexisting asymmetry of the arms, not many patients note the difference and this can be a source of medicolegal matters in the future. The physician then evaluates the quality of the skin, subcutaneous tissue, and muscle. A person who has very thin tissues or significant hypoplasia of the biceps may not be able to adequately accommodate a large implant. Also, a person with thin tissues may have to be counseled about the possible need for a submuscular placement of the prosthesis. This should be accompanied by a discussion of the increased risks associated with biceps augmentation in the submuscular plane.

Next, the patient's arms are measured in circumference at the midportion of the arm, with the patient in flexed and neutral positions. These measurements are primarily used in the postoperative period to demonstrate the results of augmentation. Another measurement is taken with the patient flexing their biceps muscle. The proximal point of

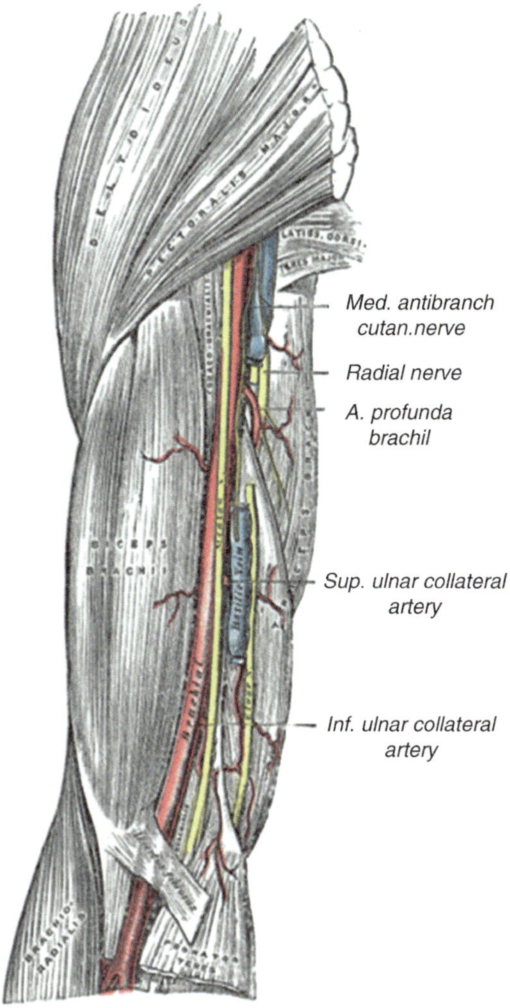

Fig. 3.5 Anatomic location of medial antebrachial cutaneous nerve. Note close proximity of medial antebrachial cutaneous nerve to major neurovascular structures on the medial aspect of the arm, high near the initial entry point for surgery (axilla)

the muscle belly is palpated and marked as is the distal portion of the muscle belly and then measured. Having this second measurement allows one to assess the maximum length of implant that can be accommodated in the biceps region. Next, the width of the muscle belly is measured from its medial to lateral extent while the patient's muscle is flexed. Based on these latter measurements, the surgeon can choose the implant that would best suit the patient's body habitus (Fig. 3.6).

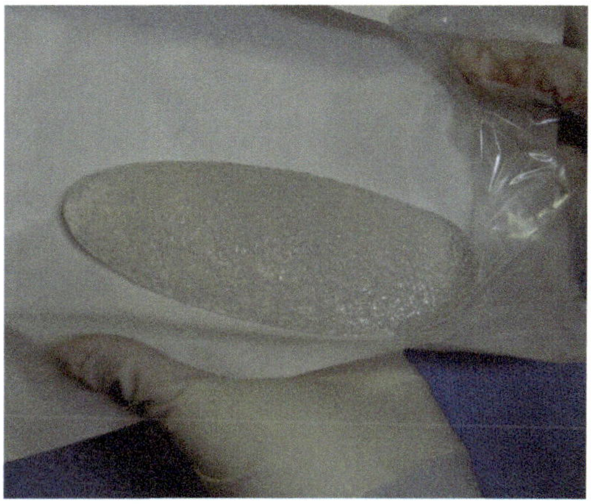

Fig. 3.6 Biceps implant (style 8, size 1)

Available Implants (Table 3.1)

Preoperative Planning and Marking

The biceps contour is marked out with a surgical marking pen, taking special care to also mark the apex of the biceps. A marking is then made in the axillary region for the initial incision in the axilla (Fig. 3.7).

Operative Technique

Subfascial Placement (Standard)

The incision is made in the axillary region with a number 15 blade, and the skin is dissected out by sharp and blunt dissection (Fig. 3.8). With gentle digital pressure, the tissues are displaced until the bicipital fascia is exposed (Fig. 3.9). The bicipital fascia is then incised with a # 15 blade, and 3-0 nylon stay sutures are placed on each side into the fascia for retraction (Figs. 3.10 and 3.11). A pocket is dissected in the subfascial plane, exposing the biceps muscle fibers. The authors' standard of practice is to place the implant in a subfascial plane to avoid many of the complications that can arise from damage to neurovascular structures in a submuscular plane.

Table 3.1 Available biceps implants (Aesthetic and Reconstructive Technologies, Inc., Reno, NV)

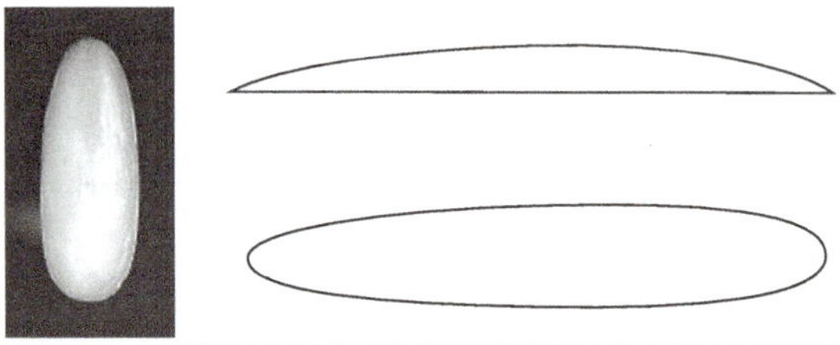

Size	Catalog #	Width	Length	Projection	Volume (cc)
1	600–801	6.2	16.3	2.3	151
2	600–802	5.8	13.3	2.0	60
3	600–803	5.9	13.3	2.4	86

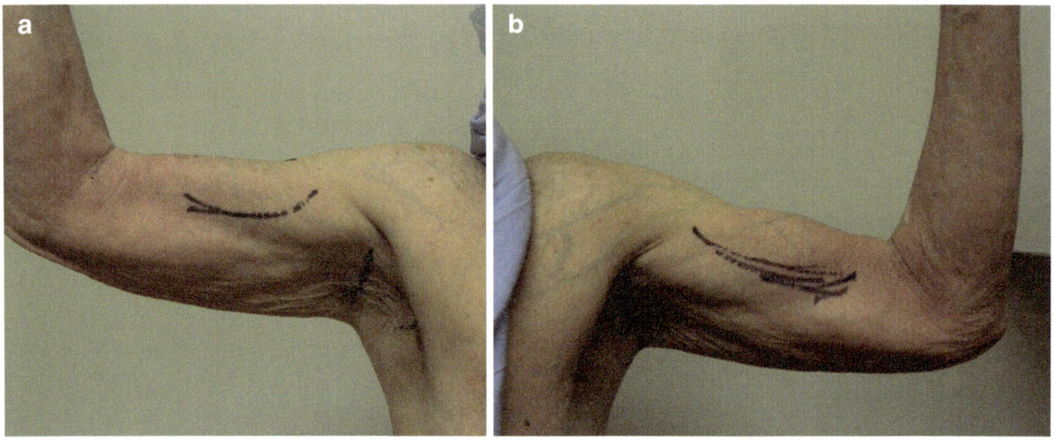

Fig. 3.7 Preoperative markings for biceps augmentation taking care to mark borders of biceps muscle and axillary incision. (**a**) Patient's right arm (**b**) Patient's left arm

If proceeding with a subfascial approach to augmentation, the surgeon will use a combination of blunt finger dissection and spatula dissection to create a subfascial pocket that encompasses the biceps muscle as previously marked (Fig. 3.12). Care is taken not to over-dissect the pocket as a pocket that is over-dissected can lead to greater problems with implant migration and possible seroma formation. The pocket is then packed with a lap sponge and the same procedure is repeated on the contralateral side. At this point the packs are removed and hemostasis is achieved with electrocautery as needed. The pocket is irrigated with a solution containing saline, Betadine, 1 g of cefazolin, and 80 mg of gentamicin. This is aspirated from the pocket. Then, 10 mL of 0.5 % Marcaine is instilled into the pocket for postoperative analgesia. A custom Chugay bicipital implant (AART Corp) is placed into the subfascial pocket (Fig. 3.13). Symmetry is now assessed. If symmetry is not achieved, then pocket manipulation is performed as needed. Once symmetry is noted, closure is begun. The bicipital fascia is repaired with 2-0 Vicryl suture. 3-0 Vicryl suture is used to approximate the deep dermis and then the skin is closed with subcuticular 4-0 Monocryl suture. Collodion is applied to the suture line with Robbins tape as a dressing. The arms are wrapped in Coban to minimize postoperative edema. The patient is then returned to the recovery room and monitored before discharge home.

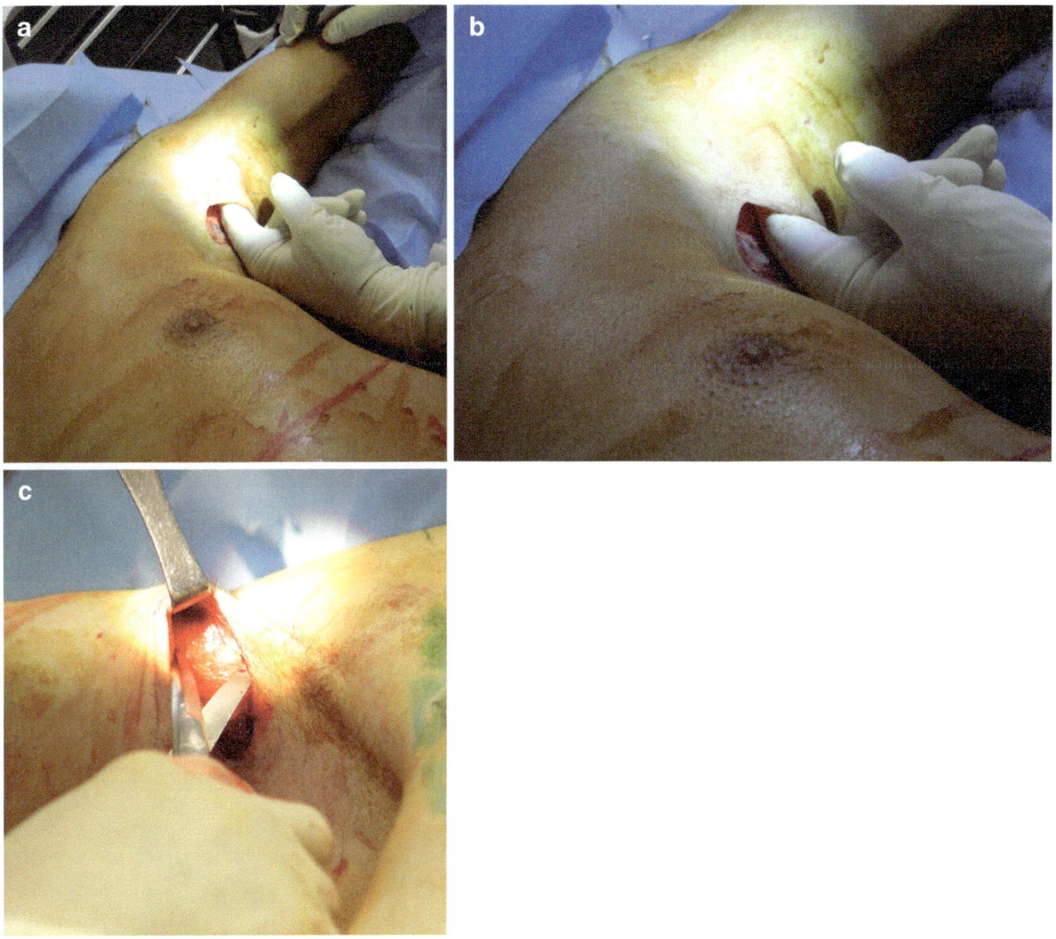

Fig. 3.8 Dissection through subcutaneous tissues using blunt finger dissection and scissors in a spreading manner. (**a**) Blunt finger dissection in the subcutaneous plane using the surgeon's digit. (**b**) Close up view of blunt dissection with the operator's digit. (**c**) Blunt dissection through the subcutaneous tissue with scissors

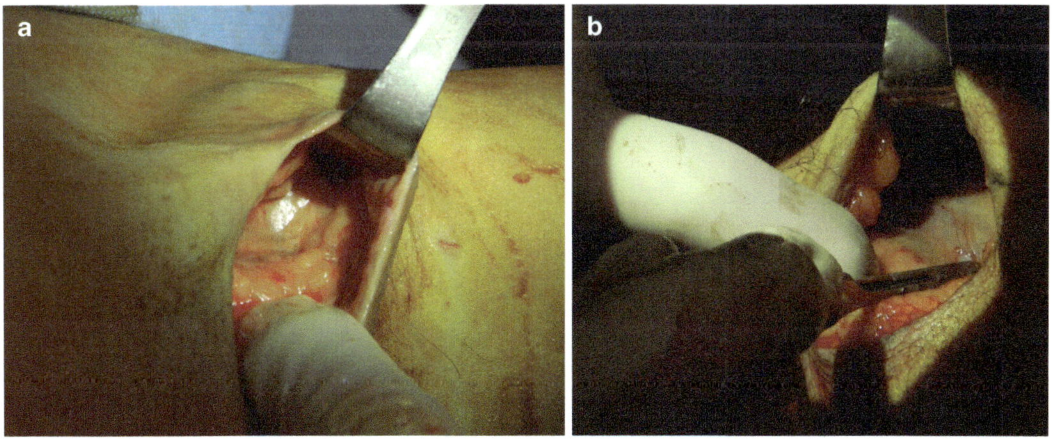

Fig. 3.9 (**a**) Biceps fascia shown in the left axilla (glistening). (**b**) Biceps fascia identified in right axilla (glistening) and being pointed to with scalpel

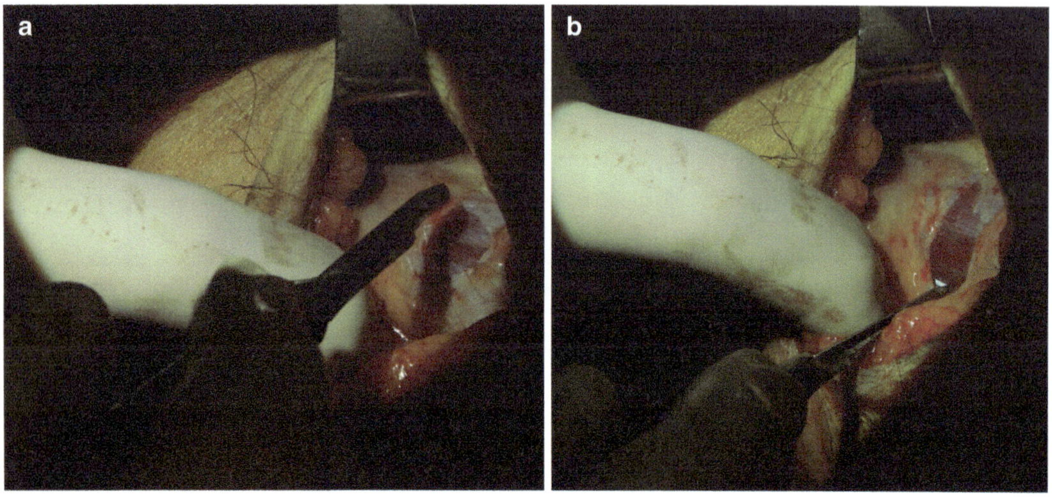

Fig. 3.10 (**a**) Incision started in bicipital fascia. (**b**) Incision completed in biceps fascia

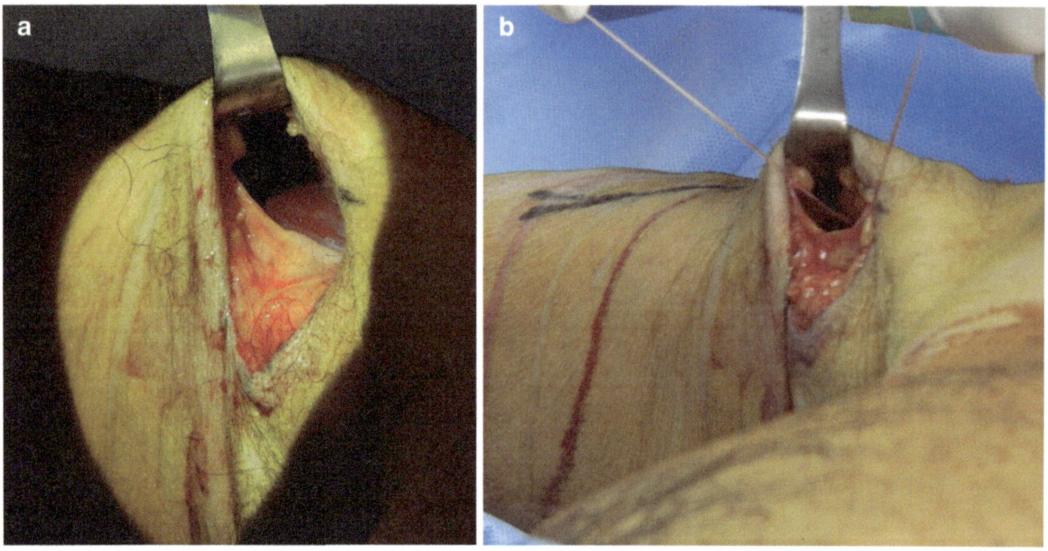

Fig. 3.11 (**a**) Biceps muscle identified and fascia elevated. (**b**) Stay sutures placed in both ends of the biceps fascia, to be used for reapproximation after placement of the implant

Submuscular Approach

If placing the implant in a submuscular plane, the procedure is performed as described above until the biceps muscle is identified. At this point, the muscle fibers are gently spread in a longitudinal fashion with a curved hemostat, and a pocket is dissected underneath the biceps muscle digitally with a spatula dissector (Fig. 3.14). The pocket is packed with a lap sponge and the same procedure is repeated on the contralateral side. At this point the packs are removed and hemostasis is achieved with electrocautery as needed. The pocket is irrigated with a solution containing saline, Betadine, 1 g of cefazolin, and 80 mg of gentamicin. This is aspirated from the pocket. Then, 10 mL of 0.5 % Marcaine is instilled into the pocket for postoperative analgesia. A custom Chugay bicipital implant (AART Corp) is placed into the submuscular pocket. Symmetry is now assessed. If symmetry is not achieved, then pocket manipulation is performed as needed. Once symmetry is noted, closure is begun. In the case of

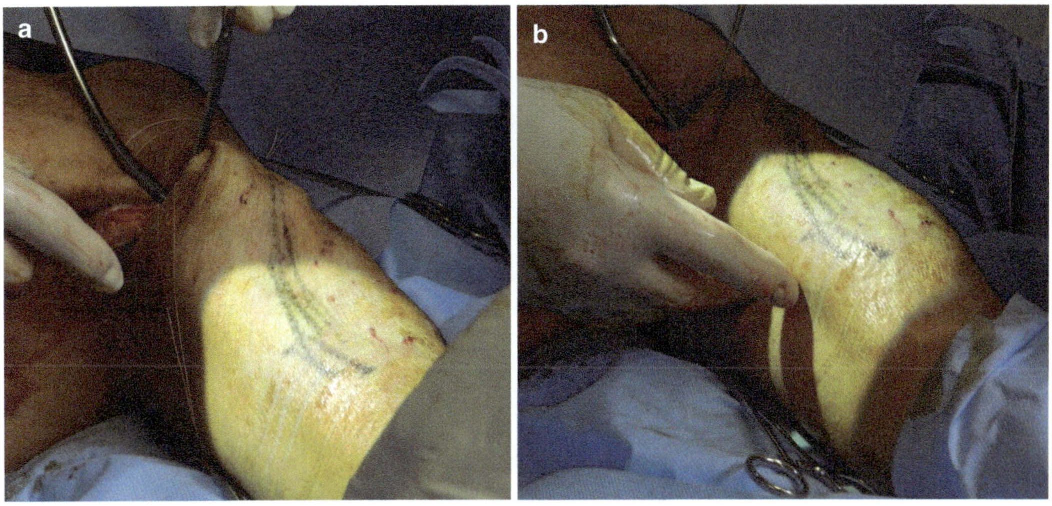

Fig. 3.12 (**a**) Spatula being used to dissect subfascial plane. (**b**) Spatula further being used to dissect plane with finger pointing to location of spatula tip, at the edge of the biceps fascia where it joins the medial intermuscular septum

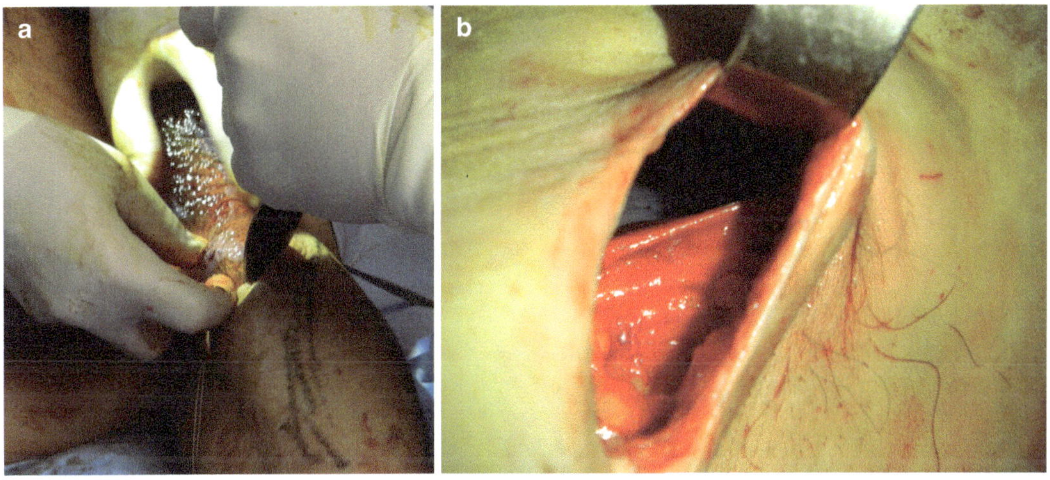

Fig. 3.13 (**a**) Biceps implant being placed with a folding-over method (like a taco). (**b**) Biceps implant in position with fascia overlying

a submuscular implant, the biceps muscle is reapproximated with 2-0 Vicryl sutures, with buried knots. The remainder of the closure is as noted above in the subfascial approach.

Postoperative Care/Instructions

On discharge from the office on the day of surgery, the patients have their arms wrapped in elastic compression sleeves to diminish the amount of swelling and potential for seroma formation. These sleeves are removed on the first postoperative day and a compression garment is applied that is to be worn at all times for a period of 4 weeks. Patients may remove the sleeves to shower and to wash the sleeves as needed. Patients may begin showering the day after surgery, taking care to dry the elastic tape over their incisions with a hair dryer on a low heat setting. The patient is instructed postoperatively to limit the use of the upper extremities and to avoid exertion or any heavy lifting. Patients may begin to use their arms as tolerated

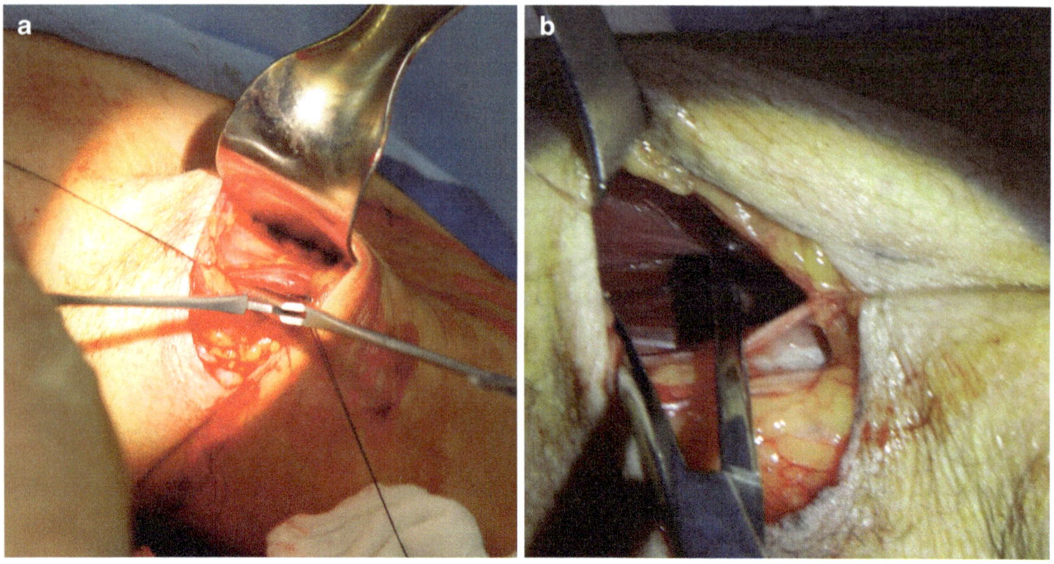

Fig. 3.14 (**a**) Biceps muscle being split in line with its fibers using a hemostat. (**b**) Biceps muscle being elevated to demonstrate the submuscular plane

immediately after surgery but are restricted from heavy lifting or vigorous activity for 4–6 weeks postoperatively.

Complications

In performing biceps augmentation, there is a host of potential complications that can arise (Table 3.2).

Table 3.2 Potential complications of biceps augmentation

Potential complications of biceps augmentation surgery
1. Infection
2. Seroma
3. Hematoma
4. Asymmetry
5. Implant visibility
6. Hypertrophic scarring
7. Hyperpigmentation of the scar
8. Capsular contracture
9. Wound dehiscence
10. Nerve injury (permanent or temporary; motor or sensory)
11. Compartment syndrome

Infection

Infection, either superficial or deep, is a possibility in biceps augmentation surgery. Our own work in this field has demonstrated an infection rate of 1.3 % (3/220) [12, 13]. Species identified in the authors' experiences were isolated to *Staphylococcus aureus* and *Staphylococcus epidermidis*, relatively common skin flora. Prior to making incision, standard practice should be the administration of 2 g of Ancef IV (or 300 mg intravenous (IV) clindamycin in a penicillin- or cephalosporin-allergic patient). During the procedure, irrigation of the pocket with a standard antibiotic solution containing normal saline, Betadine, Ancef, and gentamicin should be performed. Postoperatively, a 5–10 day regimen of oral antibiotics covering the normal skin flora should be administered. If a deep infection occurs, the standard of practice is removal of the implant, closure, and possible reimplantation in 3–6 months. There are reports in other forms of implant surgery (i.e., breast augmentation surgery) that conservative management and implant salvage are possible. This should be left to the discretion of the surgeon and performed with careful counseling of the patient.

Seroma

Seromas are statistically the most common complication occurring in implant surgery. In our own series of patients, we have noted a seroma rate of 1.3 % (3/220). They typically present as new-onset pain, swelling, or asymmetry. The treatment of choice remains percutaneous aspiration. This complication is best prevented with patient compliance with compression sleeves and proper implant placement at the time of surgery, thereby minimizing dead space. In the senior author's (NVC) experience, it is noncompliance with compression garments and postoperative early return to vigorous activity that result in seroma formation rather than technical issues.

Hematoma

Although a rare occurrence due to the relatively avascular plane of dissection for the biceps augmentation procedure, a hematoma is always possible if damage is done to the vessels that perforate the investing fascia of the arm. Of note the cephalic vein, because of its superficial course in the lateral aspect of the arm, can be damaged and care should be taken when performing a subfascial dissection of the lateral biceps region. In the event of a hematoma, rapid evacuation, pocket irrigation, and reimplantation are the mainstays of therapy. This complication is best prevented by meticulous hemostasis at the time of surgery and good compression of the arm postoperatively to prevent potential space creation.

Asymmetry

This can occur as a product of preexisting variability in the patient's arms or variability in dissection of the pocket bilaterally. This is best minimized by good preoperative photography and noting any asymmetries preoperatively. To avoid creation of asymmetry, it is important to maintain the same pattern of dissection and pocket creation bilaterally. Ideally, the pocket created should be tight and minimize the chance of implant migration. Should a pocket be over-dissected and patients note postoperative asymmetry due to a pocket's over-dissection, the patient may require a return to the operating room to adjust the pocket. A revision case should be planned for no sooner than 3 months postoperatively, allowing a capsule to form around the implant. On return to the OR, then, the capsule can be tailored to more appropriately fit around the implant, producing a more snug fit and bringing greater symmetry to the arms. In our own series of 220 cases, we have noted a rate of asymmetry of 5 % (11/220). Only two of the 11 required operative intervention to tighten the implant pocket and bring about symmetry to the arms.

Implant Visibility

Regardless of position below the muscle or below the fascia, implant visibility is a rare complication. However, those patients that have very thin and atrophic arms to begin with may suffer from implant palpability and visibility. Patients should be counseled on this fact preoperatively if there is a feeling that the patient could be at risk. If a patient is determined to be thin and have minimal development of the biceps brachii muscle, the surgeon may elect for placement of the implant in a submuscular plane to better camouflage the implant. However, a discussion must be had with the patient regarding the increased risk of neurovascular injury and a greater potential for muscle injury and compartment syndrome.

Implant Dislodgment/Migration

In the authors' series of 220 patients, one case of implant extrusion occurred. This was noted in a 23-year-old male patient. The patient had an uneventful operation. He presented to the office

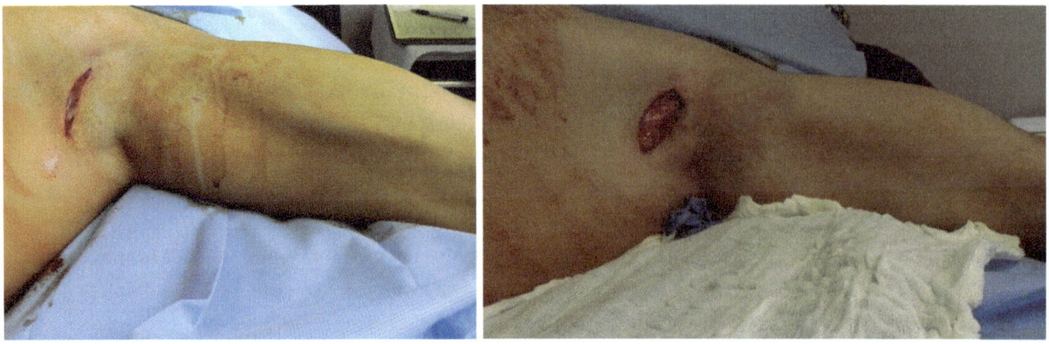

Fig. 3.15 A 23-year-old male patient. The patient had an uneventful operation. He presented to the office 1.5 months postoperatively complaining of a noticeable protrusion around the site of operation. On examination, the patient was noted to have the outline of the implant visible in the subcutaneous tissue that was flipped upside down. (*Left*) Preoperative. (*Right*) Postoperative after implant position was corrected

1.5 months postoperatively complaining of a noticeable protrusion around the site of operation. On examination, the patient had the outline of the implant visible in the subcutaneous tissue that was flipped upside down (Fig. 3.15). He was taken to the operating room for repositioning of the implant as it could not be done manually. He later elected to have the implants removed. When asked about his activity level in the time postoperatively, the patient admitted to beginning his workout regimen in the third postoperative week, demonstrating noncompliance with the postoperative instructions. As scar tissue had not sufficiently formed, the implant was able to work its way upside down with excessive movement.

Scar Hyperpigmentation and Hypertrophy

Scar hyperpigmentation was noted in two cases (0.09 %). This complication occurred in one African American patient and one Hispanic patient. The higher Fitzpatrick level may have played into this complication. Also, the movement of the arms and tension at the level of the axilla may further play into this complication's incidence. The key to reduction of these problems is careful layered closure. The authors also stress the need for scar management for the patients and silicone sheeting is recommended beginning at 1 month after surgery, provided the incision is completely healed.

Capsule Contracture

This is a possible late sequelae of any implant placement, most frequently described in the breast augmentation literature. To date, the authors have not experienced any cases of capsular contracture, and this is possibly due to the significant use of the arms on a regular basis, making it difficult for significant scar tissue to set up around the implant.

Wound Dehiscence

Wound dehiscence is a product of poor wound closure under too much tension typically. In order to prevent this, meticulous closure in three layers is paramount: fascia, deep dermis, and skin. To date, the authors have not experienced any wound dehiscence.

Nerve Injury

Due to the avascular and relatively structure free dissection performed in the vast majority of cases, permanent nerve injury is rarely a problem. It is quite common for patients to complain of some numbness over the area of the biceps and in the axilla at the site of incision; however, this returns within 1–3 months postoperatively. This risk can be minimized by performing the majority of dissection bluntly with the operator's digit rather than using dissectors and potentially creating greater traction injury. Major motor and sensory deficits can accompany compartment syndrome, and this must be ruled out immediately if any significant deficits are appreciated. In their work with stacked implants, Abadesso and Serra [15] reported a 6.25 % incidence of neuropathic pain and paresthesia. These patients had resolution of their symptoms within 4 months, necessitating the use of oral pain medicine, stellate ganglion blockade, and physiotherapy in the immediate post-injury period. In the authors' series of submuscular augmentations, there were 6/220 (2.7 %) patients who presented with numbness over the distribution of the lateral antebrachial cutaneous nerve (radial aspect of the forearm). However, these complaints were transient and sensation returned to normal after 6 weeks with no intervention.

Compartment Pressure Problems/ Compartment Syndrome

Volkman [20], who first described the phenomenon of compartment syndrome, believed that the pathophysiology was related to massive venous stasis associated with simultaneous occurrence of arterial insufficiency. This in turn prevents proper circulation of blood to the muscles and nerves in a given compartment of an extremity, as tissue pressure increases. Nerve and muscle cells start to die within 4–8 h. Compartment syndrome typically presents as a tensely swollen compartment with extreme pain, out of proportion to examination, on palpation. This is sometimes accompanied by referred pain to the affected compartment with passive stretch of muscles distal to the compartment. There may or may not be a neuropathy, typically described as a burning or prickling sensation, appreciated over the skin of the affected region. Finally, the patient may experience frank pulselessness or paralysis of muscles in the affected compartment. However, the patient who presents with these final findings has typically progressed beyond the point of muscle salvage.

In patients with a compatible history and a tense extremity, clinical diagnosis may be sufficient. If the diagnosis is in doubt, compartment pressures may be measured with a handheld Stryker device. An absolute pressure greater than 30 mmHg in any compartment, a pressure within 30 mmHg of the diastolic blood pressure in hypotensive patients, and a patient with a concerning history who demonstrates the constellation of signs and symptoms of compartment syndrome are all possible indications for surgical compartment release via fasciotomy [21]. In the authors' experience, there was one case of compartment syndrome and one case of near-compartment syndrome with rhabdomyolysis.

Case 1

Compartment Syndrome

A 38-year-old male patient initially presented for consultation to attain greater definition in his extremity as he had been born with a neuromuscular condition producing a frozen elbow in his left upper extremity. This produced a hypoplasia of his biceps and triceps muscles on the affected side that was not correctable with physical therapy and routine exercise. He underwent simultaneous biceps and triceps implantation, using the smallest implants that could be possibly constructed to achieve symmetry with the unaffected side. Four days postoperatively, the patient presented with pain in his left upper extremity that had been quite severe. He subsequently had an opening of his initial incision with serosanguineous drainage being expelled. On physical examination, there was a dusky appearance to the skin over the bicipital region with significant tension noted in the tissues of the area. Serosanguineous drainage was noted from the axillary incision site. He was taken to the operating room, where the initial incision was opened and dissection was carried down to the bicipital fascia. On opening the bicipital fascia, the tension in the bicipital region was relieved with serosanguineous drainage being expressed. The biceps implant was removed and the fascia closed. The skin was closed and the patient recovered without incident. He returned 6 months later for minor fat grafting (50 mL) to the affected limb to bring about greater symmetry between the arms. He is currently happy with the aesthetic result and has no long-term sequelae.

In this patient, it is clear that the placement of biceps and triceps implants in such a hypoplastic upper extremity may have been overzealous. Obviously, the addition of so much mass to the upper extremity and lack of room for stretch produced a potentially catastrophic situation in which the patient may have been at risk of losing the upper extremity. The surgeon, therefore, must be careful to not use overly large implants in the region nor add too much bulk to the area without allowing room for adequate stretching of the compartment. Currently, for those patients that present for triceps and biceps augmentation, our standard practice is to perform an augmentation of either the triceps or biceps region with augmentation of the second muscle group after a period of 3–6 months, allowing for accommodation of the added volume in the arm. If patients are adamant about wanting a simultaneous augmentation and one-stage procedure, we will perform the procedure so long as the patient understands that the augmentation achieved may be smaller than that which could be achieved with an isolated augmentation/staged procedure.

Case 2

Near-Compartment Syndrome with Rhabdomyolysis

A 48-year-old male body builder presented for simultaneous pectoral and biceps augmentation as he felt that he did not have sufficiently large pectoralis and biceps despite an aggressive workout regimen. His preoperative blood work demonstrated a BUN of 37 (normal range 6–20 mg/dL) and creatinine of 1.79 (normal range 0.7–1.3 mg/dL). It was agreed upon that the patient could proceed with surgery with plans for aggressive fluid administration intraoperatively. The patient underwent a routine operation with placement of style 2, size 3 implants into the pectoral region and style 8, size 1 implants into the biceps region (submuscular position). The operation was uneventful and the patient was discharged home the same day of surgery. On the following morning, the patient presented for postoperative evaluation claiming to feel weak, having fever, and being short of breath. He did complain also of some weakness in the right hand as compared to the left. At this point, auscultation of the lungs demonstrated decreased breath sounds at the bases and there was concern of a possible pneumothorax. The examination of the arms did not demonstrate any skin changes or excessively tight compartments, but there was note of some decreased strength in grip and range of motion in the right hand by comparison to the left. The patient was urgently sent to the emergency room for CXR and laboratory testing. Laboratory studies demonstrated a white blood cell count of 11.9 (normal range 4.3–10.0), BUN 113 (normal range 6–20 mg/dL), creatinine 5.61 (normal range 0.7–1.3 mg/dL), CPK 16201 (normal 32–294 mcg/L), and myoglobin 5413 (normal 0–110 ng/mL). A chest x-ray demonstrated no pneumothorax but significant atelectasis with a small basilar effusion. The patient was admitted to the medical service for rhabdomyolysis and basilar atelectasis. His treatment plan included aggressive IV fluid hydration and alkalinization of the urine to prevent further significant damage to the kidneys. Pulmonary toilet was also instituted to help expand the lower poles of the lungs.

Two days into his hospitalization, the patient was showing improvement in renal function, his lungs were better inflated, and he no longer had leukocytosis. However, it was noted that the patient had not had any improvement in the function of his right hand in comparison to the left. A neurology consult was requested and surgery was asked to evaluate the patient for compartment syndrome. On evaluation of the arms, the axillary incisions were healing well. There was no evidence of infection. The radial and ulnar arteries had palpable pulses bilaterally. The arms were more tense than normal but this was consistent with the recent augmentation and postoperative edema. After admission to the hospital, the patient had been without his arm compression wraps as was instructed in routine postoperative orders, making the swelling more dramatic. On neurologic examination, there was a clear weakness of the right hand when compared to the left with weakness in the ability to pronate the right forearm, weakness in opposing the thumb. No obvious compartment syndrome was appreciated by surgery or by neurology. Continued neurovascular checks were performed to monitor the situation. A CT scan was ordered of the arm and brachial plexus. There was no evidence of implant impingement on structures, and there was no evidence of hematomas or seromas within the substance of the arm. There was some stranding of the biceps muscle noted, consistent with postoperative inflammation. There was note of a semiocclusive thrombus in the right axillary vein. The patient was started on heparin and subsequently transitioned to Coumadin for treatment on discharge. After 7 days in the hospital, the patient was discharged with the creatinine back at baseline, no pulmonary issues, and Coumadin for 3 months to treat the semiocclusive thrombus. The patient's hand, still with weakness, was felt to be associated with the implant surgery and possible traction on the median nerve. Outpatient physical therapy and neurology follow-up were ordered. After 1 month, the patient had minor improvement in the function of the right hand and the patient requested to have the biceps implants removed. At the time of surgery, the muscle was noted to be viable and not in any way compromised, which would not have been the case if the patient had suffered compartment syndrome and myonecrosis. The neurovascular bundle was not visualized in the dissection. The implants were removed in their entirety without difficulty. Five months postoperatively, the patient is continuing with physical therapy to the arm and has noticed slow but steady progress in his strength.

It is felt that the patient may have had an early pre-compartment syndrome which could have produced rhabdomyolysis in addition to the trauma to the muscle produced by the actual surgical procedure. This caused a shower of myoglobin to the kidneys, producing acute renal failure. Of note, the patient's preoperative creatinine indicated renal insufficiency. Measures such as aggressive intraoperative hydration and alkalinization may have prevented renal injury, in hind sight. Also, admission to the hospital for preoperative hydration may have been considered to improve the patient's creatinine. After surgery, in retrospect, the patient and his primary physician had noticed a worsening of his creatinine, which is a common occurrence in body builders according to the literature and the patient's physician [22, 23]. It is now the authors' standard practice to advise all patients with borderline creatinine of the risk of rhabdomyolysis and renal insufficiency. Also, those patients that wish to proceed with surgery despite this warning are given aggressive intraoperative hydration to prevent significant renal injury. His median nerve injury is likely attributable to traction injury on the nerve at the time of surgery or by pressure exerted on the nerve by an adjacent implant. It seems that removal of the implant has had a beneficial result for the patient and further supports this theory. For this reason, the authors are reluctant to place implants in a submuscular plane as clearly there is an increased risk of potential neurovascular injury.

Adjunct Procedures for Upper Extremity Contouring

Patients seeking contouring of the upper extremity can present with a constellation of problems including lipodystrophy, skin laxity, and muscle hypoplasia. In addition to treating the hypoplastic muscle with biceps implants, a patient may require some combination of liposuction of the arm, fat grafting to the arm, and/or excision of excess skin with formal brachioplasty. Overzealous tissue manipulation at the time of biceps augmentation is avoided, and it is recommended that any liposuction, fat grafting, or skin excision be performed at a separate procedure (before or after an implant surgery) as excessive swelling associated with these procedures when combined with the swelling produced by biceps augmentation may precipitate a compartment syndrome.

In patients that present with significant lipodystrophy of the arm but with little in the way of laxity of skin, isolated liposuction of the arm may be sufficient [24, 25]. The surgeon must be careful in performing circumferential and superficial liposuction of the arms as it may lead to unaesthetic irregularities particularly in the anterior and medial aspects of the arm [24]. Best results are had with liposuction in the deeper layer of adipose tissue, using small-diameter cannulas no larger than 2.5–3 mm. Chamosa even goes so far as to recommend taking some of this harvested fat and grafting to the deltoid region to improve the contour of the upper extremity, placing the maximum width of the arm at the deltoid region.

With advances in bariatric procedures, there has been an increase in the number of patients presenting to the cosmetic surgeon with laxity of skin in the arms after massive weight loss. While adding volume with implants can at times camouflage the overall volume loss in the arm and liposuction can take care of stubborn fat deposits, at times excision of skin is the only way to produce an aesthetic result in the upper extremity. Appelt et al. [25] recommend an algorithmic approach to upper arm contouring to help surgeons best manage the spectrum of patients who present for improvement in arm contour. Using the skin pinch test as a starting point, patients with greater than 1.5 cm of fat detectable with the pinch test could potentially benefit from liposuction. However, the surgeon must take into account skin laxity to assess if liposuction alone is the best option. Rohrich [26] has devised a three-tier classification system that has been modified to better define issues of skin laxity and fat excess in the upper extremity, helping surgeons determine which procedures may be applicable to the patient seeking upper arm contouring. His initial classification described three classifications of upper extremity dystrophy: (I) minimal skin excess and moderate fat excess, (II) moderate skin excess with minimal fat excess, and (III) moderate skin excess with moderate fat excess. Based on his system, Rohrich recommends upper arm contouring with liposuction alone for class I patients. He emphasizes the need for long, uniform strokes to prevent contour irregularities. Patients with type II dystrophy have moderate skin laxity with minimal fat excess and are best treated with some form of brachioplasty and excision of the excess skin. Patients who are type III suffer from moderate skin excess and moderate fat excess and are best treated with a multimodality therapy (liposuction and brachioplasty) in either a single-stage or staged approach [26].

Combined Biceps and Triceps Augmentation

Very frequently, patients will present to the practice wishing to add volume to both the triceps and biceps regions. In the authors' early practice, we were much more willing to perform this procedure. However, having encountered some patients with near-compartment syndrome, the practice has been to avoid doing both biceps and triceps augmentation simultaneously. In the cases where simultaneous augmentations recently were performed, it has been the authors' preference to achieve a smaller augmentation in both muscle groups (rather than larger augmentation in an isolated muscle group) to possibly avoid complications such as compartment syndrome.

Biceps Augmentation with Fat Grafting

Recently, a few patients have requested fat grafting for muscle augmentation. To date, the authors have not yet performed this procedure as it is felt that there is not adequate nutritional support for grafted fat in the area of the upper extremity. Also, due to the rich network of blood vessels and nerves, there is a concern for possible trauma to these structures. Due to the inconsistency of fat take after grafting, the authors do not believe that sufficient and reliable augmentations can be achieved as seen with biceps augmentation with implants.

Author's Personal Results

In reviewing the primary author's (NVC) own experience with the procedure, there have been a total of approximately 220 biceps augmentations since introducing the procedure in 2004. Since that time, 100 procedures have been performed in the submuscular plane and 120 in the subfascial plane. During that time, our seroma rate cumulatively has been 1.3 % (3/220). The infection rate has also been 1.3 % (3/220). The most commonly reported complication was asymmetry, which occurred in 5 % (11/220) of cases. This was largely due to one pocket being slightly over-dissected when compared to the other. Of those patients experiencing asymmetry, only two required operative intervention due to significant asymmetry as noted by the patient and surgeon. The primary author has not had any cases of wound dehiscence or capsular contracture. Satisfaction with the procedure was noted to be 95 % (209/220) with the unhappy patients saying that they achieved an inadequate augmentation.

Patient Cases

Case 1 (Fig. 3.16)
A 27-year-old male underwent biceps and pectoral augmentation. The patient wished to have an exaggerated appearance. His pectoral implants were style 2, size 3. His biceps implants were style 8, size 1.

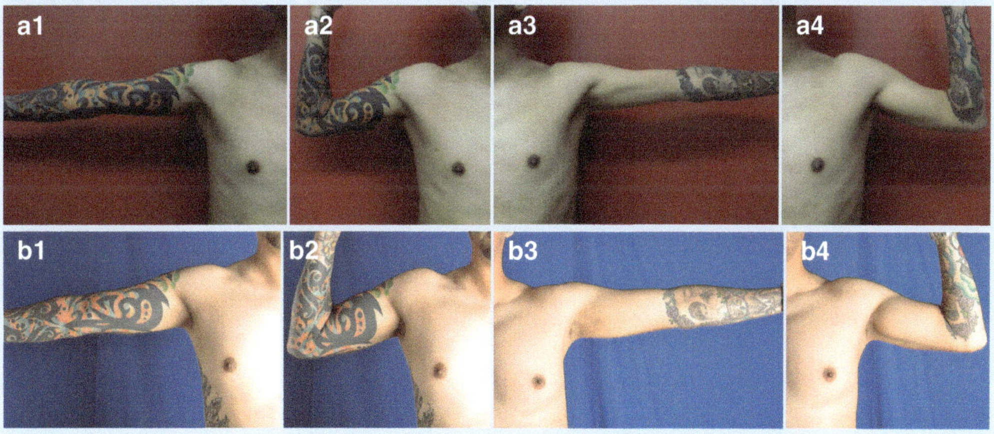

Fig. 3.16 Case 1. (**a**) Preoperative. (**b**) Postoperative

Case 2 (Fig. 3.17)

A 45-year-old male wanted a more defined physique and underwent pectoral, biceps, and triceps augmentation. A style 8, size 25 triceps implant was placed. He had style 8, size 1 biceps implants placed. He also had a style 2, size 3 pectoral augmentation. In addition, liposuction was performed on the chest with excision of glandular tissue in both sides of the chest for gynecomastia.

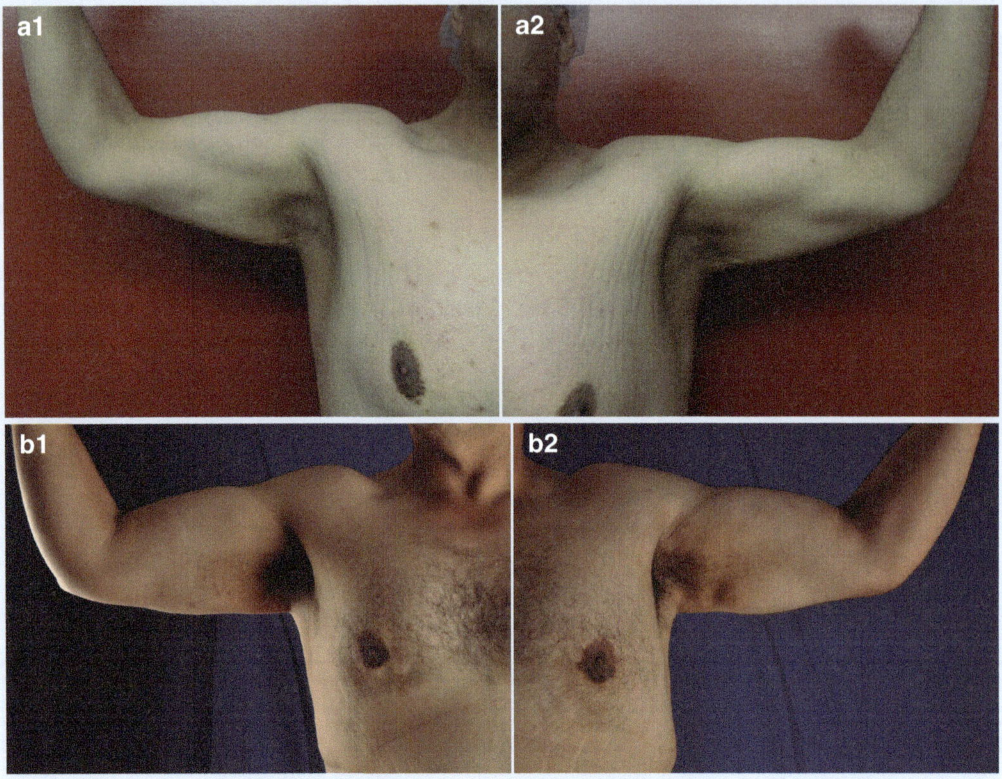

Fig. 3.17 Case 2. (**a**) Preoperative. (**b**) Postoperative

Case 3 (Fig. 3.18)

A 45-year-old male underwent biceps augmentation with style 8, size 1 implants.

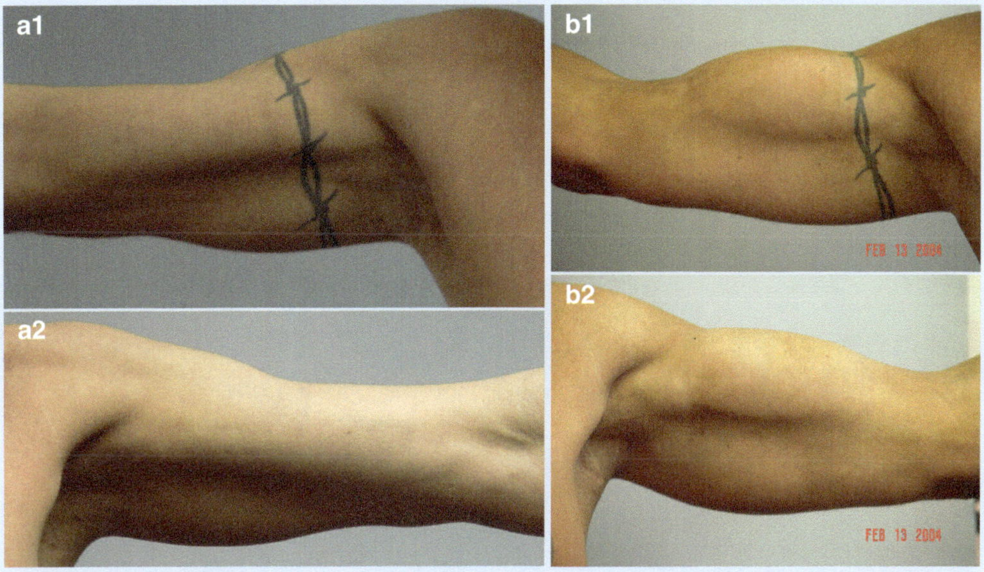

Fig. 3.18 Case 3. (**a**) Preoperative. (**b**) Postoperative

Case 4 (Fig. 3.19)
A 44-year-old male underwent simultaneous biceps augmentation (style 8, size 3) along with triceps augmentation (style 8, size 25).

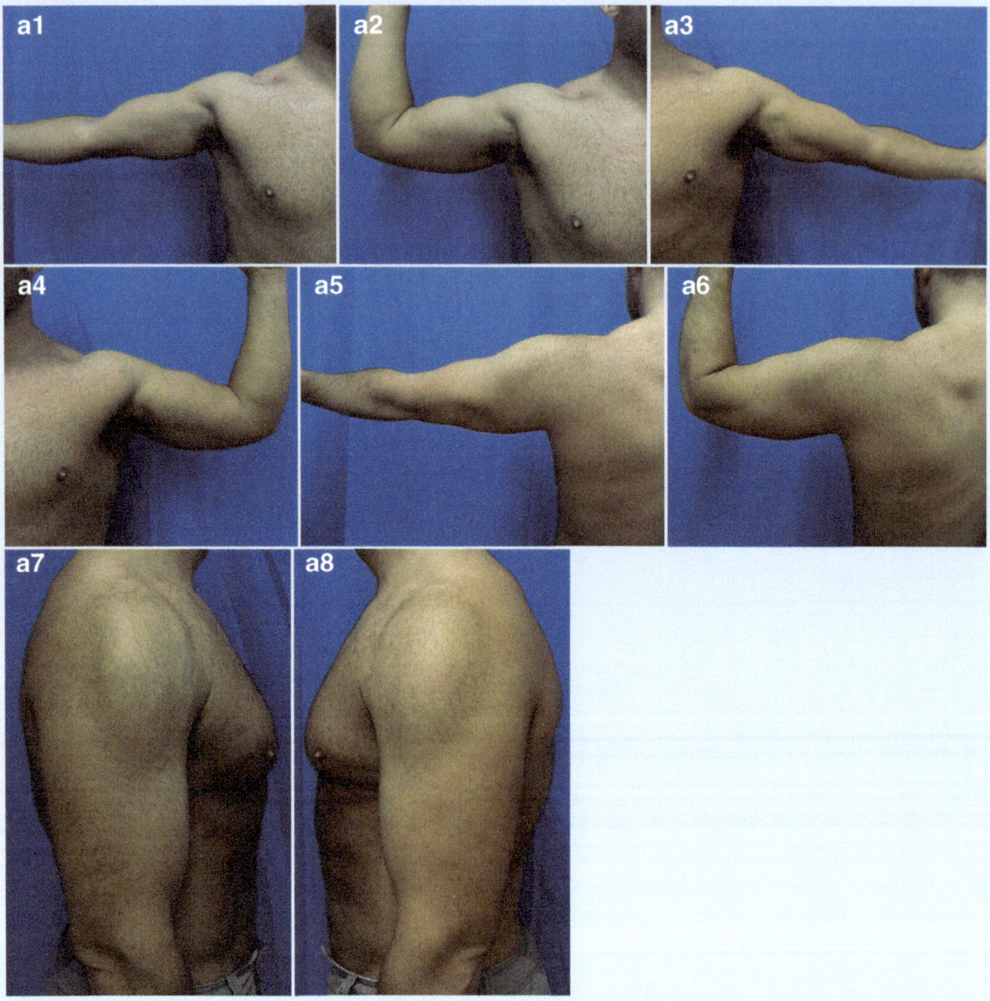

Fig. 3.19 Case 4. (**a**) Preoperative. (**b**) Postoperative

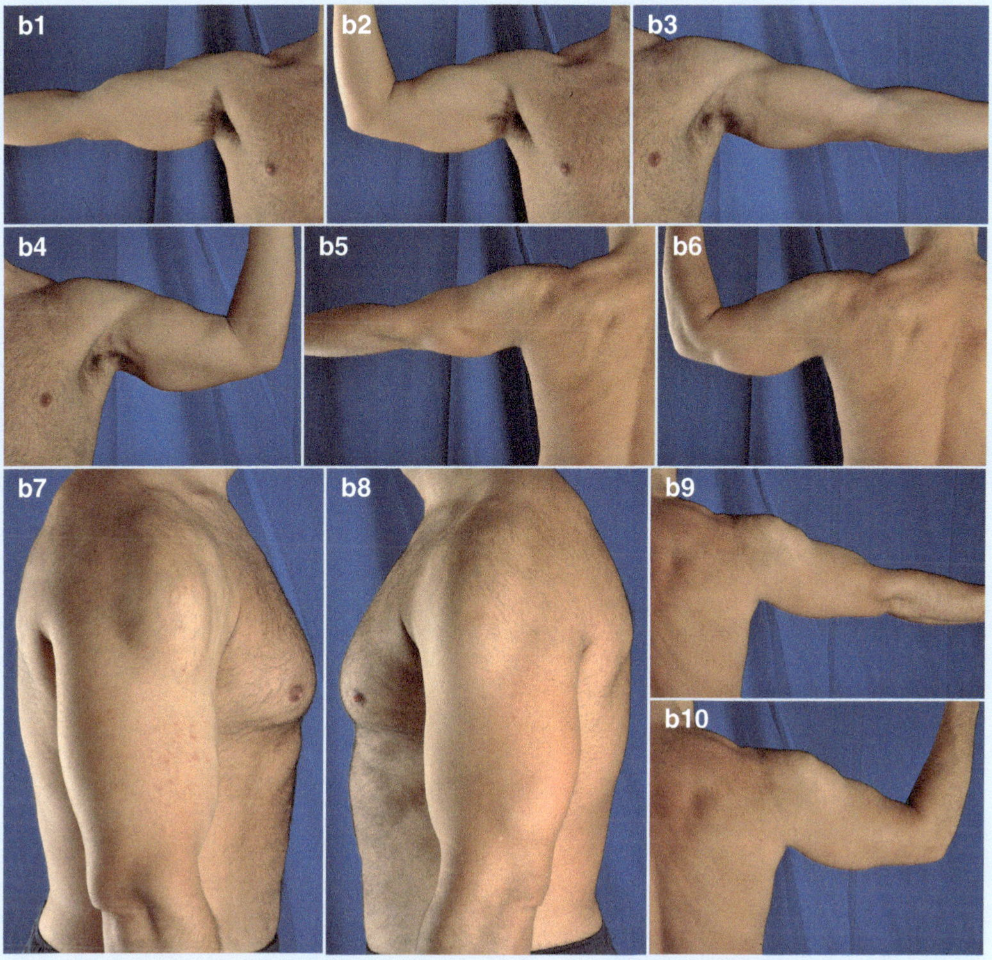

Fig. 3.19 (continued)

Case 5 (Fig. 3.20)

A 54-year-old male underwent biceps augmentation with style 8, size 1 implants.

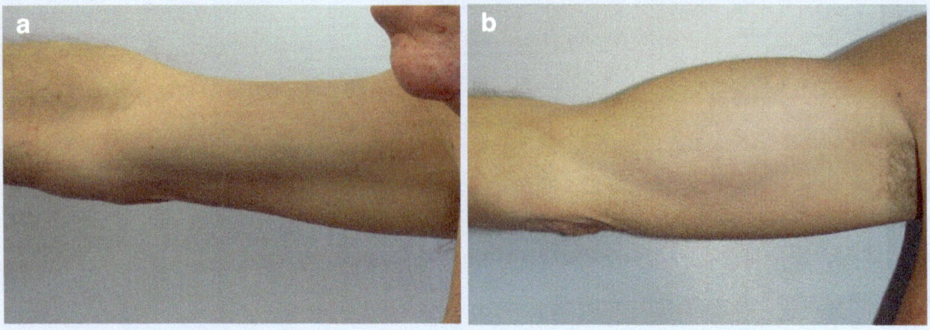

Fig. 3.20 Case 5. (**a**) Preoperative. (**b**) Postoperative

Case 6 (Fig. 3.21)

A 42-year-old male underwent biceps augmentation with style 8, size 1 implants.

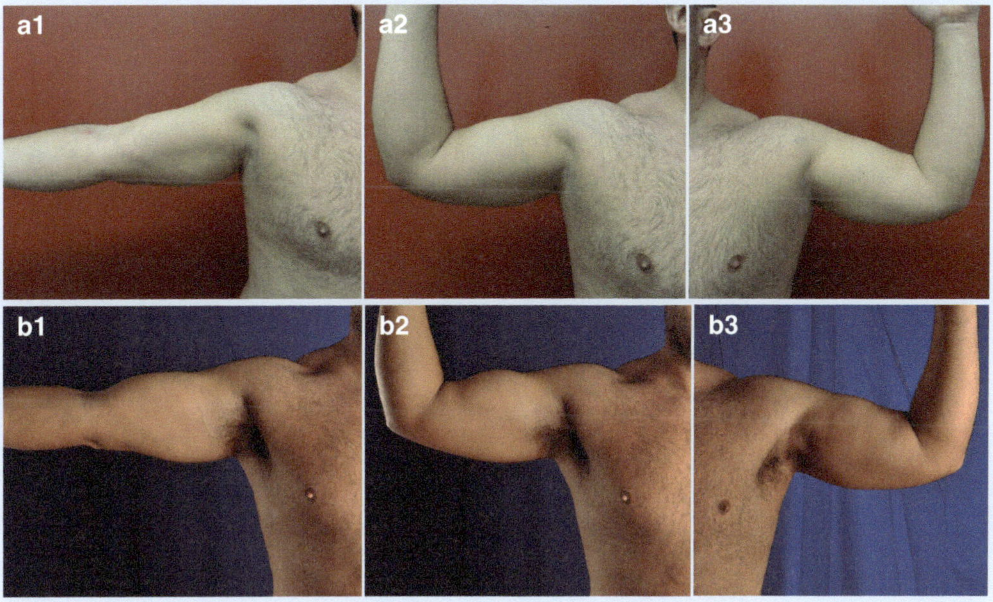

Fig. 3.21 Case 6. (**a**) Preoperative. (**b**) Postoperative

Case 7 (Fig. 3.22)
A 38-year-old male underwent biceps augmentation with style 8, size 1 implants and triceps augmentation with style 8, size 20 implants.

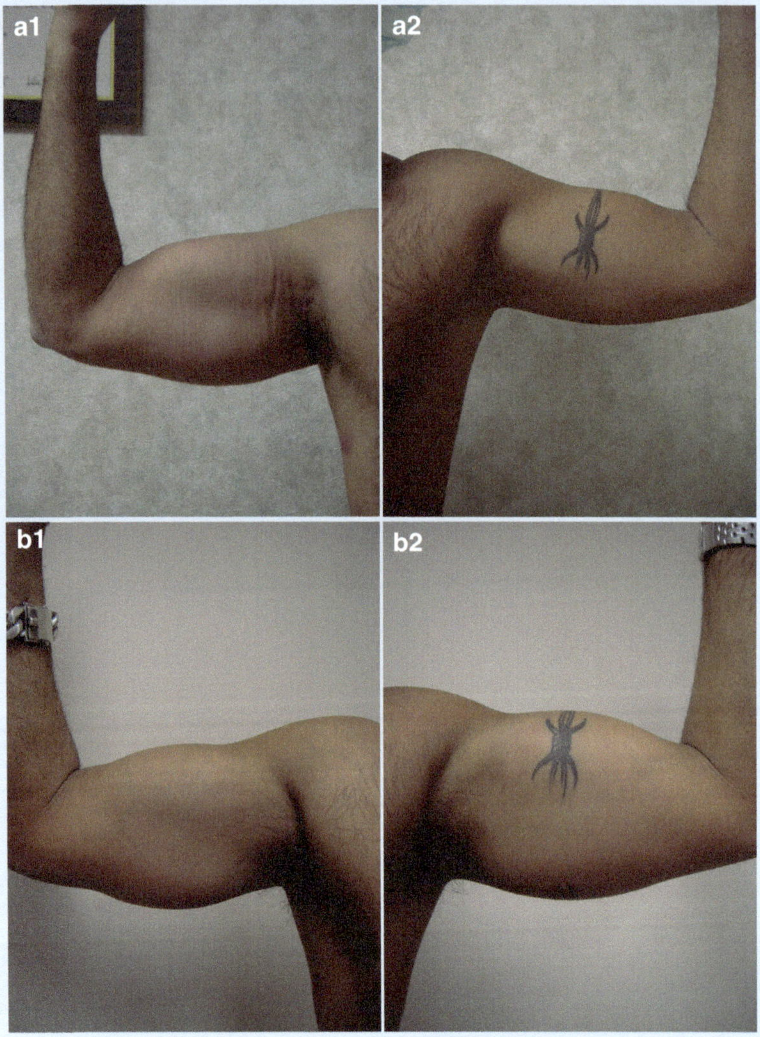

Fig. 3.22 Case 7. (**a**) Preoperative. (**b**) Postoperative

Conclusions

The biceps augmentation operation is a relatively straightforward procedure that affords great results. Prudent dissection of the pocket for the implant is essential for optimal cosmetic result and to prevent implant malposition. The vast majority of dissection during the procedure is blunt with natural tissue planes, thus preventing any damage to vital structures in the upper arm. While a submuscular plane has been achieved by the primary author and others in the past, it is the author's current practice to place the implant in a subfascial position, affording excellent cosmetic results with minimal morbidity.

References

1. Plastic surgery statistics report. 2012. http://www.plasticsurgery.org/Documents/news-resources/statistics/2012-Plastic-Surgery-Statistics/full-plastic-surgery-statistics-report.pdf. Accessed 9 May 2013.
2. American Academy of Cosmetic Surgery procedural census. 2008. http://multivu.prnewswire.com/mnr/aacs/36867/docs/36867AACS2008ProceduralSurveyResults.pdf. Accessed 9 May 2013.
3. Pope HG, Olivardia R, Gruber A, Borowiecki J. Evolving ideals of male body image as seen through action toys. Int J Eat Disord. 1999;26(1):65–72.
4. Flores-Lima G, Eppley BL. Body contouring with solid silicone implants. Aesthetic Plast Surg. 2009; 33(2):140–6.
5. Olivardia R, Pope HG, Borowiecki JJ, Cohane GH. Biceps and body image: the relationship between muscularity and self-esteem, depression, and eating disorder symptoms. Psychol Men Masculinity. 2004;5(2):112–20.
6. Leit RA, Pope HG, Gray JJ. Cultural expectation of muscularity in men: the evolution of playgirl centerfolds. Int J Eat Disord. 2001;29(1):90–3.
7. Phillips KA. Body image and body dysmorphic disorder. In: Cash T, Smolak L, editors. Body image: a handbook of science, practice, and prevention. 2nd ed. New York: The Guilford Press; 2011. p. 305–13.
8. Pope HG, Gruber AJ, Mangweth B, Bureau B, deCol C, Jouvent R, Hudson JI. Body image perception among men in three countries. Am J Psychiatry. 2000;157(8):1297–301.
9. Cafri G, Thompson JK, Riccciardelli L, McCabe M, Smolak L, Yesalis C. Pursuit of the muscular ideal: physical and psychological consequences and putative risk factors. Clin Psychol Rev. 2005;25(2):215–39.
10. Bonnecarrere ER, Butler B. Case report: upper extremity soft-tissue reconstruction by alloplastic implant: long-term result and follow-up. Ann Plast Surg. 1997;38(1):74–6.
11. Hodgkinson DJ. Contour restoration of the upper limb using solid silicone implants. Aesthetic Plast Surg. 2006;30(1):53–8.
12. Chugay N, Racanelli J, Hsu J, Chugay P. Bicipital augmentation. Am J Cosmet Surg. 2006;23(1):33–6.
13. Chugay N, Chugay P. Bicipital augmentation: a retrospective review of 94 patient cases. Am J Cosmet Surg. 2009;26(4):241–5.
14. Dini GM, Ferreria LM. Augmentation brachioplasty with cohesive silicone gel implants. In: Shiffman MA, Di Giuseppe A, editors. Body contouring: art, science, and clinical practice. Berlin: Springer; 2010. p. 327–30.
15. Abadesso I, Serra F. Augmentation brachioplasty: surgery for improving the appearance of the arms. Rev Bras Cir Plast. 2012;27(1):97–101.
16. Gray H. Anatomy of the human body. Philadelphia: Lea & Febiger; 1918.
17. Toomayan GA, Robertson F, Major NM, Brigman BE. Upper extremity compartmental anatomy: clinical relevance to radiologists. Skeletal Radiol. 2006;35(4):195–201.
18. Mazurek MT, Shin AY. Upper extremity peripheral nerve anatomy. Clin Orthop Relat Res. 2001;383:7–20.
19. Dailiana ZH, Roulot E, Le Viet D. Surgical treatment of compression of the lateral antebrachial cutaneous nerve. J Bone Joint Surg Br. 2000;82(3):420–3.
20. Amendola A. Compartment syndromes. In: Browner BD, Jupiter JB, Levine AM, Trafton BG, Krettek C, editors. Skeletal trauma: basic science, management, and reconstruction. Philadelphia: Saunders; 2003.
21. Cothren CC, Biffl WL, Moore EE. Trauma. In: Brunicardi FC, Andersen DK, Billiar TR, Dunn DL, Hunter JG, Matthews JB, Pollock RE, editors. Schwartz's principles of surgery. New York: McGraw-Hill Professional; 2010.
22. Clarkson PM, Kearns AK, Rouzier P, Rubin R, Thompson PD. Serum creatine kinase levels and renal function measures in exertional muscle damage. Med Sci Sports Exerc. 2006;38(4):623–7.
23. Daher EF, Silva Júnior GB, Queiroz AL, Ramos LM, Santos SQ, Barreto DM, Guimarães AA, Barbosa CA, Franco LM, Patrocínio RM. Acute kidney injury due to anabolic steroid and vitamin supplement abuse: report of two cases and a literature review. Int Urol Nephrol. 2009;41(3):717–23.
24. Chamosa M, Murillo J, Vazquez T. Lipectomy of arms and lipograft of shoulders balance the upper body contour. Aesthetic Plast Surg. 2005;29(6):567–70.
25. Appelt EA, Janis JE, Rohrich RJ. An algorithmic approach to upper arm contouring. Plast Reconstr Surg. 2006;118(1):237–46.
26. Rohrich RJ, Beran SJ, Kenkel JM. Back and arms. In: Rohrich RJ, Beran SJ, Kenkel JM, editors. Ultrasound assisted liposuction. 1st ed. St Louis: Quality Medical Publishing; 1998. p. 231–51.

4 Triceps Augmentation

Introduction

As men are increasingly becoming interested in cosmetic surgery, surgeons have to modify procedures and create new ones to meet the needs of the male population [1, 2]. With the advent of the biceps augmentation in 2004, the introduction of the triceps augmentation procedure was a natural progression. Many patients presented for muscle augmentation surgery and wanted a circumferential upper extremity augmentation. As there was no established procedure or formal implant in use, it was necessary to construct an implant that would easily fit below the long head of the triceps or under the deep investing fascia of the arm, depending on the patient's needs. This implant had to be pliable and yet sturdy enough to resist the constant movement of the arm and contraction of the upper extremity musculature. Using the Chugay Biceps Prosthesis as a starting point, a custom-designed triceps prosthesis was developed to help achieve augmentation in the triceps area for reconstructive and cosmetic needs.

Body Dissatisfaction in Males

It stands to emphasize that many men have some element of body dysmorphic disorder and wish to have a more muscular and "built" physique in order to be better accepted in society and by the opposite sex [3–8]. Society has created an idealistic model of the male that is oftentimes hard to attain with simple diet and exercise alone. For this reason, muscle augmentation surgery of the upper extremity, both biceps and triceps augmentation, gives a male the opportunity to achieve this ideal.

History of the Procedure

Triceps augmentation really takes its early steps in the work done by various surgeons to augment the bicipital region. The biceps implant, as mentioned previously, was initially used by surgeons to help in the reconstruction of soft tissue defects of the upper extremity left by significant trauma or post-oncologic surgery [9]. Hodgkinson further added to the literature on the use of solid silicone implants for restoration of symmetry and addition of volume to traumatized extremities [10]. In his paper from 2006, he discusses the use of silicone implants to add volume to the upper extremity after ruptures of triceps and biceps muscles and in cases of axillary nerve injury that showed degeneration of the deltoid muscle.

Using his experience with biceps augmentation and having a good understanding of the upper extremity musculature and neurovascular structures, the primary author sought to begin performing triceps augmentation not only for restoration of volume following traumatic injury or as a result of congenital abnormalities but to aid those patients who wished to increase the volume of the triceps region purely for vanity [11, 12]. In 2010, the primary author published his work on

N.V. Chugay et al., *Body Sculpting with Silicone Implants*,
DOI 10.1007/978-3-319-04957-1_4, © Springer International Publishing Switzerland 2014

14 patients that received triceps augmentation from 2008 to 2010 [13]. All of the initial procedures were performed via an incision in the axilla and placement of the implant primarily in the submuscular plane. In the primary author's experience, greater risks for complications were possible with placement of the implant under the muscle, as in biceps augmentation, and for that reason the author routinely uses the subfascial plane for augmentation in the vast majority of cases. With placement solely beneath the fascia, the improved contour was similarly noted but without the increased risk of damage to vital neurovascular structures.

In 2012, Abadesso and Serra [14] published their work on 32 cases of biceps augmentation for improving the cosmetic appearance of the arms. They used calf implants in the submuscular plane to achieve the desired augmentation. Although the majority of their cases were performed for biceps augmentation, the authors do note that they were able to achieve a triceps augmentation in one patient who very much liked the aesthetics of his biceps augmentation. Using two stacked calf implants secured by a 3-0 nylon suture as they did for biceps augmentation, the authors placed this stacked set of implants beneath the triceps muscle to achieve a triceps augmentation. The incision used is the same one described for their biceps augmentation, namely, an S-shaped incision in the midarm region over the intermuscular septum.

Indications

Initially, triceps augmentation was introduced as a means to treating asymmetries in the arm region left due to congenital anomalies and trauma producing atrophy of muscles in the upper extremity and in those patients who suffered volume deficits secondary to trauma or post-oncologic surgery. Triceps augmentation, for purely aesthetic reasons, is indicated for the patient who has hypoplasia in the area of the triceps muscle. It can be used in the patient who has a condition from birth resulting in hypoplasia or may be applied to a patient who is unsuccessful in achieving the desired volume in the region of the triceps, despite aggressive weight training (e.g., bodybuilders).

Contraindications

While not every male presenting for triceps augmentation suffers from muscle dysmorphia/body dysmorphic disorder, the surgeon must be aware of this and take it into consideration when considering a patient for muscle augmentation surgery. A patient who seems unrealistic in the goals of his surgery should be turned away.

Limitations

In any initial triceps augmentation, patients are instructed on the fact that they can achieve an augmentation of approximately 1 inch in added circumference of the arm. Larger augmentations may require a second operation with larger, custom implants. Also, patients are instructed that while biceps and triceps augmentations can be performed, it is safer to separate this into two separate surgeries to avoid the risk of compartment syndrome in the upper extremity.

Relevant Anatomy

The technique described herein is ideal in that it avoids major neurovascular structures in the upper extremity. The posterior compartment of the arm is relatively devoid of major structures in the superficial planes. However, for completeness sake we will review some of the basic anatomy that is pertinent to the discussion of triceps augmentation.

An axial section through the midarm shows much of the relevant anatomy for triceps augmentation (Fig. 4.1). Two distinct muscular compartments (anterior and posterior) exist and are separated by the medial and lateral intermuscular septa and humerus [15]. The medial and lateral intermuscular septa arise from the humerus and insert into the brachial fascia, which covers the superficial muscles of the anterior compartment. The anterior compartment is composed of the biceps brachii, brachialis, and coracobrachialis.

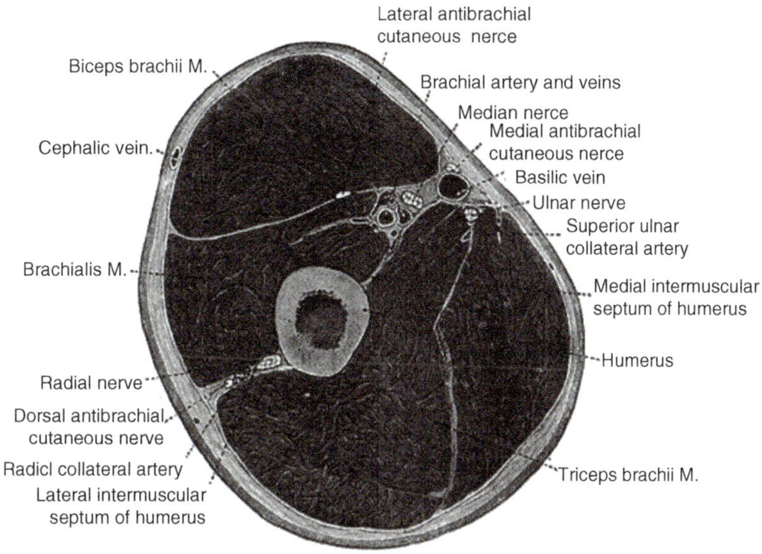

Fig. 4.1 Axial cross section of the arm showing the humerus with medial and lateral intermuscular septa that separate anterior from posterior compartments of the arm. The anterior compartment is composed of the biceps brachii, brachialis, and coracobrachialis. The posterior compartment is composed of the triceps muscle. Major neurovascular structures are primarily localized to the medial aspect of the arm

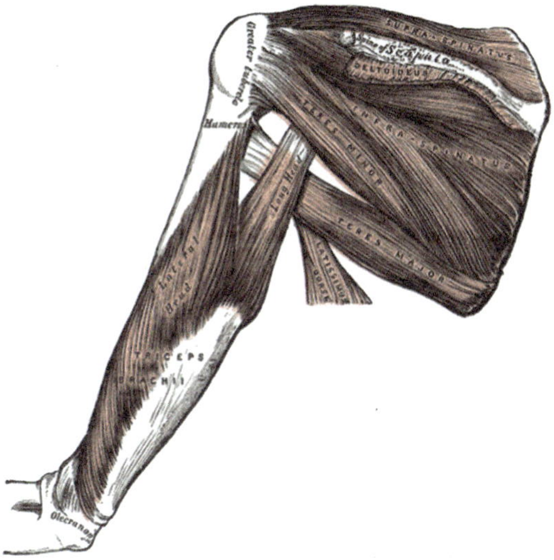

Fig. 4.2 Diagram depicting the triceps muscle, focusing on the lateral and long heads of the triceps which are most superficial and pertinent to the dissection for triceps augmentation. The medial head of the triceps is not visualized

The posterior compartment, also covered by extensions of the intermuscular septa, is comprised of the triceps muscle, which acts in extension of the forearm. The triceps brachii is composed of three heads (Fig. 4.2). The long head arises by a flattened tendon from the infraglenoid tuberosity of the scapula. The lateral head arises from the posterior surface of the body of the humerus. The medial head arises from the posterior surface of the body of the humerus, below the groove for the radial nerve. The three heads then converge into one triceps tendon which begins about the middle of the muscle and inserts into the posterior portion of the olecranon of the ulna. Most superficial of these three heads is the long head of the triceps. Also in a very superficial position, but more laterally, is the lateral head of the triceps muscle. The medial head is found deeper, adjacent to the medial aspect of the humerus.

The major neurovascular structures of the arm are located in an extracompartmental location on the medial aspect of the arm (Fig. 4.3). The basilic vein plays a major role in the superficial venous drainage of the upper extremity. It runs upward along the medial border of the biceps brachii; perforates the deep fascia slightly below the middle of the arm; and, ascending on the medial side of the brachial artery to the lower border of the teres major, continues onward as the axillary vein. The brachial artery (a continuation of the axillary artery) commences at the lower margin of the tendon of the teres major and, passing down the arm, ends about 1 cm below the bend of the elbow, where it divides into the radial and ulnar arteries. At first, the brachial artery lies medial to the humerus; however, it gradually moves in front of the bone as it runs down the arm, and at the bend of the elbow, it lies midway between its two epicondyles. The brachial artery is the major supplier of blood flow to

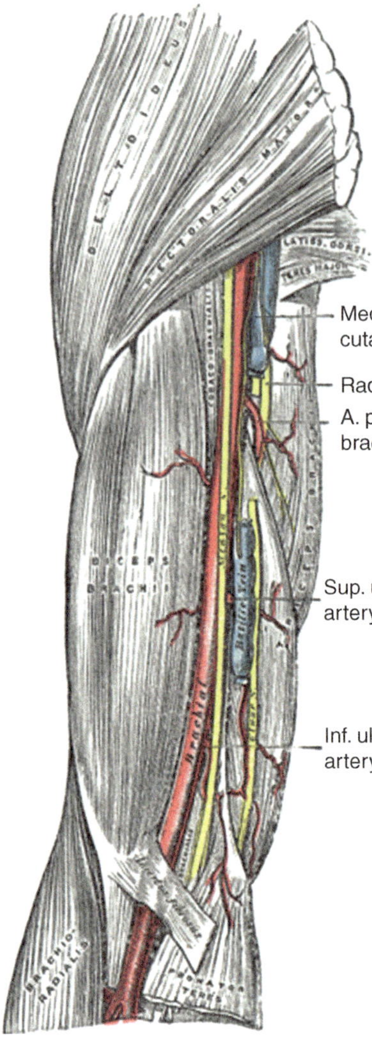

Fig. 4.3 Major neurovascular structures located in medial aspect of the arm in the extracompartmental space

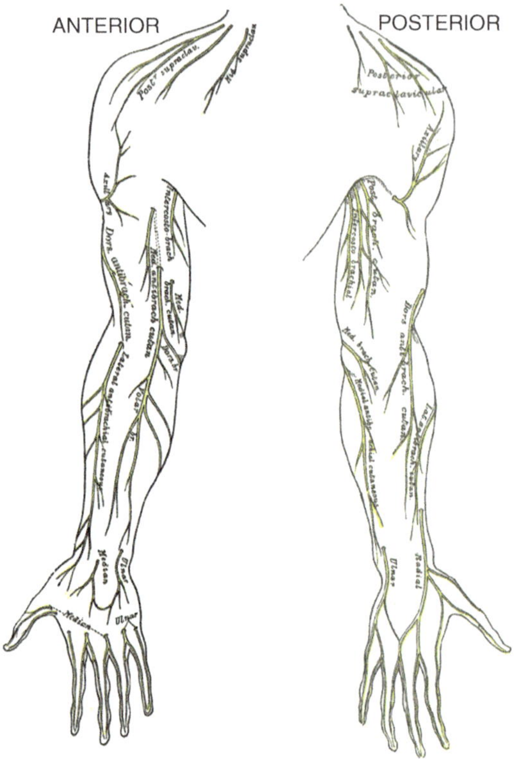

Fig. 4.4 Major sensory nerves of the arm and their distribution

the upper extremities. Because this artery is superficial throughout its entire extent, being covered in front by the integument and the superficial and deep fascia, great care should be taken to preserve its integrity. The ulnar nerve is similarly located in this medial extracompartmental location. It arises from the medial cord of the brachial plexus and descends on the posteromedial aspect of the humerus. The nerve supplies motor function to the forearm and hand. It is only with extensive submuscular dissection that any of these major neurovascular structures can be encountered as they are removed from the proposed planes of dissection for triceps augmentation, particularly when performed in the subfascial position.

When considering triceps augmentation, structures that are significantly at risk of injury are the radial nerve and two of its smaller cutaneous branches, the posterior cutaneous nerve of the arm (posterior brachial cutaneous nerve) and the dorsal antebrachial cutaneous nerve (posterior cutaneous nerve of the forearm) (Fig. 4.4). The radial nerve occupies a position deep within the posterior compartment in close proximity to the posterior aspect of the humerus and medial head of the triceps, approximately 97–142 mm distal to the acromion [15, 16] (Fig. 4.5). The radial nerve is responsible for the innervation of the triceps and arises from the seventh and eighth cranial nerves. It is really only of note in patients receiving submuscular placement of the triceps implant. In this case, overaggressive dissection near the humerus may put the radial nerve at

Cross-section of the arm

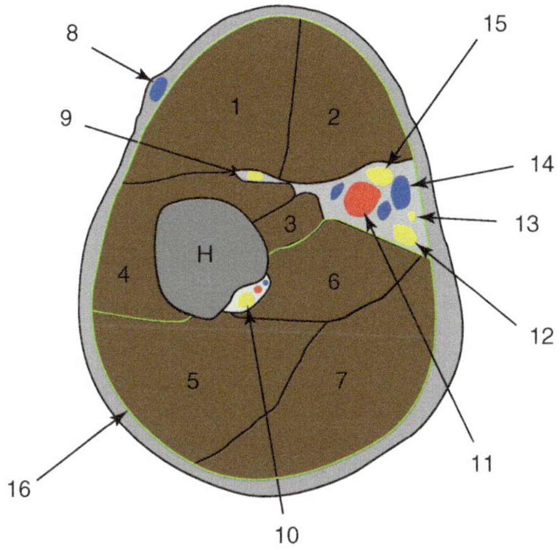

H- Humerus
1. m. biceps brachii, caput longum
2. m. biceps brachii, caput breve
3. m. coracobrachialis
4. m. brachialis
5. m. triceps brachill, caput laterale
6. m. triceps brachill, caput mediale
7. m. triceps brachill, caput longum
8. v. cephalica
9. n. musculocutaneus
10. n. radialis, a.+v. profunda brachii
11. a.+vv. Brachii
12. n. ulnaris
13. n. cutaneus antebrachii medilais
14. v. basilica
15. n. medianus
16. fascia brachii + septum intermusculare brachii mediale et laterale (green)

Fig. 4.5 Radial nerve in its position deep within the arm and giving off two of its major cutaneous branches at risk for injury in triceps augmentation: posterior cutaneous nerve of the arm and the dorsal antebrachial cutaneous nerve

risk of injury. Immediately adjacent to the radial nerve course some of its cutaneous branches, namely, the posterior cutaneous nerve of the arm and the dorsal antebrachial cutaneous nerve. The posterior cutaneous nerve of the arm provides sensory innervation for much of the skin on the back of the arm (Fig. 4.6). The dorsal antebrachial cutaneous nerve, also a branch of the radial, provides sensation to the posterior aspect of the forearm. Typically the cutaneous branches are at greater risk as they are smaller and more fragile nerves. Injuries, when encountered, are the result of traction injury rather than transection. Traction injuries result in a temporary neurapraxia with loss of sensation in the posterior arm (posterior cutaneous nerve of the arm) or the forearm (dorsal antebrachial cutaneous nerve). Generally these nerves are avoided in the dissection of the subfascial plane and are really only at risk in submuscular augmentation cases.

Consultation/Implant Selection

The consultation begins with a thorough medical history of the patient. Special attention is taken to ask specifically about trauma to the extremity, history of vascular insufficiency which may put blood flow at risk, history of venous insufficiency or arm swelling, and any history of nerve damage or sensory deficits as may be seen in patients with diabetes mellitus. Also, patients with histories of nerve entrapment disorders should be asked about the current state of those nerves and any long-term sequelae. At the time of consultation, the patient is asked what specifically about their arm bothers them as it may be necessary to combine muscle augmentation surgery with adjunct procedures such as liposculpture or brachioplasty to achieve the patient's goals. Preoperative goals are assessed at this point. A patient who has unrealistic expectations and is unable to comply with the strict postoperative instructions is deemed a poor candidate for augmentation. Patients who have congenital anomalies, a significant size disparity between the two arms, or bilateral hypoplasia are informed that several surgeries may be required to attain symmetry and achieve the augmentation they desire. Patients are also asked about their current level of activity and muscle building history, taking care to inform the patient of the need to take at least 1 month of time to recover before resuming any vigorous arm building regimens.

After completion of the history, the patient's arms are evaluated. First, symmetry of the two sides is assessed and any disparity is brought to the attention of the patient. Although the majority of patients present with a preexisting asymmetry

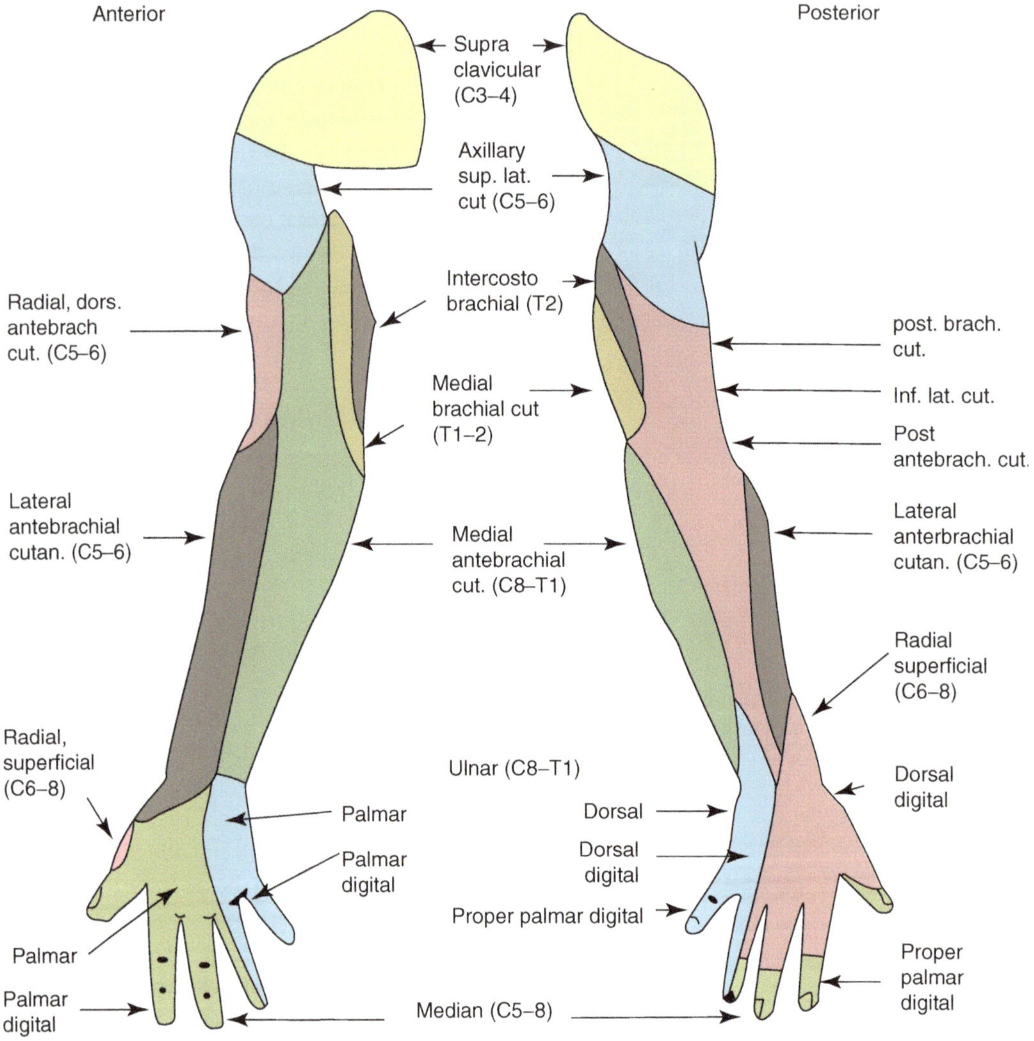

Fig. 4.6 Dermatomes of major sensory nerves of the arm

of the arms, not many patients note the difference, and this can be a source of medicolegal matters in the future. The physician then evaluates the quality of the skin, subcutaneous tissue, and muscle. A person who has very thin tissues or significant hypoplasia of the triceps may not be able to adequately accommodate a large implant. Also, a person with thin tissues may have to be counseled about the possible need for a submuscular placement of the prosthesis. This should be accompanied by a discussion of the increased risks associated with triceps augmentation in the submuscular plane.

Next, the patient's arms are measured in circumference at the midportion of the arm, with the patient in flexed and neutral positions. These measurements are primarily used in the postoperative period to demonstrate the results of augmentation. Another measurement is taken with the patient flexing their triceps muscle. The proximal point of the muscle belly is palpated and marked as is the distal portion of the muscle belly and this is measured. Having this second measurement allows one to assess the maximum length of implant that can be accommodated in the triceps region. The width of the muscle belly is measured from its medial to lateral extent while the patient's muscle is flexed. Based on these latter measurements, the surgeon can choose the implant that would best suit the patient's body habitus.

Available Implants (Table 4.1)

Table 4.1 Triceps implants (Aesthetic and Reconstructive Technologies, Inc., Reno, NV)

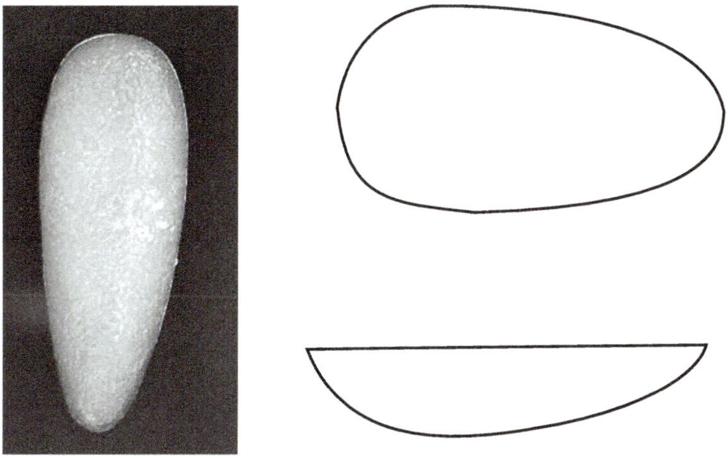

size	Catalog #	Width	Length	Projection	Volume (cc)
1	600–820	10.0	5.0	2.2	
2	600–825	15.0	6.0	2.2	

Preoperative Planning and Marking

The triceps contour is marked out with a surgical marking pen, taking special care to also mark the apex of the triceps on contraction as the implant must be centered under this point. A marking is then made in the axillary region for the initial incision in the axilla.

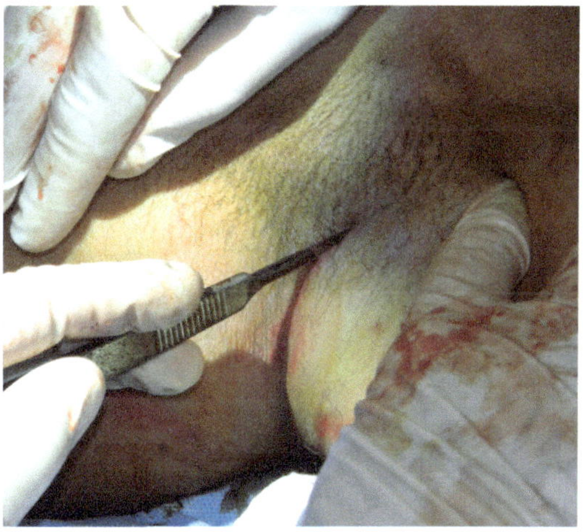

Fig. 4.7 Axillary incision being made

Operative Technique

The patient is brought to the operating room, prepped, and draped in the usual supine position with the arms extended. A 3–4 cm incision is made in the axillary region with a number 15 blade scalpel (Fig. 4.7). The skin is elevated by sharp using Metzenbaum scissors and blunt finger dissection (Fig. 4.8). The fascia overlying the long head of the triceps muscle is identified. Next, an incision is made in the fascia with a number 15 blade scalpel in the direction of the muscle fibers (Fig. 4.9). The long head of the triceps is then visualized (Fig. 4.10). Stay sutures are then placed into the muscle fascia to aid in closure at the end of the procedure (Fig. 4.11). If the patient is to have placement of the implant below the triceps muscle, it is at this point that the long head of the triceps is split with a hemostat in line with its fibers. A submuscular plane can then be developed below the long head of the triceps muscle primarily, but also below the lateral head. This plane seats the implant squarely on the humerus. The authors' preference is to create a subfascial pocket for implant placement. Blunt dissection is performed using the operator's digit underneath the fascia overlying the

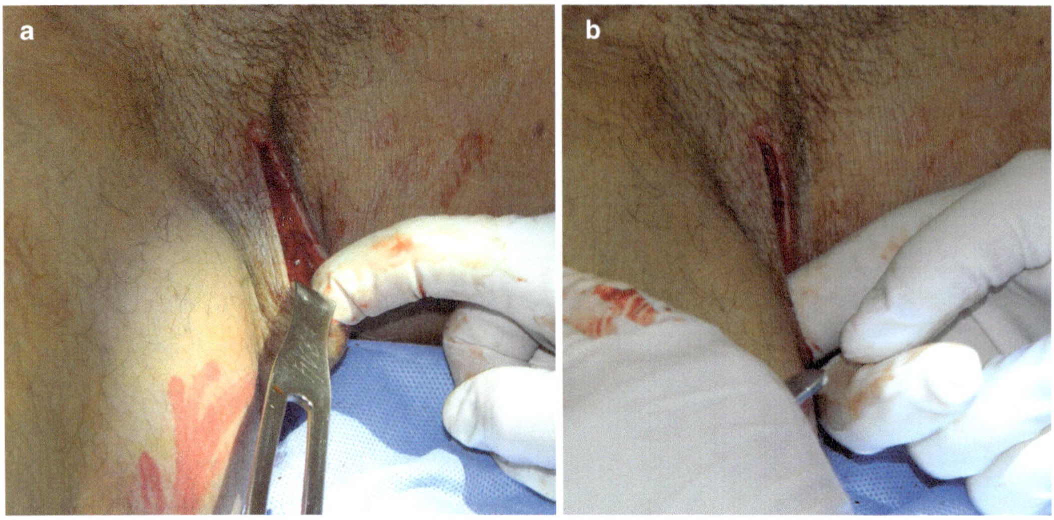

Fig. 4.8 (**a**, **b**) Blunt finger dissection down to triceps fascia with use of army navy retractor to provide adequate exposure

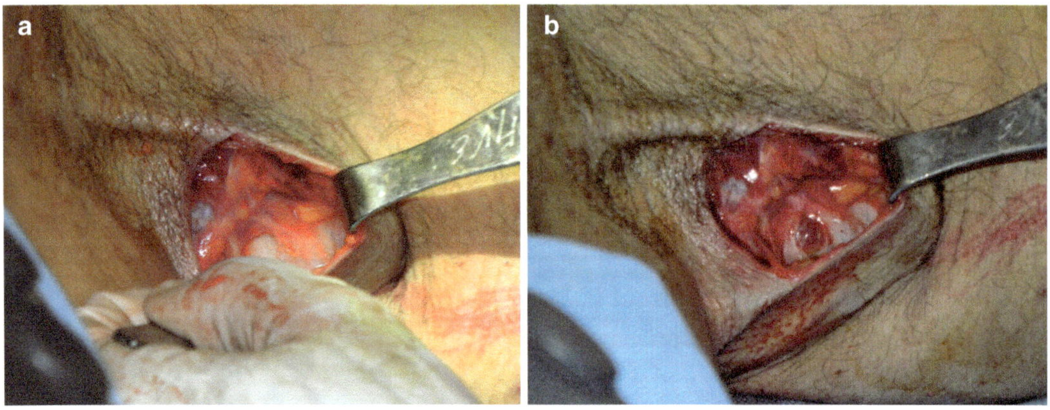

Fig. 4.9 (**a**) Exposed triceps fascia at 3–5 o'clock position (*glistening white*). (**b**) Incision in the triceps fascia

long head of the triceps muscle. Once the pocket dissection is well underway, a spatula dissector is placed underneath the fascia, and the dissection of the pocket is completed (Fig. 4.12). The plane of dissection is continued distally toward the elbow until resistance is met. The pocket is packed with a sponge and attention is turned to the contralateral side to perform the same procedure. Once both sides have been dissected, the lap sponges are removed and hemostasis is achieved as necessary with electrocautery. The pocket is irrigated with a solution containing cefazolin, gentamicin, Betadine, and normal saline. This solution is then aspirated. Then, 10 mL of 0.5 % Marcaine is instilled into the pocket for postoperative analgesia. A custom-made, solid silicone triceps prosthesis is placed underneath the fascia of the long head of the triceps muscle or below the muscle in cases of submuscular augmentation (Fig. 4.13). Once the position of the implant is deemed satisfactory, closure in layers is begun. The fascia is repaired with 3-0 Vicryl suture (Fig. 4.14). The subcutaneous tissues are then reapproximated using 4-0 Vicryl suture. The skin is then closed in subcuticular fashion using 4-0 Monocryl suture. The incision is covered with collodion and Robbins tape. Elastic

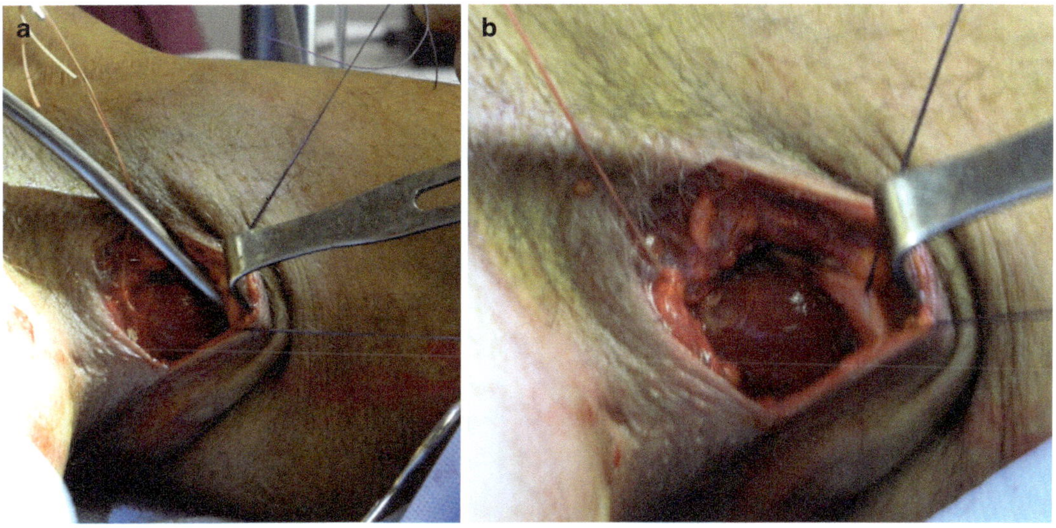

Fig. 4.10 (**a**) Exposed triceps long head. (**b**) Closer view of the exposed triceps long head

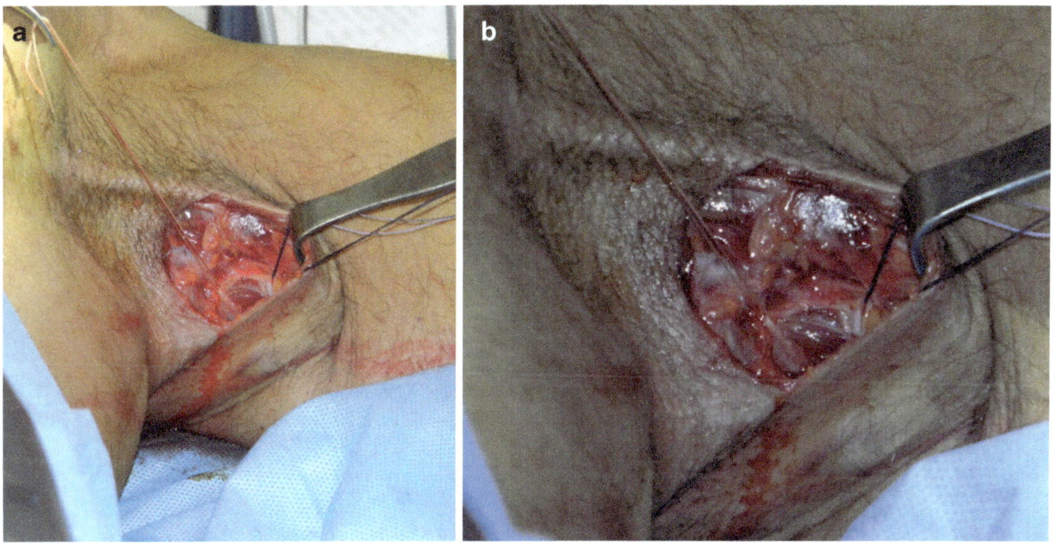

Fig. 4.11 (**a**) Stay sutures in place for use at closure in both ends of the fascia. The authors prefer to use dark sutures as the distal/down and the light, undyed Vicryl as the proximal/up suture. (**b**) Close-up of sutures in triceps fascia

compression wraps are applied to the arms at this time. The patient is then returned to the recovery room and monitored before discharge home.

Postoperative Instructions

On discharge from the office on the day of surgery, the patients have their arms wrapped in elastic compression sleeves to diminish the amount of swelling and potential for seroma formation. These sleeves are to be worn at all times for a period of 4 weeks. Patients may remove the sleeves to shower and to wash the sleeves as needed. Patients may begin showering the day after surgery, taking care to dry the elastic tape over their incisions with a hair dryer on a low heat setting. The patient is instructed postoperatively to limit the use of the upper extremities and to avoid exertion or any heavy lifting.

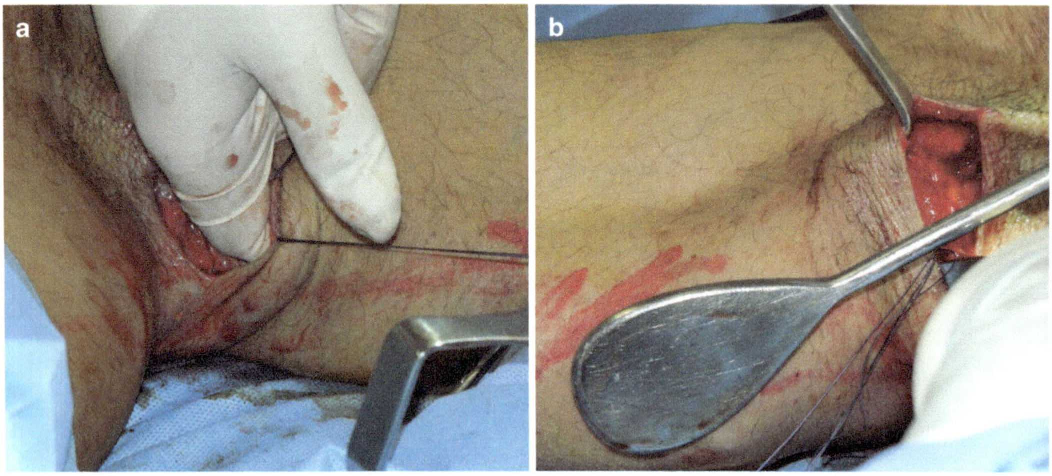

Fig. 4.12 (**a**) Dissection of the subfascial pocket is begun with blunt finger dissection. (**b**) Further dissection of the pocket is performed with the spatula dissector

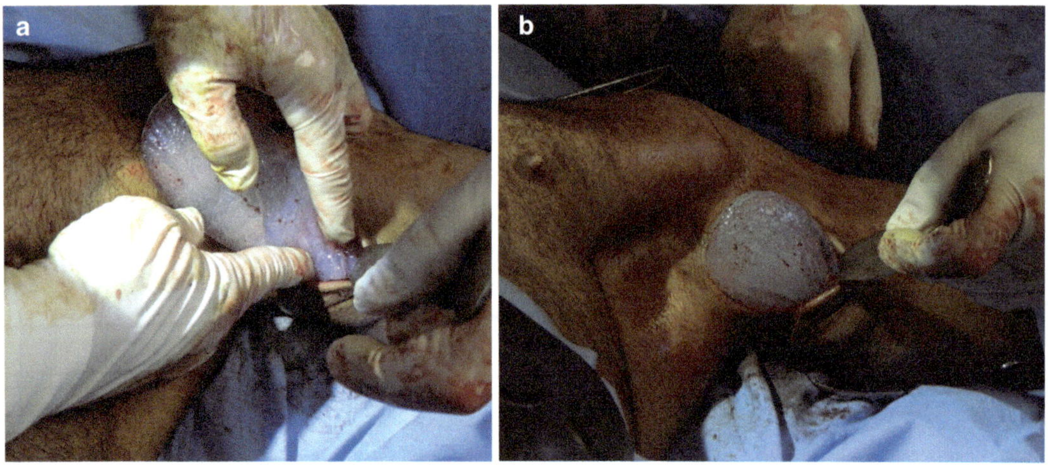

Fig. 4.13 (**a**) Placement of the triceps implant using a folding over technique. (**b**) Triceps implant 50 % introduced

Patients may begin to use their arms as tolerated immediately after surgery but are restricted from heavy lifting or vigorous activity for 4–6 weeks postoperatively.

Complications

In performing triceps augmentation, there is a host of potential complications that can arise (Table 4.2).

Infection

Infection, either superficial or deep, is a possibility in triceps augmentation surgery. The authors' series of 30 patients has demonstrated only one superficial skin infection that grew *Staphylococcus aureus* (MSSA), giving an incidence of 3.3 %. The patient was a health-care provider and presented 1 week after surgery with erythema around the incision with minor serous drainage. Prior to making the incision, standard practice should be

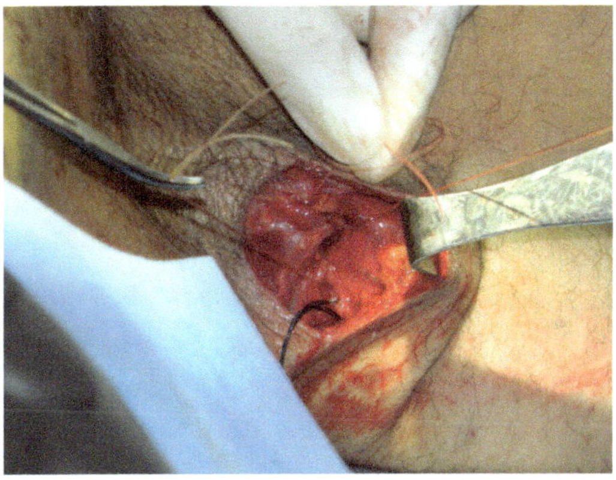

Fig. 4.14 Closure of the triceps fascia over the implant, completely locking away the implant and hence preventing superficial implant migration

Table 4.2 Potential complications of triceps augmentation

Potential complications of triceps augmentation surgery
Infection
Seroma
Hematoma
Asymmetry
Implant visibility
Hypertrophic scarring
Hyperpigmentation of the scar
Capsular contracture
Wound dehiscence
Nerve injury (permanent or temporary, motor or sensory)
Compartment syndrome

the administration of 2 g of Ancef IV (or 300 mg IV clindamycin in a penicillin or cephalosporin allergic patient). During the procedure, irrigation of the pocket with a standard antibiotic solution containing normal saline, Betadine, Ancef, and gentamicin should be performed. Postoperatively, a 5–10-day regimen of oral antibiotics covering normal skin flora should be administered. If a deep infection occurs, the standard of practice is removal of the implant, closure, and possible reimplantation in 3 6 months. There are reports in other forms of implant surgery that conservative management and implant salvage are possible. This should be left at the discretion of the surgeon and performed with careful counseling of the patient.

Seroma

Seromas are statistically the most common complication occurring in implant surgery. In the authors' series of patients, a seroma rate of 3.3 % (1/30) was noted. They typically present as new onset pain, swelling, or asymmetry. The treatment of choice remains percutaneous aspiration. This complication is best prevented with patient compliance with compression sleeves and proper implant placement at the time of surgery, thereby minimizing dead space. In the senior author's experience, it is noncompliance with compression garments and postoperative early return to vigorous activity that result in seroma formation rather than technical issues.

Hematoma

Although a rare occurrence due to the relatively avascular plane of dissection for the triceps augmentation procedure, a hematoma is always possible. In the event of a hematoma, rapid evacuation, pocket irrigation, and reimplantation are the mainstays of therapy. This complication is best prevented by meticulous hemostasis at the time of surgery and good compression of the arm postoperatively to prevent potential space creation.

Asymmetry

This can occur as a product of preexisting variability in the patient's arms or variability in dissection of the pocket bilaterally. This is best minimized by good preoperative photography and noting any asymmetries preoperatively. To avoid creation of asymmetry, it is important to maintain the same pattern of dissection and pocket creation bilaterally. Ideally, the pocket created should be tight and minimize the chance of implant migration. Should

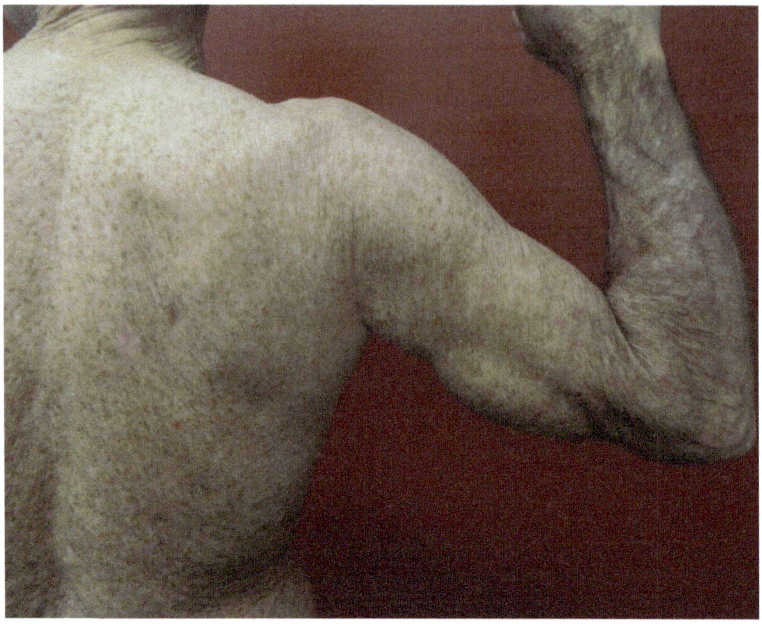

Fig. 4.15 A 64-year-old HIV-positive patient (RS) underwent triceps augmentation with custom triceps implants for poor definition in the triceps area. He presented 3 weeks after surgery with a distally displaced implant on the right arm after resuming exercise early in his postoperative period

a pocket be overdissected and patients note postoperative asymmetry due to a pocket's overdissection, the patient may require a return to the operating room to adjust the pocket. A revision case should be planned for no sooner than 3 months postoperatively, allowing a capsule to form around the implant. On return to the operating room (OR), the capsule can be tailored to more appropriately fit around the implant, producing a more snug fit and bringing greater symmetry to the arms. In the authors' series of cases, there was one such case with one implant being more distal in the underarm region than the contralateral side. The patient was taken to the operating room where a lighted retractor was used to collapse the pocket distally and prevent distal displacement of the implant. The roof of the capsule was sewn down to the underlying triceps muscle with a 2-0 Vicryl suture. After surgery, the patient experienced no further issues.

Implant Visibility

Regardless of position below the muscle or below the fascia, implant visibility is a rare complication. However, those patients that have very thin and atrophic arms to begin with may suffer from implant palpability and visibility. Patients should be counseled on this fact preoperatively if there is a feeling that the patient could be at risk. If a patient is determined to be thin and have minimal development of the triceps muscle, the surgeon may elect for placement of the implant in a submuscular plane to better camouflage the implant. However, a discussion must be had with the patient to discuss the increased risk of neurovascular injury and a greater potential for muscle injury and compartment syndrome.

Implant Dislodgment/Migration

In the authors' series there were two cases of implant extrusion/migration (6.6 %). The two cases were noted in patients who began vigorous activity before the recommended 4–6-week cutoff point. In both cases, the patients noted that the implants were shifted out of position, one being flipped on itself and the other migrating distally (Fig. 4.15). The flipped implant was manually manipulated into its correct position with subsequent resumption of compression garments to the arm. This patient had no further sequelae. The patient with the distally migrated implant opted for the removal of the implants to avoid future issues.

Scar Hyperpigmentation and Hypertrophy

There were no any cases of hypertrophic scarring for triceps augmentation in the authors' series. The key to reduction of these problems is careful layered closure.

Capsular Contracture

This is a possible late sequela of any implant placement, most frequently described in the breast augmentation literature. To date, the authors have not experienced such a complication. This may be due to the short experience with the procedure and small number of cases. However, if it were to occur, the patient would likely be started on Accolate 10 mg orally BID for 3 months in the hope of softening the capsule. If this was unsuccessful, then a return to the OR would be warranted for capsulotomies. A capsulectomy would be difficult to perform in triceps augmentation cases as the arm's position may be prohibitive for attaining good visualization to perform such a procedure.

Wound Dehiscence

Wound dehiscence is a product of poor wound closure under too much tension typically. In order to prevent this, meticulous closure in three layers is paramount: fascia, deep dermis, skin. To date, the authors have not experienced any wound dehiscence in triceps augmentation.

Nerve Injury

Permanent nerve injury is rarely a problem with this procedure as the majority of dissection is performed in a blunt, atraumatic fashion. It is quite common for patients to complain of some numbness over the area of the triceps; however, this returns within 1–3 months postoperatively. This risk can be minimized with the dissection being performed bluntly with the operator's digit rather than using dissectors and potentially creating greater traction injury. Major motor and sensory deficits can accompany compartment syndrome, and this must be ruled out immediately if any significant deficits are appreciated.

The authors experienced one case of neurapraxia. A 32-year-old male, who underwent a unilateral triceps augmentation to correct a congenital defect, presented the day after surgery with weakness in the hand on the operative side, with difficulty writing. His compartments were appropriately swollen. A palpable pulse was appreciated at the radial and ulnar arteries. Gross sensation in the distal hand was intact, except for numbness in the fourth and fifth digit. The patient was noted to have a weak grip with difficulty grasping objects. This was consistent with ulnar nerve injury. Conservative management was decided on with patient consultation. The patient's condition spontaneously resolved within 3 weeks of surgery, suggesting a traction injury. Admittedly, this was one of the first patients who underwent triceps augmentation, and the dissection performed was more aggressive than is currently the authors' practice. This may have put unnecessary tension on the ulnar nerve resulting in neurapraxia in the distal distribution of the nerve, affecting the muscles of the hand. In this patient, the prosthesis was placed in a submuscular plane beneath the long head of the triceps muscle. It is now the authors' practice to perform subfascial placement of the prosthesis to prevent excessive dissection, decrease the incidence of bleeding complications, and decrease the incidence of neurapraxia due to nerve injury. The authors had two cases of neurapraxias consistent with traction injury of the dorsal antebrachial cutaneous nerve, resulting in numbness over the posterior aspect of the forearm. These resolved spontaneously within the first 3 months postoperatively and had no further sequelae. These three neurapraxias have given us an incidence of temporary nerve injury of 10 % (3/30).

Compartment Pressure Problems/ Compartment Syndrome

Volkmann, who first described the phenomenon of compartment syndrome, believed that the pathophysiology was related to massive venous stasis associated with simultaneous occurrence of arterial insufficiency [17]. This in turn prevents proper circulation of blood to the muscles and nerves in a given compartment of an extremity, as tissue pressure increases. Nerve and muscle cells start to die within 4–8 h. Compartment syndrome typically presents as a tensely swollen compartment with extreme pain, out of proportion to examination, on palpation. This is sometimes accompanied by referred pain to the affected compartment with passive stretch of muscles distal to the compartment. There may or may not be a neuropathy, typically described as a burning or prickling sensation, appreciated over the skin of the affected region. Finally, the patient may experience frank pulselessness or paralysis of muscles in the affected compartment. However, the patient who presents with these final findings has typically progressed beyond the point of muscle salvage.

In patients with a compatible history and a tense extremity, clinical diagnosis may be sufficient. If the diagnosis is in doubt, compartment pressures may be measured with a handheld Stryker device. An absolute pressure greater than 30 mmHg in any compartment, or a pressure within 30 mmHg of the diastolic blood pressure in hypotensive patients, or a patient with a concerning history who demonstrates the constellation of signs and symptoms of compartment syndrome are all possible indications for surgical compartment release via fasciotomy [18].

In the authors' experience in triceps augmentation, this complication did not occur. However, the clinician must always have this diagnosis in the back of his mind with any patient in the immediate postoperative period who presents with neurovascular issues in the treated extremity, particularly when pain is out of proportion to examination and poorly controlled with prescribed medications.

Adjunct Procedures for Upper Extremity Contouring/Treatment of Skin Laxity in the Triceps Region

Patients seeking contouring of the upper extremity can present with a constellation of problems including lipodystrophy, skin laxity, and muscle hypoplasia. In addition to treating the hypoplastic muscle with triceps implants, a patient may require some combination of liposuction of the arm and/or excision of excess skin with formal brachioplasty. The authors avoid overzealous tissue manipulation at the time of triceps augmentation and would recommend that any liposuction or skin excision be performed at a separate procedure (before or after an implant surgery) as excessive swelling associated with these procedures when combined with the swelling produced by triceps augmentation may precipitate a compartment syndrome.

In patients that present with significant lipodystrophy of the arm but with little in the way of laxity of the skin, isolated liposuction of the arm may be sufficient [19, 20]. The surgeon must be careful in performing circumferential and superficial liposuction of the arms as it may lead to unaesthetic irregularities particularly in the anterior and medial aspects of the arm [19]. Best results are had with liposuction in the deeper layer of adipose tissue, using small-diameter cannulas no larger than 2.5–3 mm. Chamosa even goes so far as to recommend taking some of this harvested fat and grafting to the deltoid region to improve the contour of the upper extremity, placing the maximum width of the arm at the deltoid region.

Although the authors have used muscle implants to augment the triceps region in patients with laxity of the skin in the underarm region, either due to aging or after massive weight loss, the results have been mixed. The authors rarely recommend triceps augmentation for pure skin laxity in the underarm region as it tends to produce a hanging mass rather than a filling out of the lax tissue. This pathology is best treated with some form of brachioplasty and direct skin excision to better contour the extremity.

Case 1 (Fig. 4.16)
A 78-year-old female presented for significant laxity to the underarm region. It was recommended that she undergo brachioplasty for correction of this problem. However, the patient did not wish to have significant scars. As an alternative, triceps augmentation was offered in the hope of filling out the underarm region. After augmentation, the patient complained of having a significant weight in the underarm region without a feeling of significant improvement. For this reason, the author has elected to be very selective in patients receiving triceps implants for skin laxity correction. The patient is shown preoperatively and 2 weeks after surgery with an improvement in overall contour and better filling of the skin envelope.

With advances in bariatric procedures, there has been an increase in the number of patients presenting to the cosmetic surgeon with laxity of the skin in the arms after massive weight loss. While adding volume with implants can at times camouflage the overall volume loss in the arm and liposuction can take care of stubborn fat deposits, at times excision of skin is the only way to produce an aesthetic result in the upper extremity. Appelt et al. [20] recommend an algorithmic approach to upper arm contouring to help surgeons best manage the spectrum of patients who present for improvement in arm contour. Using the skin pinch test as a starting point, patients with greater than 1.5 cm of fat detectable with the pinch test could potentially benefit from

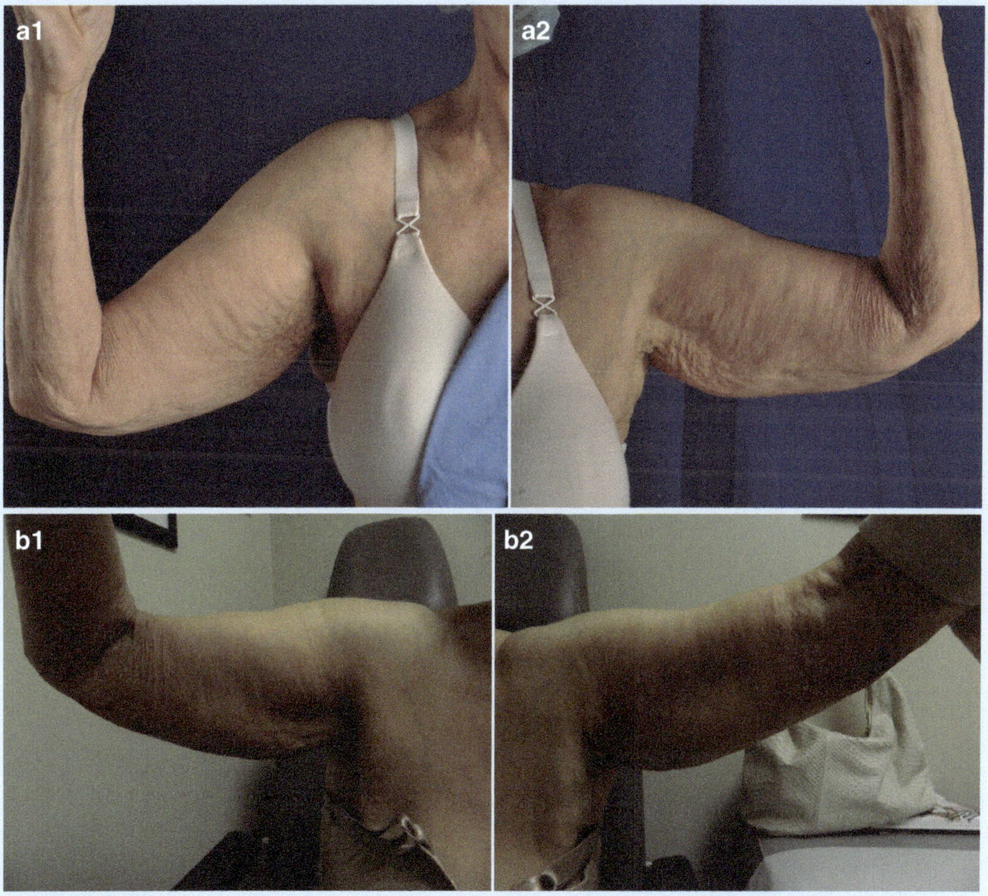

Fig. 4.16 (**a**) Preoperative. (**b**) Postoperative

liposuction. However, the surgeon must take into account skin laxity to assess if liposuction alone is the best option. Rohrich [21] has devised a three-tier classification system that has been modified to better define issues of skin laxity and fat excess in the upper extremity, helping surgeons determine which procedures may be applicable to the patient seeking upper arm contouring. His initial classification described three classifications of upper extremity dystrophy: (I), minimal skin excess and moderate fat excess; (II), moderate skin excess with minimal fat excess; and (III), moderate skin excess with moderate fat excess. Based on his system, Rohrich recommends upper arm contouring with liposuction alone for class I patients. He emphasizes the need for long, uniform strokes to prevent contour irregularities. Patients with type II dystrophy have moderate skin laxity with minimal fat excess and are best treated with some form of brachioplasty and excision of the excess skin. Patients who are type III suffer from moderate skin excess and moderate fat excess and are best treated with a multimodality therapy (liposuction and brachioplasty) in either a single stage or staged approach [21].

The surgeon may elect to augment the biceps and triceps region at the same time. In cases that have been performed, the relative augmentation to each muscle group is small compared to an isolated biceps or triceps augmentation. This smaller augmentation is performed to avoid complications associated with compartment syndrome. The surgeon may elect to offer both procedures at the same time but must always err on the side of caution to avoid major complications with excessive addition of volume to the arms.

Triceps Augmentation with Fat Grafting

Work in autologous fat grafting has prompted patients to ask about fat grafting to the triceps region. While it might be possible to achieve some augmentation in the biceps region due to the greater muscle mass in the anterior compartment, it is our belief that fat grafting to the posterior compartment of the arm would likely not take well but may also result in an unaesthetic result. For that reason, we do not recommend or perform fat grafting to the triceps region.

Authors' Personal Results

In reviewing the primary author's (NVC) own experience with the procedure, there have been a total of approximately 30 triceps augmentations performed since introducing the procedure in 2008. There has been an overall satisfaction rate of 96.7 % (29/30). The patient who was dissatisfied underwent triceps augmentation for severe skin laxity in the underarm region. She did not wish to undergo any form of brachioplasty, even though it was recommended that she undergo a traditional, long incision brachioplasty. As an alternative, the patient was offered a small triceps implant to give volume to the area and perhaps fill in all of the loose skin. While she had a moderate improvement, the patient felt that the arm now appeared more bulky and had hanging skin on top of it.

Since starting the procedure, ten procedures have been performed in the submuscular plane and 20 in the subfascial plane. During that time, the seroma rate cumulatively has been 3.3 % (1/30). The infection rate has also been 3.3 % (1/30). Asymmetry was also noted in one case, giving an incidence of 3.3 % (1/30). There were two cases of implant migration in the group of 30 patients (6.7 %). There were three cases of neurapraxia in patients receiving a submuscular triceps implant (10 %). There have been no cases of wound dehiscence or capsular contracture.

Patient Cases

Case 2 (Fig. 4.17)
A 38-year-old female presented for biceps and triceps augmentation secondary to mild underdevelopment. Bilateral style 8, size 3 biceps implants were placed along with custom triceps implants (style 8, size 20). She also underwent breast augmentation with 400 mL Mentor moderate plus silicone gel implants.

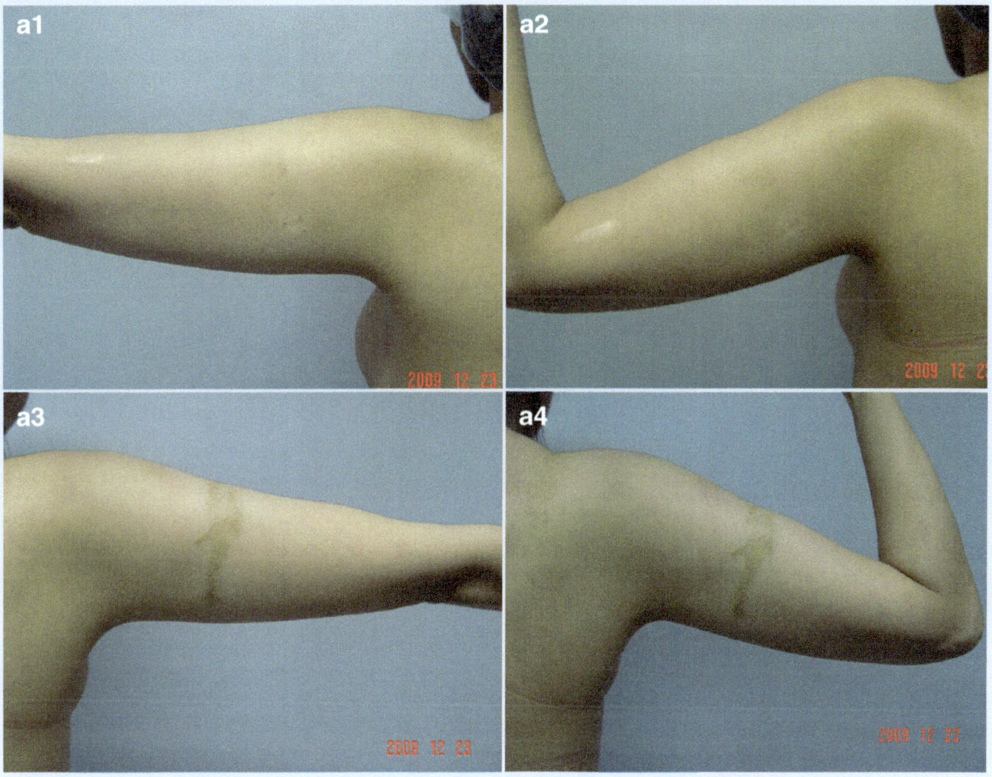

Fig. 4.17 (**a**) Preoperative. (**b**) Postoperative

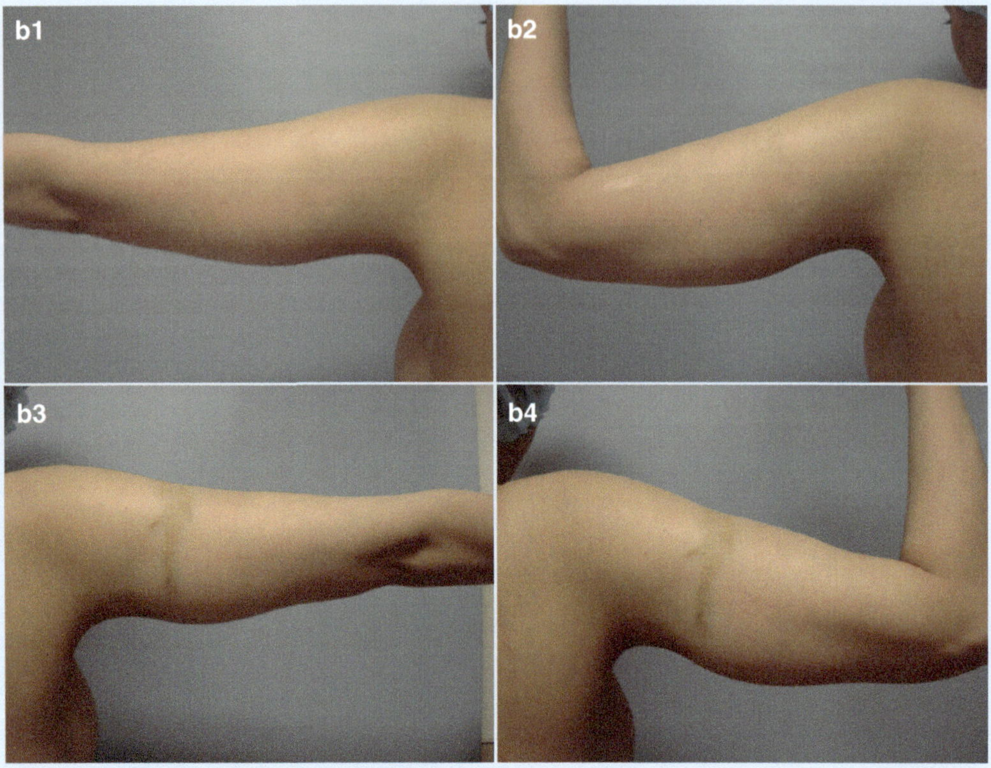

Fig. 4.17 (continued)

Case 3 (Fig. 4.18)
A 29-year-old male underwent biceps and triceps augmentation with custom implants. The biceps implants were style 8, size 1 and the triceps implants were style 8, size 20.

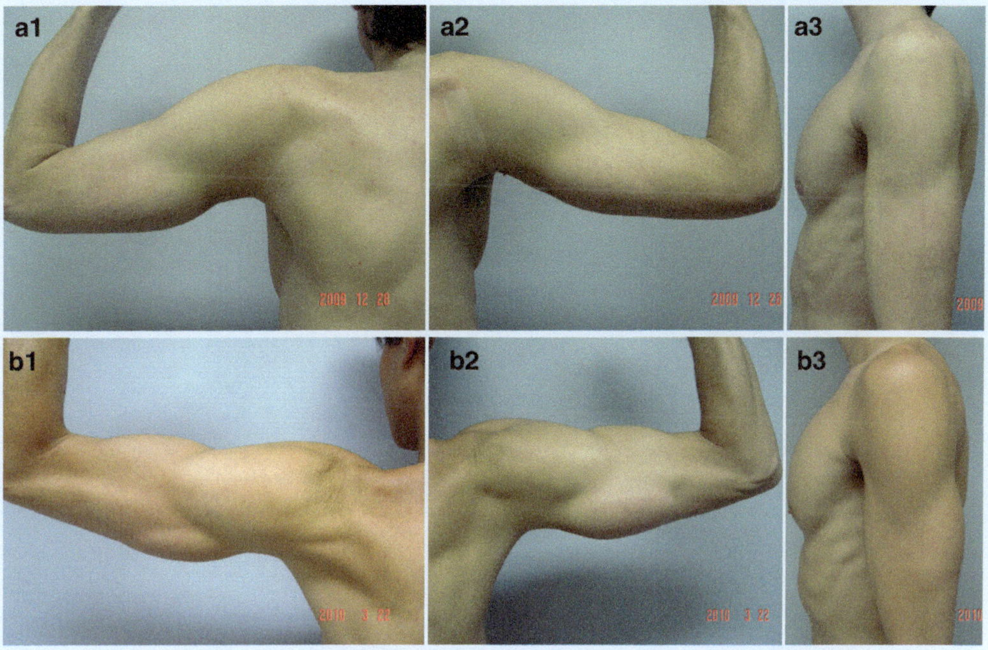

Fig. 4.18 (**a**) Preoperative. (**b**) Postoperative

Case 4 (Fig. 4.19)
A 24-year-old male underwent triceps augmentation with a custom triceps implant. He complained primarily of a poorly developed triceps muscle despite a rigorous weight training program.

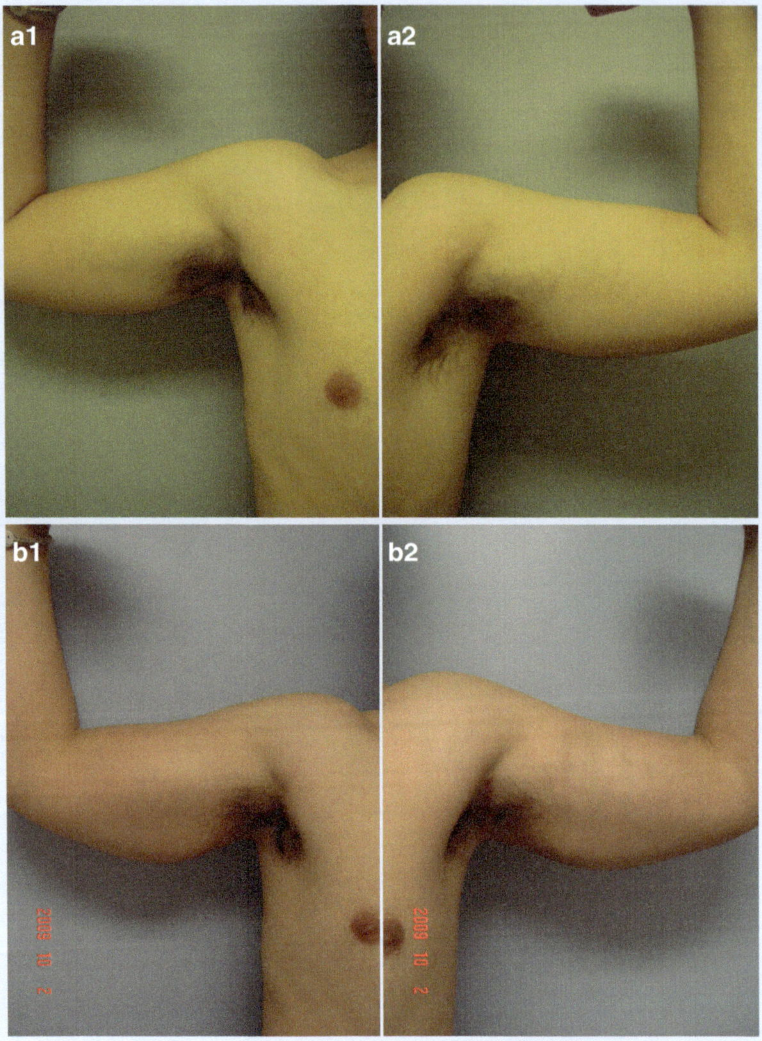

Fig. 4.19 (**a**) Preoperative. (**b**) Postoperative

Case 5 (Fig. 4.20)
A 44-year-old male underwent liposuction of the abdomen with bilateral biceps, pectoral, and triceps augmentation. The patient received style 2, size 1 pectoral implants (not demonstrated). He received style 8, size 1 biceps implants. Lastly, style 8, size 20 triceps implants were placed.

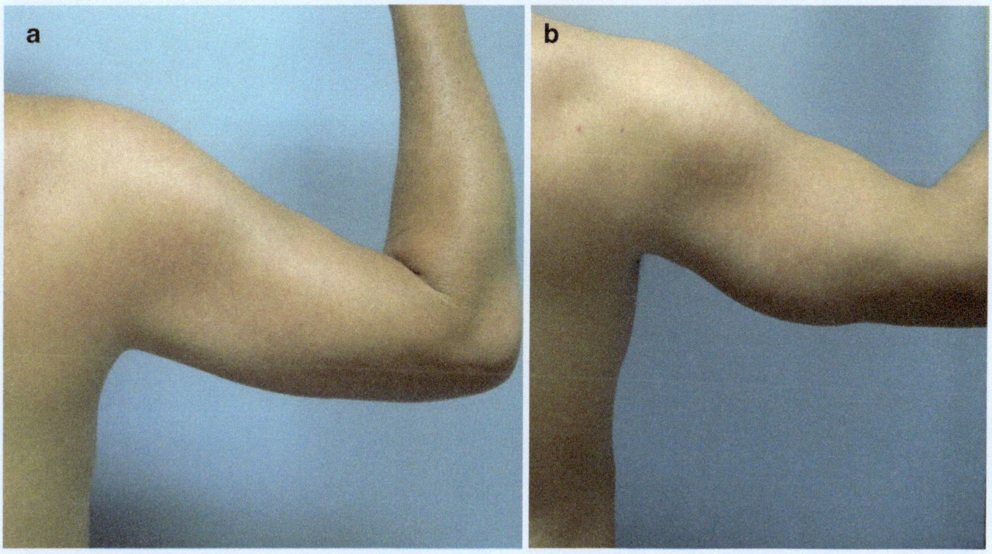

Fig. 4.20 (**a**) Preoperative. (**b**) Postoperative

Case 6 (Fig. 4.21)
A 27-year-old male underwent triceps augmentation with style 8, size 25 triceps implants as he was unable to develop adequate triceps definition with conventional workouts.

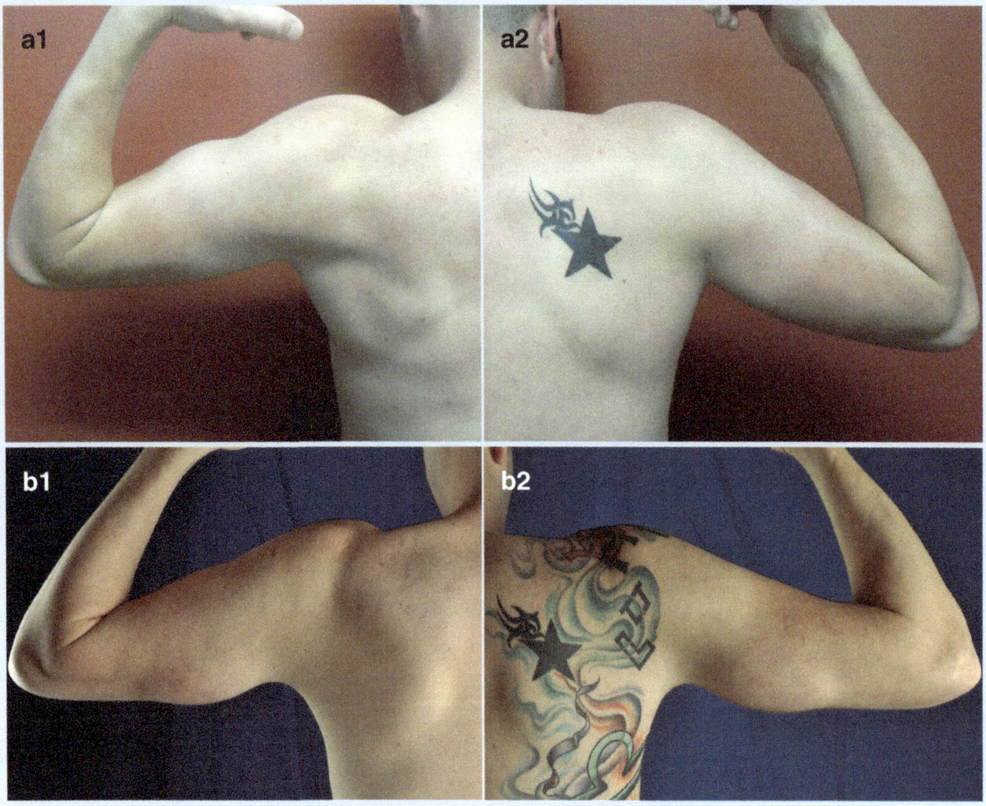

Fig. 4.21 (**a**) Preoperative. (**b**) Postoperative

Case 7 (Fig. 4.22)
A 44-year-old male underwent biceps and triceps augmentation. He received style 8, size 25 triceps implants and style 8, size 3 biceps implants.

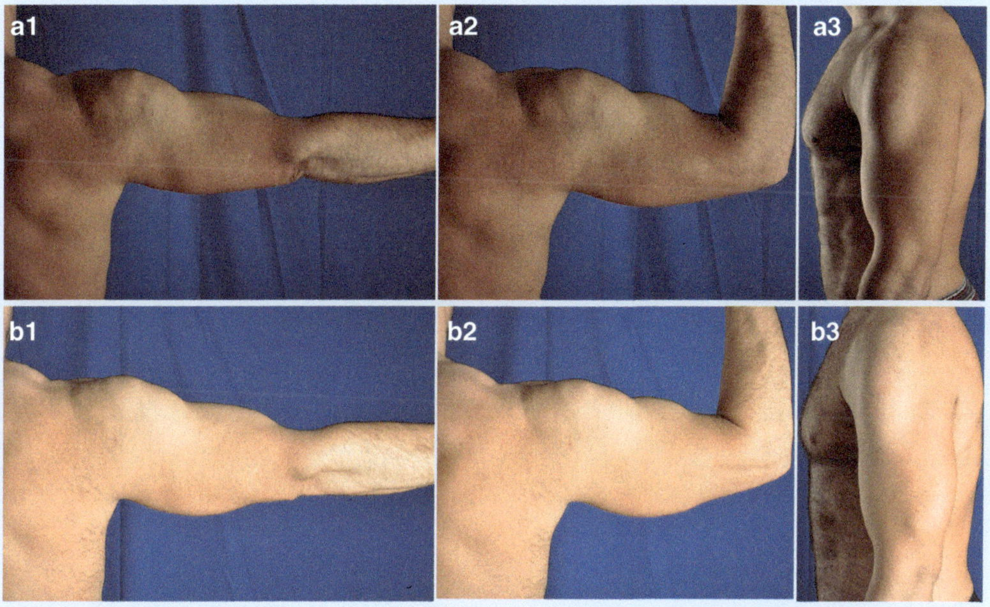

Fig. 4.22 (**a**) Preoperative. (**b**) Postoperative

Case 8 (Fig. 4.23)
A 54-year-old male underwent bilateral biceps augmentation with style 8, size 1 implants and triceps augmentation with style 8, size 25 triceps implants.

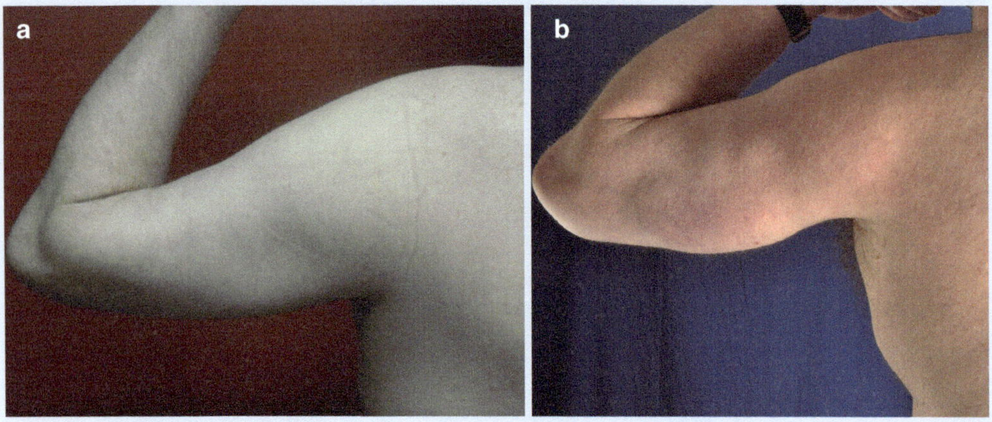

Fig. 4.23 (**a**) Preoperative. (**b**) Postoperative

Case 9 (Fig. 4.24)
A 47-year-old male underwent bilateral biceps and triceps augmentation with style 8, size 1 implants (biceps) and style 8, size 25 implants (triceps). He had normal development but wanted better definition and increased volume.

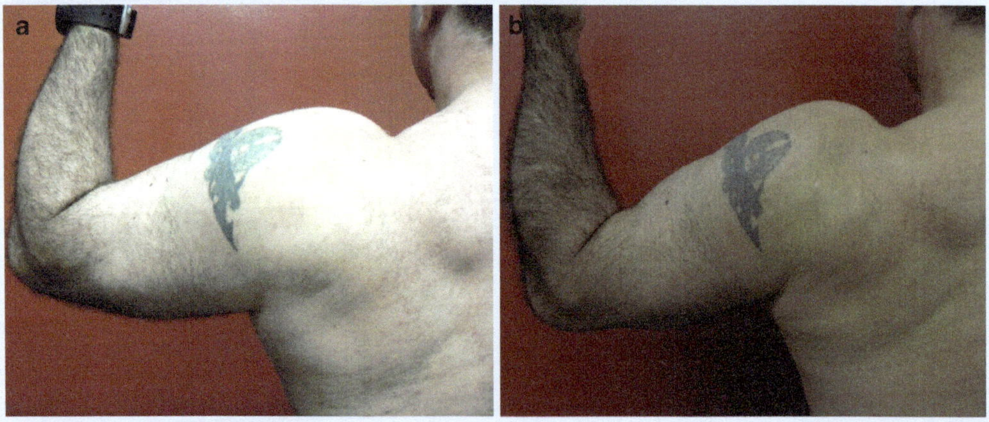

Fig. 4.24 (**a**) Preoperative. (**b**) Postoperative

Conclusions

The triceps augmentation procedure is an excellent complement to the augmentation of the biceps region. While it is not recommended to perform both augmentations at the same time due to the risk of compartment syndrome, they can very easily be performed 3–6 months apart with excellent results. Although triceps augmentation does have significant utility in the realm of reconstructive surgery to bring about greater symmetry between the two arms, it is clear that it can be successfully used to augment a hypoplastic triceps region, giving the patient a more musculature and defined upper extremity.

References

1. Plastic surgery statistics report. 2012. http://www.plasticsurgery.org/Documents/news-resources/statistics/2012-Plastic-Surgery-Statistics/full-plastic-surgery-statistics-report.pdf. Accessed 9 Jun 2013.
2. American Academy of Cosmetic Surgery Procedural Census. 2008. http://multivu.prnewswire.com/mnr/aacs/36867/docs/36867AACS2008ProceduralSurveyResults.pdf. Accessed 9 Jun 2013.
3. Phillips KA. Body image and body dysmorphic disorder. In: Cash TL, Smolak L, editors. Body image: a handbook of science, practice, and prevention. 2nd ed. New York: The Guilford Press. 2012, p. 305–13.
4. Pope HG, Gruber AJ, Mangweth B, Bureau B, deCol C, Jouvent R, Hudson JI. Body image perception among men in three countries. Am J Psychiatry. 2000; 157(8):1297–301.
5. Olivardia R, Pope HG, Borowiecki JJ, Cohane GH. Biceps and body image: the relationship between muscularity and self-esteem, depression, and eating disorder symptoms. Psychol Men Masculinity. 2004; 5(2):112–20.
6. Leit RA, Pope HG, Gray JJ. Cultural expectation of muscularity in men: the evolution of playgirl centerfolds. Int J Eat Disord. 2001;29(1):90–3.
7. Cafri G, Thompson JK, Riccciardelli L, McCabe M, Smolak L, Yesalis C. Pursuit of the muscular ideal: physical and psychological consequences and putative risk factors. Clin Psychol Rev. 2005;25(2):215–39.
8. Pope HG, Olivardia R, Gruber A, Borowiecki J. Evolving ideals of male body image as seen through action toys. Int J Eat Disord. 1999;26(1):65–72.
9. Bonnecarrere ER, Butler B. Case report: upper extremity soft-tissue reconstruction by alloplastic implant: long-term result and follow-up. Ann Plast Surg. 1997;38:74–6.
10. Hodgkinson DJ. Contour restoration of the upper limb using solid silicone implants. Aesthetic Plast Surg. 2006;30(1):53–8.
11. Chugay N, Racanelli J, Hsu J, Chugay P. Bicipital augmentation. Am J Cosmet Surg. 2006;23(1):33–6.
12. Chugay N, Chugay P. Bicipital augmentation: a retrospective review of 94 patient cases. Am J Cosmet Surg. 2009;67(4):241–5.
13. Chugay NV, Chugay PN. Triceps augmentation: early experience with the procedure. Am J Cosmet Surg. 2010;27(4):200–3.
14. Abadesso I, Serra F. Augmentation brachioplasty: surgery for improving the appearance of the arms. Rev Bras Cir Plast. 2012;27(1):97–101.
15. Toomayan GA, Robertson F, Major NM, Brigman BE. Upper extremity compartmental anatomy: clinical relevance to radiologists. Skeletal Radiol. 2006;35(4):195–201.
16. Mazurek MT, Shin AY. Upper extremity peripheral nerve anatomy. Clin Orthop Rel Res. 2001;383:7–20.
17. Amendola A. Compartment syndromes. In: Browner BD, Jupiter JB, Levine AM, Trafton BG, Krettek C, editors. Skeletal trauma: basic science, management, and reconstruction. Philadelphia: Saunders; 2003.
18. Cothren CC, Biffl WL, Moore EE. Chapter 7. Trauma. In: Brunicardi FC, Andersen DK, Billiar TR, Dunn DL, Hunter JG, Matthews JB, Pollock RE, editors. Schwartz's principles of surgery. New York: McGraw-Hill Professional; 2010.
19. Chamosa M, Murillo J, Vazquez T. Lipectomy of arms and lipograft of shoulders balance the upper body contour. Aesthetic Plast Surg. 2005;29(6):567–70.
20. Appelt EA, Janis JE, Rohrich RJ. An algorithmic approach to upper arm contouring. Plast Reconstr Surg. 2006;118(1):237–46.
21. Rohrich RJ, Beran SJ, Kenkel JM. Back and arms. In: Rohrich RJ, Beran SJ, Kenkel JM, editors. Ultrasound assisted liposuction. 1st ed. St Louis: Quality Medical Publishing; 1998. p. 231–51.

5 Pectoral Augmentation

Introduction

Initially developed for surgical repair of deficiencies, such as congenital pectoral aplasia, pectoral implants can be used to improve the appearance of patients with an undeveloped or disproportionate chest. Over the past decade, there has been increased interest in sculpting the ideal male form, as exemplified by provocative ads of men showing off defined abdomens and muscular pectoral regions. An adequate chest wall is psychologically very important for males, denoting fitness, strength, and power. Men are becoming a larger part of the pool of cosmetic surgery patients as noted in studies by the American Society of Plastic Surgeons and the American Academy of Cosmetic Surgery [1, 2]. For all of these reasons above, pectoral augmentation has become more prevalent among men seeking cosmetic surgery as they continue to further define their physique. Men want to be able to show their chests proudly rather than covering when confronted with events that reveal the upper torso, such as physical activity (i.e., sports) or simply relaxing at the beach. Using preformed silicone pectoral prostheses, the aesthetic surgeon is able not only to correct volume deficits but provide reliable augmentation of the pectoral region, giving men a more defined and muscular appearance.

Body Dissatisfaction in Males

Although discussed in greater depth in the previous chapters, it stands to emphasize that many men have some element of body dysmorphic disorder and wish to have a more muscular and "built" physique in order to be better accepted in society and by the opposite sex [3–8]. Society has created an idealistic model of the male that is oftentimes hard to attain with simple diet and exercise alone. For this reason, muscle augmentation surgery gives a male the opportunity to achieve this ideal. While augmentations for biceps and triceps are still in their infancy [9–11], pectoral augmentation has long been present as a means of enhancing the male physique. A man with a well-developed chest is seen as being fit, strong, and powerful [12]. The advent of pectoral implants gave a male with an underdeveloped chest something of an option to enhance his chest and allow him to strut proudly like a peacock.

History of the Procedure

Since the 1970s, reconstructive surgeons have used solid silicone prostheses to reconstruct chest wall defects as a result of Poland's syndrome [13]. In 1988, Sorenson [14] described his use of silicone prostheses in a subcutaneous plane to

N.V. Chugay et al., *Body Sculpting with Silicone Implants*,
DOI 10.1007/978-3-319-04957-1_5, © Springer International Publishing Switzerland 2014

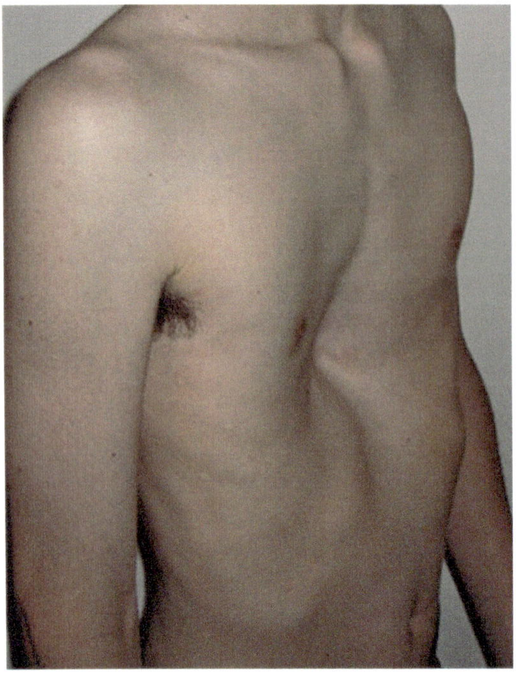

Fig. 5.1 An example of pectus excavatum in a male

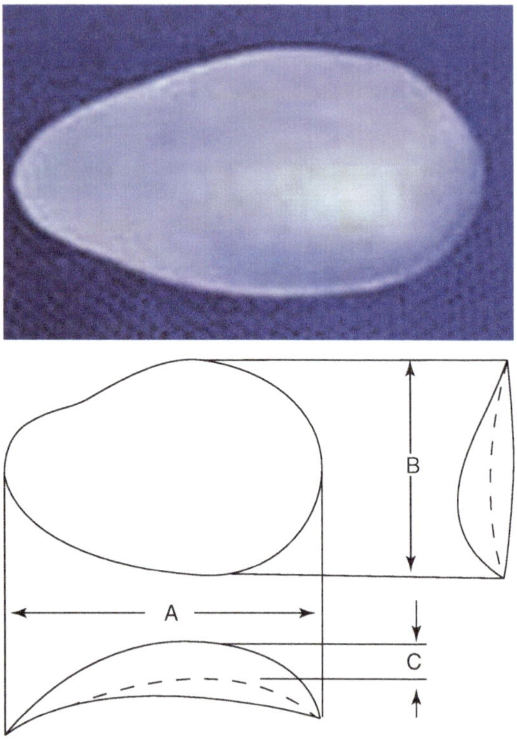

Fig. 5.2 Aiache implant

correct deformity left as a result of pectus excavatum (Fig. 5.1).

In 1991, Aiache [15] introduced his technique for aesthetic augmentation of the chest with cohesive silicone gel implants that have an anatomic design. The Aiache pectoral implant augments the sternal and costal lower two-thirds of the chest (Fig. 5.2) [15, 16]. In the same year, Novack released his extensive discussion on alloplastic implants for men, describing his work with various augmentation procedures using silicone elastomer implants (Fig. 5.3) [17]. The implants that bear his name are a more square-shaped implant that provides a more "blocky" result with less lateral fullness and increased posteroanterior projection.

Hodgkinson, in 1997 [16], reviewed his experience of 15 years using silicone implants to correct a wide range of chest wall deformities, including muscular insufficiency, Poland syndrome, pectus excavatum, and pectoralis muscle tears. His work demonstrates the true versatility of the implant in being able to correct multiple deformities of the chest. Hodgkinson further elaborates on the use of pectoral implants to correct deformities left by pectoralis muscle tears, rarely discussed in prior publications on pectoral implants. He notes that patients on occasion presented years after injuries from high-impact sports, motorcycle racing, weight lifting, and body building [16]. Although orthopedic surgeons will sometimes reattach the pectoralis tendon back to the humerus, oftentimes the injury goes untreated in the early phase and causes patients to present once there is an obvious deformity that is more prominent in the flexed position [18–20]. Hodgkinson recommends a possible resection of the bulging protuberant muscle and suture repair of the groove produced with contraction of the pectoralis. When this is impossible, a custom silicone prosthesis can be used to camouflage the abnormality. Aside from treating defects, Hodgkinson goes on to discuss his work in pectoral augmentation surgery for treatment of muscle insufficiency. Through a 5–6 cm incision in the axilla, he describes his technique of placement of a silicone implant below the pectoralis major muscle.

In 1999, the primary author (NVC) published his work on pectoral augmentation in 16 patients

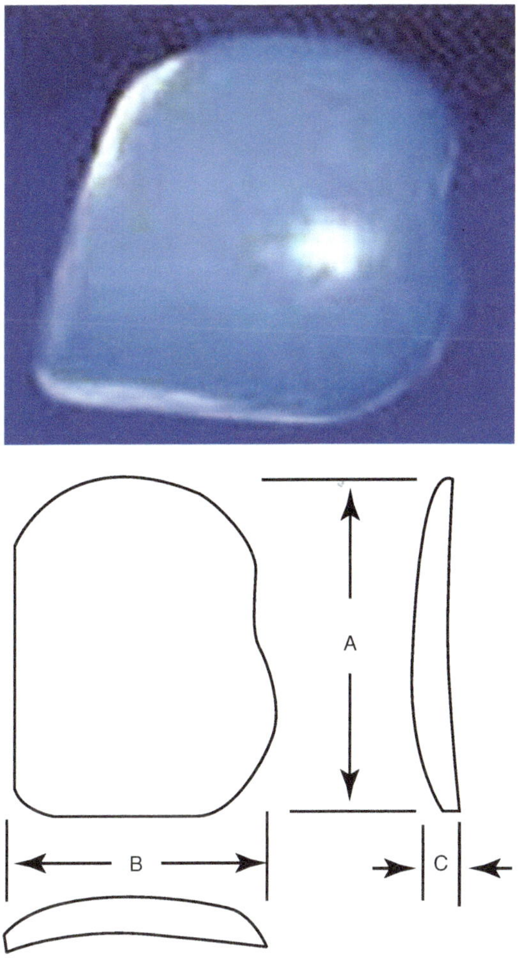

Fig. 5.3 Novack implant

for purely aesthetic purposes [21]. Describing his experience with 16 patients served as one of the largest early evaluations of pectoral augmentation along with its risks and benefits.

In 2002, Horn [22] further added to the literature on pectoral augmentation. In 12 patients, he performed pectoral augmentation with implants made of a cohesive silicone gel. His implant was created to more closely mirror the pectoral muscle, being rectangular in shape and having an axillary extension. In addition to ten cases of straightforward augmentation, Horn describes two patients who underwent pectoral augmentation after having undergone liposuction of the chest for treatment of gynecomastia and ended up dissatisfied by sagging skin in the chest. This was one of the first cases to describe volumizing an empty chest, making pectoral augmentation an option for treatment of loose and hanging skin in men that have lost significant amounts of weight in the chest region.

Ruiz introduced the use of buttock implants for male chest enhancement in 2003 [23] and 2008 [24]. Using the same technique as previously described by Aiache, he placed buttock implants into the subpectoral space, achieving good to excellent results with significant patient satisfaction.

Indications

Initially, pectoral augmentation was introduced as a means to treating asymmetries in the pectoral region left due to congenital anomalies (e.g., Poland's syndrome and pectus excavatum) and in those patients who suffered volume deficits secondary to trauma or post-oncologic surgery. Pectoral augmentation, for purely aesthetic reasons, is indicated for the patient who has hypoplasia in the area of the chest muscle and is unable to achieve the desired projection despite vigorous exercise or muscle building. The last group of patients that may benefit from pectoral augmentation are those that have suffered some injury to the pectoral region, leaving them with an asymmetry and defect in the anterior chest.

Contraindications

While not every male presenting for pectoral augmentation suffers from muscle dysmorphia/body dysmorphic disorder, the surgeon must be aware of this and take it into consideration when considering a patient for muscle augmentation surgery. A patient who seems unrealistic in the goals of his surgery should be turned away.

Limitations

In any case of pectoral augmentation, realistic expectations should be had by the prospective patient. A patient who has preexisting asymmetry has to understand that despite augmentation there will likely be a persistent asymmetry (i.e., nipple position or volume). Patients who are severely hypoplastic or have some congenital defect may require more than one procedure with larger custom implants at a second setting to achieve dramatic augmentation as an overly aggressive augmentation in one setting may put the patient at risk of compartment syndrome.

Relevant Anatomy

The pectoralis major is a thick, fan-shaped muscle that makes up the large part of the volume of the anterior thorax and is responsible for adducting and drawing the arm forward across the front of the chest (Fig. 5.4) [25]. It arises from the anterior surface of the sternal half of the clavicle, from the sternum, from the cartilages of all the true ribs with the exception of the first or seventh or both, and from the external oblique muscle of the abdomen. All of these muscle fibers join in a flat tendon that is about 5 cm broad and inserts into the greater tubercle of the humerus. The pectoralis is covered by a very thin pectoral fascia that is continuous with the rectus abdominis fascia below and extends cranially to the clavicles and laterally to the axilla (Fig. 5.5). The pectoralis minor sits below the pectoralis major and is a triangular-shaped muscle that depresses the point of the shoulder, drawing the scapula downward and medially toward the thorax. It arises from the upper margins and outer surfaces of the third, fourth, and fifth ribs and from the aponeuroses covering the intercostal muscles. These fibers pass upward and converge to form a tendon that inserts into the coracoid process of the scapula.

The pectoralis major muscle is supplied by the medial and lateral pectoral nerves. More recent studies have questioned the validity of this classification saying that there are in fact three pectoral nerves noted as follows: medial (inferior branch) and lateral (superior and middle branches) (Fig. 5.6) [26].

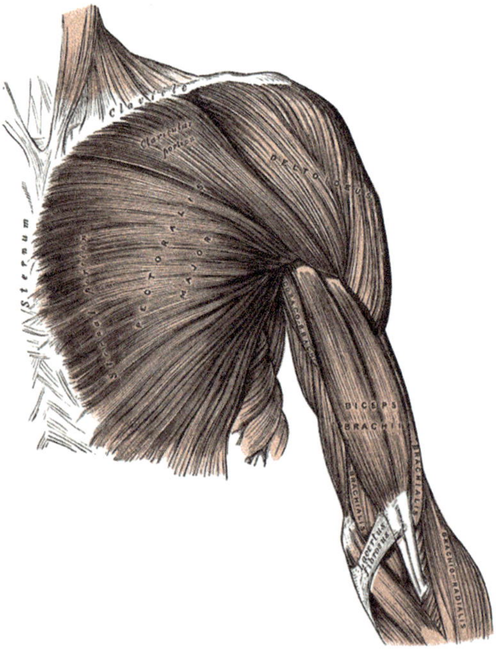

Fig. 5.4 Pectoralis major and relationship to upper extremity musculature

Medial Pectoral Nerve

The medial pectoral nerve (inferior branch) can be severed during access to the subpectoral plane [26, 27]. This results in a slight loss of the pectoralis major muscle strength. In 62 % of patients, the medial pectoral nerve (inferior branch) courses through the pectoralis minor to innervate the lower two-thirds of the pectoralis major muscle. In the other 38 %, it exits around the lateral aspect of the pectoralis minor muscle. The inferior branch of the pectoral nerve is closely associated with the lateral thoracic vessels, and care must be taken to avoid not only damage to the nerve but these vessels. Dissection with fingers and blunt instruments lessens the risk of injury to these structures.

Lateral Pectoral Nerve

The lateral branch of the pectoral nerve (superior and medial branches) is also at risk of injury with submuscular implant placement as

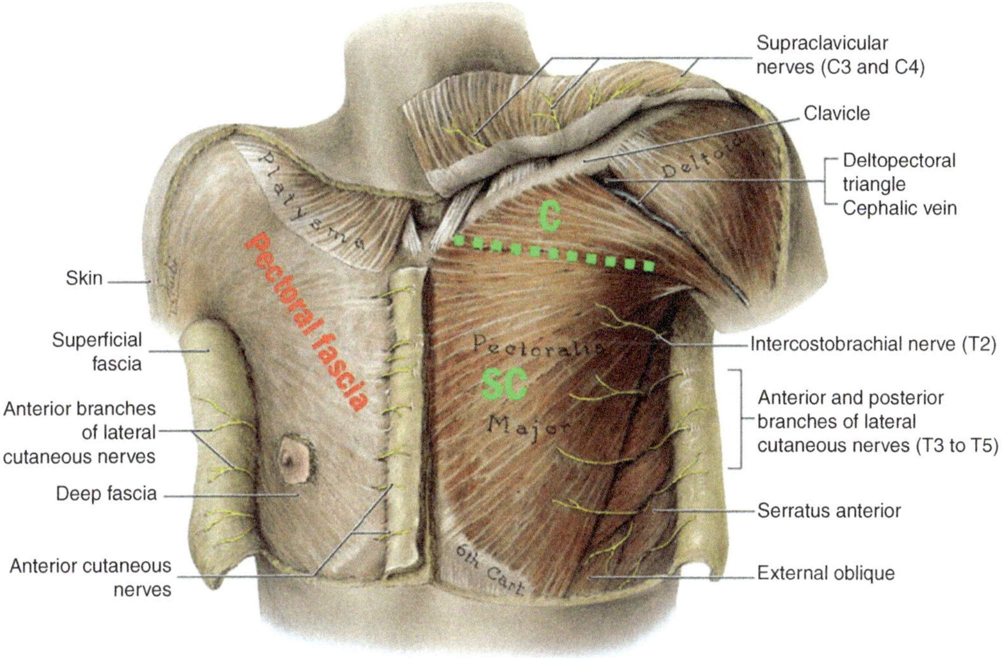

Fig. 5.5 Pectoralis fascia and cutaneous nerves depicted. Note the relationship of the pectoralis to the serratus anterior and deltoid muscle. *C* clavicle, *SC* subclavicular

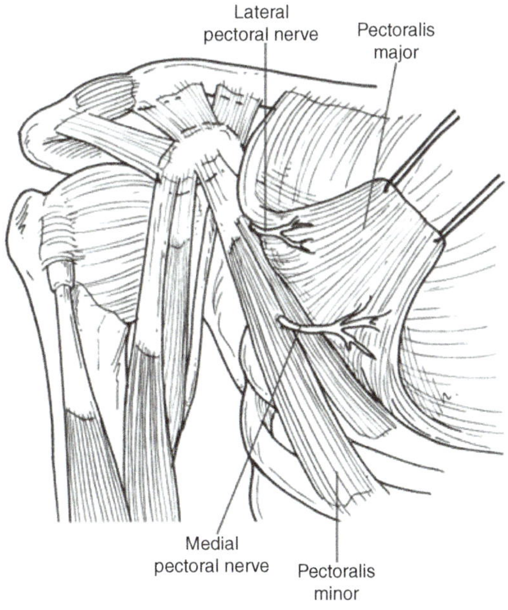

Fig. 5.6 Medial and lateral pectoral nerves and their relationship to the pectoralis major and minor

it travels on the deep surface of the pectoralis major muscle alongside the thoracoacromial artery and vein. It provides innervation to the upper one-third of the pectoralis major muscle. When injured, it produces an atrophy of the sternal aspect of the pectoralis major. Again, dissection with blunt technique helps to avoid injury to these neurovascular structures. The superior branch is relatively protected from injury due to its straight path to the clavicular portion of pectoralis major [26].

Damage to a single branch of the pectoral nerve is typically undetectable; however, injury to both the inferior and middle branches can produce significant morbidity, namely, pectoralis atrophy, fibrosis, and limitation of shoulder movement. Hoffman, in his discussion of the anatomy of the pectoral nerves, notes in patients that have undergone modified radical mastectomy that there is a possibility of injury not only to the medial pectoral nerve but also to the lateral pectoral nerve, when dissecting in the axilla [27]. Although frank transection of the lateral pectoral nerve is rare, aggressive electrocoagulation of the branches of the thoracoacromial artery and vein can cause adjacent nerve injury. For this reason, minimal dissection is advised in the axilla, primarily using blunt dissection, in the path of dissection to the lateral border of pectoralis major so as to minimize neurovascular injury.

Consultation/Implant Selection

The consultation begins with a thorough medical history on the patient. Special attention is taken to ask specifically about trauma to the torso and any history of nerve damage or sensory deficits as may be seen in patients with diabetes mellitus or patients with previous injuries. Also, patients with histories of nerve entrapment disorders should be asked about the current state of those nerves and any long-term sequelae. Preoperative goals are assessed at this point. A patient who has unrealistic expectations and is unable to comply with the strict postoperative instructions is deemed a poor candidate for augmentation. To best assess the patient's expectations, we ask the patient to supply a picture of a body builder or person who demonstrates their "ideal" chest. The surgeon is now able to assess whether or not the patient's goals are realistic. Patients who have congenital anomalies, a significant size disparity between the two sides of the chest, or bilateral hypoplasia, are informed that several surgeries may be required to attain symmetry and achieve the augmentation they desire. Patients are also asked about their current level of activity and muscle building history, taking care to inform the patient of the need to take at least 1 month of time to recover before resuming any vigorous arm building regimens.

After completion of the history, the chest is evaluated. First, symmetry of the two sides is assessed, and any disparity is brought to the attention of the patient. Although the majority of patients present with a preexisting asymmetry of the chest, not many patients note the difference and this can be a source of medicolegal matters in the future. The physician then evaluates the quality of the skin, subcutaneous tissue, and muscle. Any fatty deposits or evidence of skin laxity are noted and demonstrated to the patient. To evaluate the muscle, the patient's pectoral region is evaluated in standing natural position as well as in flexed position. The pectoralis is evaluated at its clavicular, sternal, and costal attachments, and any asymmetries should be noted at this time. Next an evaluation of the skeleton is important. This consists of assessing the symmetry of the shoulders and rib cage and evaluating the position of the sternum. The physician should evaluate the patient from the posterior aspect and evaluate the scapula and the spine itself, taking note of any asymmetries and any evidence of scoliosis as this may affect the ability to bring symmetry to the anterior thorax. The sternum is evaluated and note is made of pectus excavatum or pectus carinatum.

At this point several measurements are taken to determine the best implant for the patient. First, the width of the muscle from sternum to anterior axillary line is assessed at the lower pole of the pectoralis. This measurement is analogous to assessing the base width for patients undergoing breast augmentation surgery. Next, the height of the pectoralis muscle is assessed by measure from the clavicle to the lower border of the muscle in the midclavicular line.

Patients who suffer from Poland syndrome should have the normal side measured so as best to approximate the dimensions on the contralateral side. Custom implants can be made for patients desiring a certain look or in those that have significant chest wall abnormality. A moulage kit can be used to construct a cast which is then sent to the implant manufacturer to create the desired implant.

Available Implants (Tables 5.1, 5.2, 5.3, and 5.4)

The authors' preference is the style two square-shaped implant.

Table 5.1 Style 1 pectoral implants (Aesthetic and Reconstructive Technologies, Inc., Reno, NV)

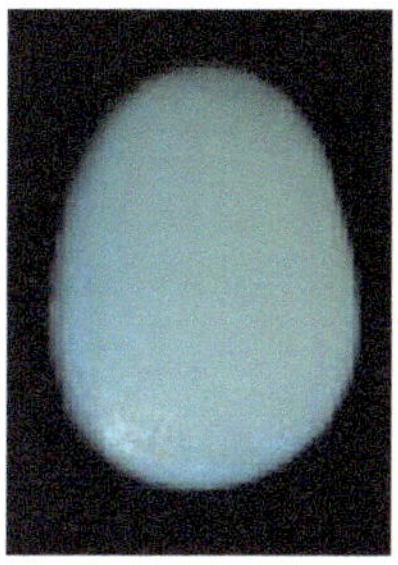

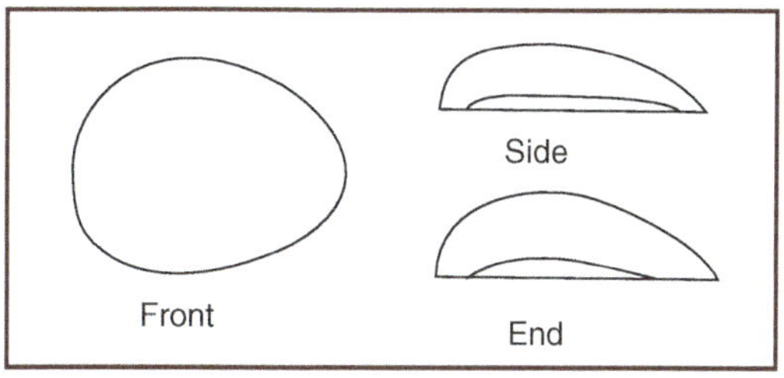

Style 1					
	Catalog #	Width	Length	Projection	Volume (cc)
Size 1	500–101	14.7	11.4	2.7	234
Size 2	500–102	15.4	12.0	3.0	273
Size 3	500–103	16.1	13.7	3.1	349
Size 4	500–104	15.5	12.0	2.1	189
Size 5	500–105	16.1	12.5	2.3	222
Size 6	500–106	17.0	14.6	2.5	289

Table 5.2 Style 2 pectoral implants (Aesthetic and Reconstructive Technologies, Inc., Reno, NV)

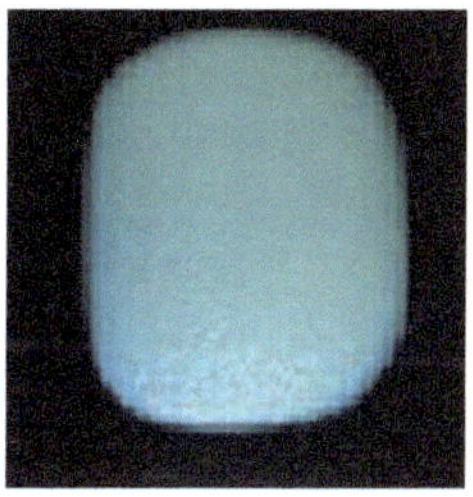

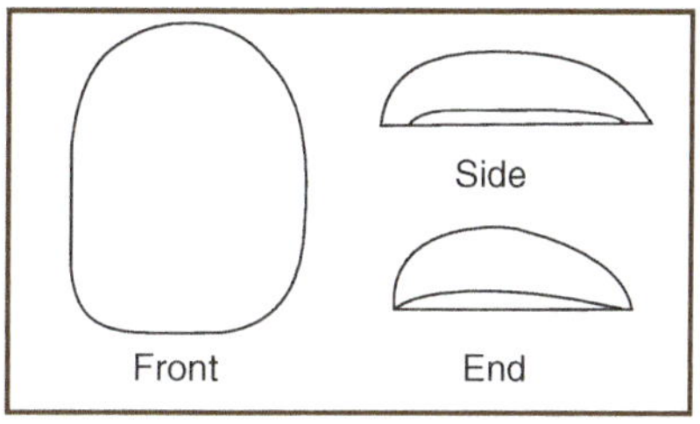

Style 2					
	Catalog #	Width	Length	Projection	Volume (cc)
Size 0	500–200	13.3	14.8	13.9	230
Size 1	500–201	13.0	15.4	2.2	294
Size 2	500–202	13.8	16.1	2.7	367
Size 3	500–203	13.9	16.6	2.9	409

Table 5.3 Style 3 pectoral implants (Aesthetic and Reconstructive Technologies, Inc., Reno, NV)

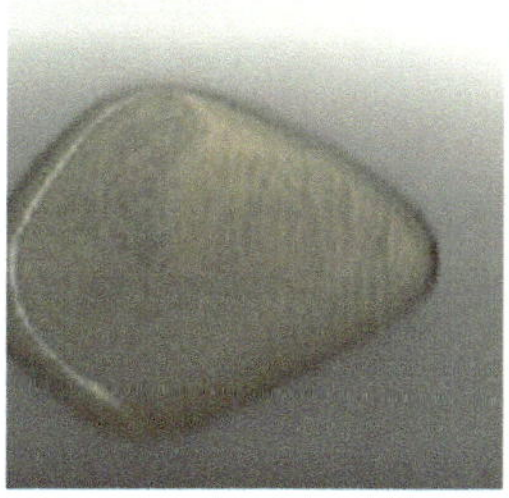

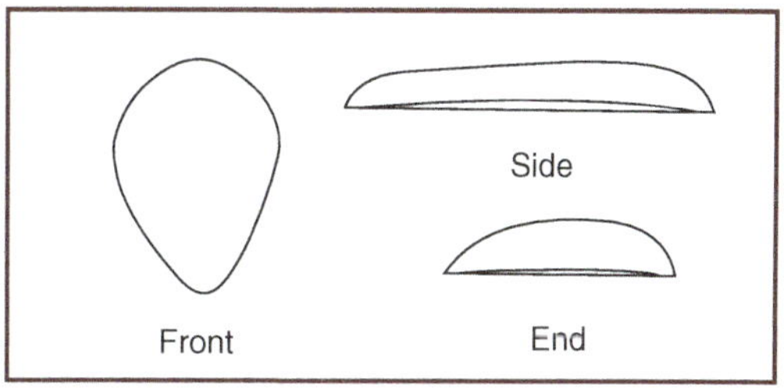

Style 3					
Catalog #	500–301	Width	Width	Projection	Volume (cc)
Size 1	500–302	13.8	18.5	2.5	300
Size 2		14.9	18.9	2.7	328

Table 5.4 Style 4 pectoral implants (Aesthetic and Reconstructive Technologies, Inc., Reno, NV)

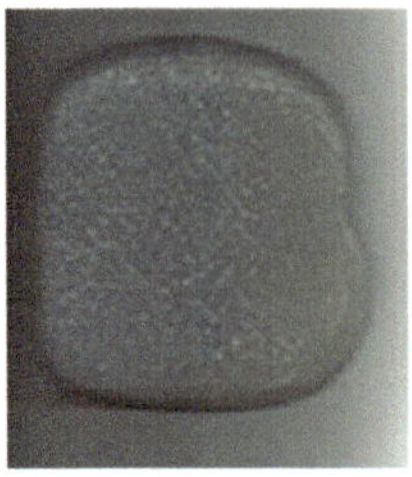

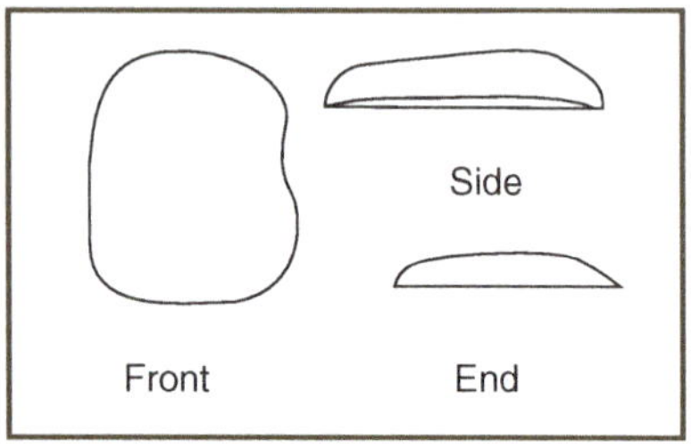

Style 4

	Catalog #	Width	Length	Projection	Volume (cc)
Size 1	500–401	11.4	16.8	2.3	231
Size 2	500–401	13.4	16.0	2.3	349
Size 3	500–403	14.5	17.0	2.5	449
Size 4	500–404	15.5	18.0	2.5	490

Preoperative Planning and Marking

With the patient in the standing position, preoperative markings can be made so as best to hide the incision. The patient's arm is abducted and then raised over the head to clearly define the lateral sweep of the pectoralis major. The patient's natural inframammary fold is also marked. The patient is then repeatedly asked to flex the pectoralis, and the borders are marked squarely on the chest to mark the proposed outline of the muscle and hence the implant position. This will help to direct dissection intraoperatively (Fig. 5.7). A 5–6 cm incision is marked in the hair bearing area of the axilla. Midline may also be marked from the level of the sternal notch down to the umbilicus (optional).

Operative Technique (Figs. 5.8, 5.9, 5.10, 5.11, 5.12, 5.13, 5.14, 5.15, and 5.16)

The patient is brought to the operating room and placed in the supine position with the arms abducted to 90°. The patient is prepped and draped in sterile fashion. Bilateral axilla and pectoral regions are anesthetized with 30–40 mL of 0.5 % lidocaine with epinephrine, taking care to place the anesthetic into the subpectoral plane primarily. A 5–6 cm incision is made in the axilla in line with preoperative markings with a #15 blade scalpel. Dissection is carried through the subcutaneous tissues using a combination of blunt finger dissection and scissor dissection. Electrocautery is used as needed for hemostasis. Dissection is carried to the edge of pectoralis major, and a subpectoral pocket is begun with blunt finger dissection. The subpectoral plane is further developed with an Agris dissector and spatula dissector. Dissection in the caudal region of the chest is limited so that there is no lowering of the inframammary fold. The dissection in the lower pole should be stopped 1–2 cm below the areola; otherwise, the implant will be positioned too low, producing a feminine appearance. Medial dissection is taken to the sternal border of the pectoralis major. This may be slowly avulsed using a serrated wheel dissector to adequately create the medial clefting desired in pectoral augmentation surgery. Care is taken not to pass the midline as this would produce one large pocket, akin to symmastia seen in breast augmentation surgery. Lateral dissection should be minimized to prevent lateral migration of the implant in the future. Once the pocket has been fully dissected, it is packed with sponges. Attention is then turned to the contralateral side and a similar process is undertaken. At this time, the previously placed packs are removed one at a time, and hemostasis is attained with the aid of cautery and a long-blade lighted retractor. If available, an endoscope may be used to evaluate for any bleeding in the medial pocket, and this can be cauterized with a

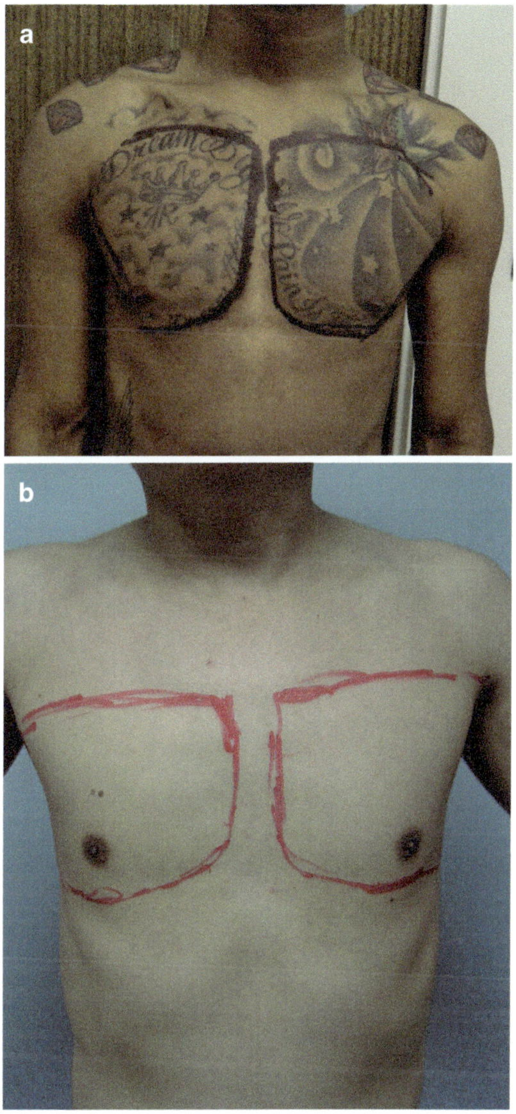

Fig. 5.7 (**a**, **b**) Preoperative markings defining the patient's natural inframammary crease, the lateral sweep of the pectoralis and borders of the palpable pectoralis when the patient was asked to flex. These markings will act as a guide to define the borders of dissection for implant placement. Over dissection can produce an improperly positioned implant

long tip cautery or bipolar forceps. The pocket is irrigated with a solution containing Betadinc, normal saline, Ancef, and gentamicin. This irrigant is then aspirated. Ten mL of 0.5 % Marcaine is instilled into the pocket for postoperative pain control. The implant is then evaluated for possible trimming. The lateral and superior portions

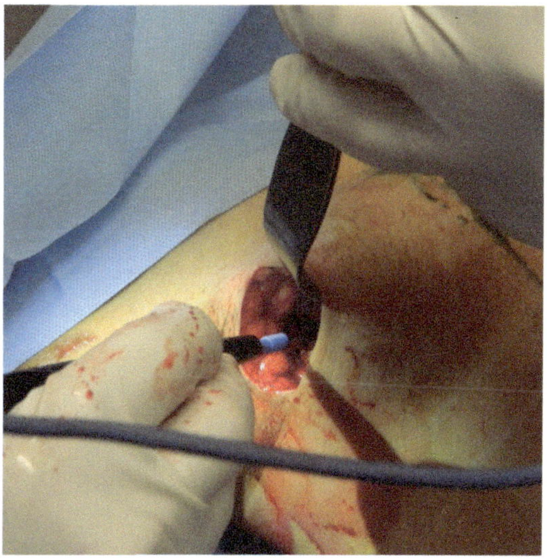

Fig. 5.8 Dissection to the edge of pectoralis major

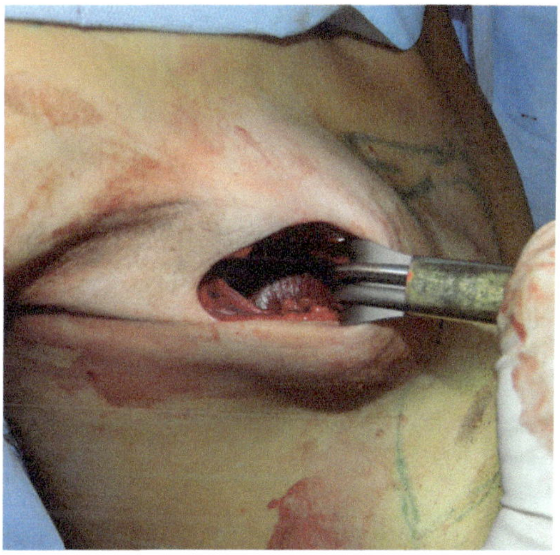

Fig. 5.9 Pectoralis major elevated with pectoralis minor (vertical fibers) noted below

of the implant may need to be trimmed sharply with scissors to prevent unnatural "show" of the implant in areas that are not well protected with muscle and subcutaneous tissue. After adjusting the contour of the implant, the implant is placed into the subpectoral pocket and aesthetics are assessed. The implant is placed by folding it in half along the long axis of the implant. The contralateral side is done and symmetry is assessed. Pocket adjustments can be performed at this time with a spatula dissector as needed. Closure is

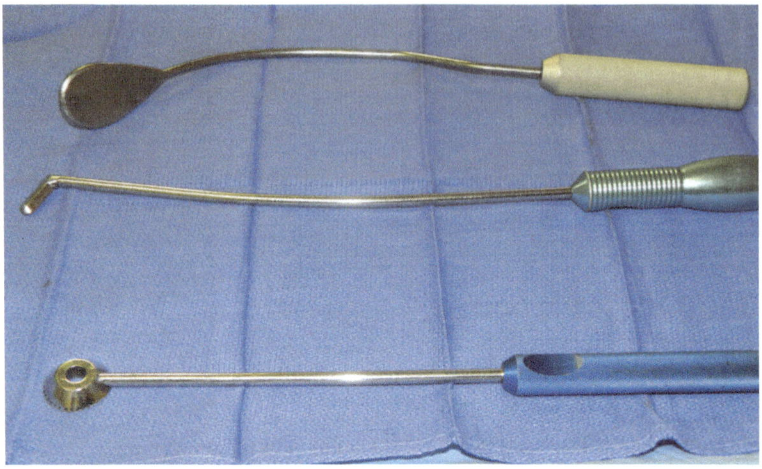

Fig. 5.10 Instruments used in creation of subpectoral plane

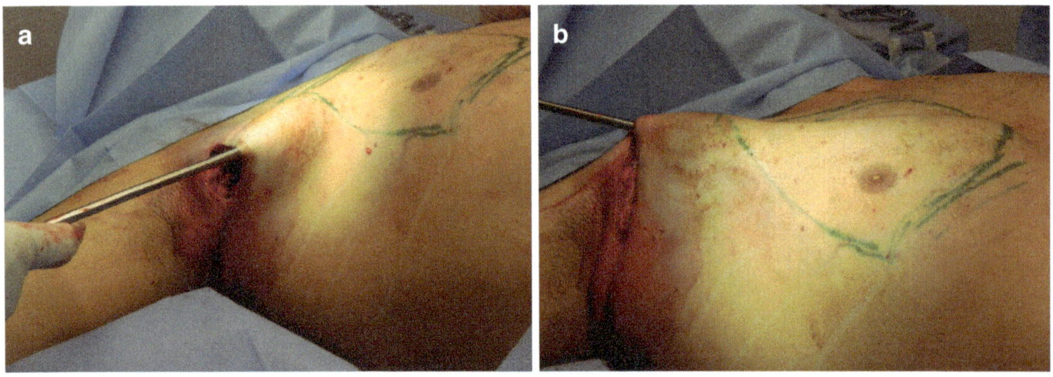

Fig. 5.11 (**a**) Spatula dissection of the pocket. (**b**) Note the medial extent of dissection to release the inferior margin of pectoralis major

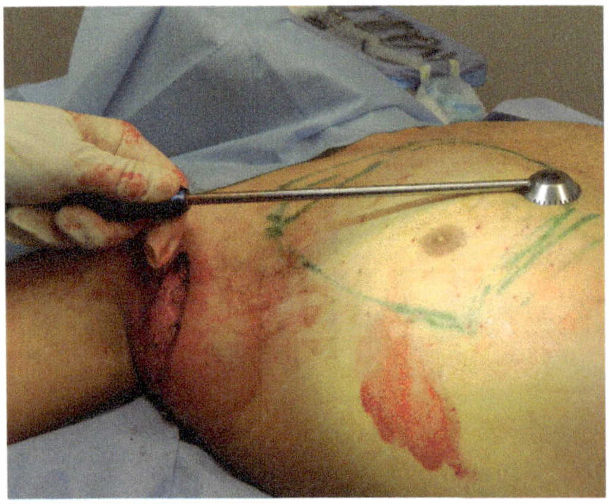

Fig. 5.12 Release of pectoralis major attachments

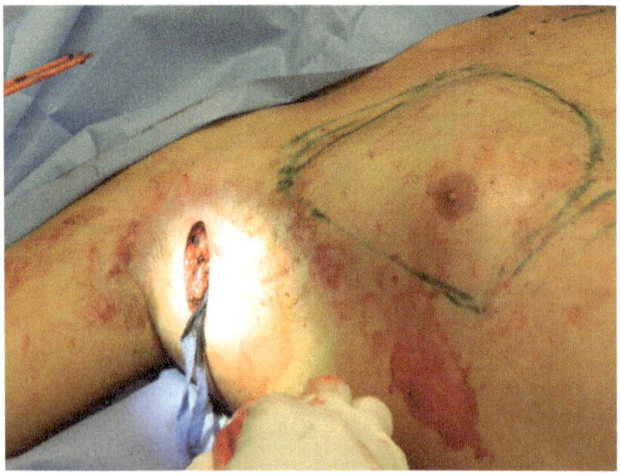

Fig. 5.13 Chest pocket packed with sponges

then begun. The lateral border of the pectoralis is sutured to the lateral thoracic wall using 1-0 Nurulon suture or some other permanent suture. This returns the normal anatomy to the area and ensures a tight pocket around the implant to prevent lateral migration. The subcutaneous tissues and deep dermis are approximated with

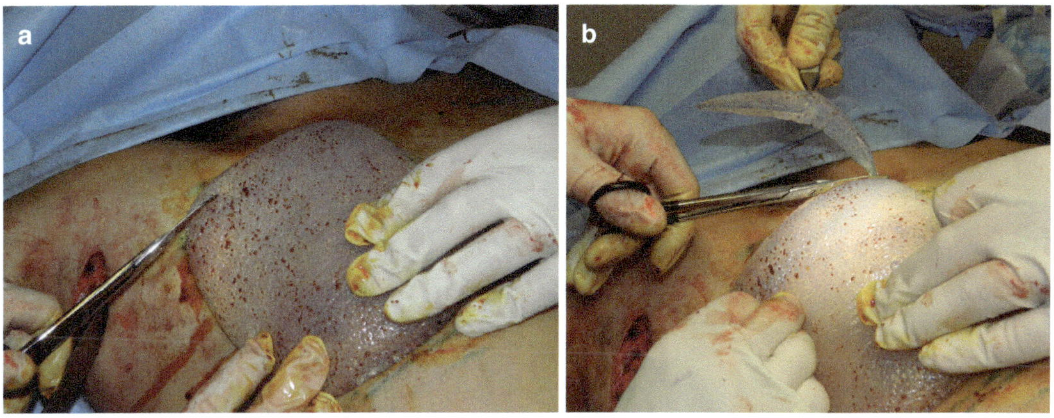

Fig. 5.14 (**a**, **b**) Trimming of the implant as needed, particularly in the cephalic area to prevent abutting the clavicle and in the lateral aspect so that the implant remains completely covered by pectoralis major

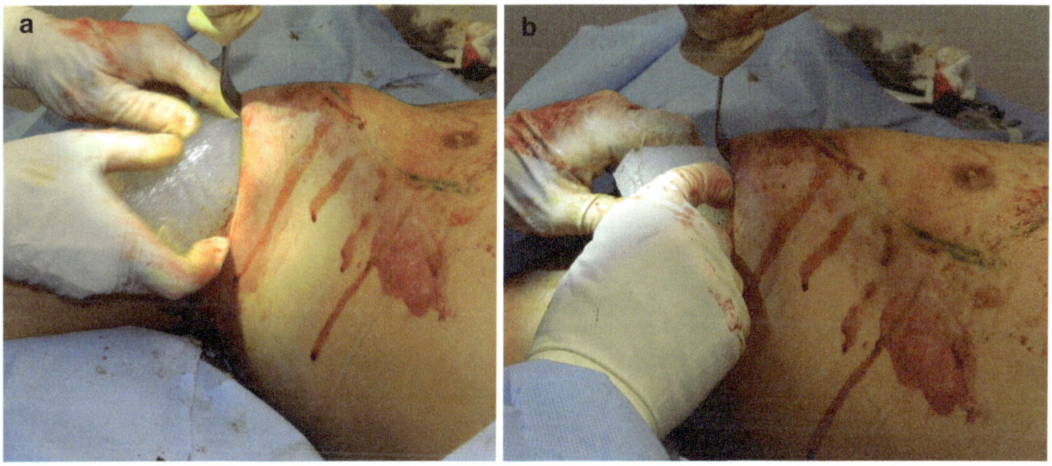

Fig. 5.15 (**a**) Implant placement. (**b**) Implant 50 % inserted

2-0 Vicryl suture. The skin in the axilla is closed in subcuticular fashion using 3-0 Vicryl suture. Collodion is applied to the incision and Robbins tape is applied as a dressing. The chest is wrapped with an elastic bandage and the patient is taken to the postanesthesia care unit (PACU).

Postoperative Care/Instructions

On discharge from the office on the day of surgery, the patients have their chest wrapped in an elastic bandage to diminish the amount of swelling and potential for seroma formation. The patient is seen the following day and the wrap is removed. The chest is placed into a tight spandex vest or has an ACE bandage wrapped around the chest. This compression garment is to be worn at all times for a period of 4 weeks. The patients may remove the compression to shower and to wash as needed. Showering begins the day after surgery, taking care to dry the tape over their incisions with a hair dryer on a low-heat setting. The patient is instructed postoperatively to limit the use of the upper extremities and to avoid exertion or any heavy lifting. Patients may begin to use their arms as tolerated immediately after surgery but are restricted from heavy lifting or vigorous chest activity for 4–6 weeks postoperatively.

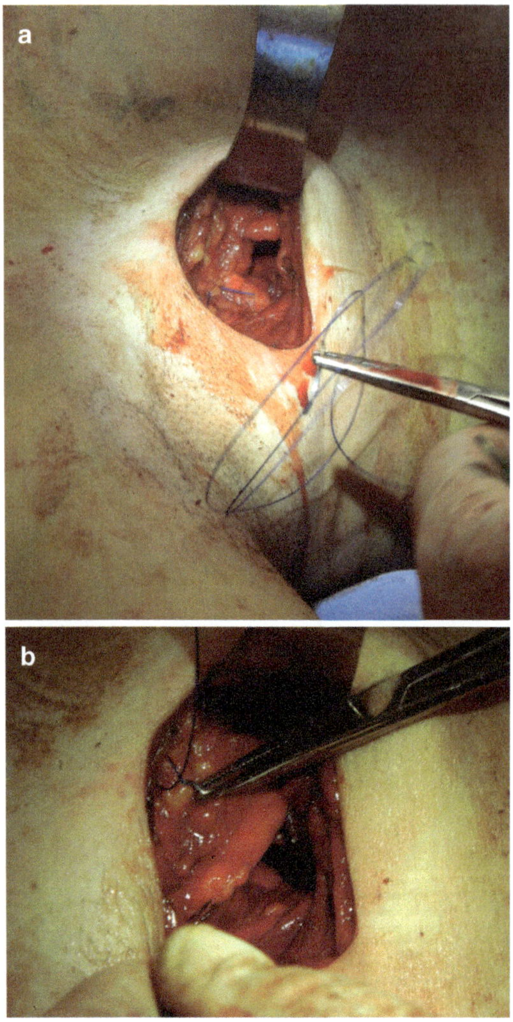

Fig. 5.16 (**a**) Fascia and pectoralis major muscle sewn down to the lateral thoracic wall with first stitch in position and remaining defect at 3 o'clock. (**b**) Pectoralis muscle being sewn down with remaining defect at 3 o'clock position (close)

Complications

In performing pectoral augmentation, there is a host of complications that can arise (Table 5.5).

Infection

Infection, either superficial or deep, is a possibility in pectoral augmentation surgery. Prior to making incision, standard practice should be the administration of 2 g of Ancef IV (or 300 mg IV clindamycin in a penicillin or cephalosporin allergic patient). During the procedure, irrigation of the pocket with a standard antibiotic solution containing normal saline, Betadine, Ancef, and Gentamicin should be performed. Postoperatively, a 5–10-day regimen of oral antibiotics covering normal skin flora should be administered. If a deep infection occurs, the standard of practice is removal of the implant, closure, and possible reimplantation in 3–6 months. There are reports in other forms of implant surgery that conservative management and implant salvage are possible. This should be left at the discretion of the surgeon and performed with careful counseling of the patient. The primary author's (NVC) experience has demonstrated an infection rate of 3.0 % (8/259). This includes both deep and superficial space infections. Only one of these cases required explantation as it was a deep space infection that occurred after multiple seroma drainages with persistent fluid accumulation despite compression and sterile drainage. The patient returned 6 months after explantation for replacement of the chest implants as he was dissatisfied by the flattening of his chest.

Table 5.5 Potential complications of pectoral augmentation

Potential complications of pectoral augmentation surgery
Infection
Seroma
Hematoma
Asymmetry
Implant visibility
Implant migration
"Double-bubble" deformity
Hypertrophic scarring
Hyperpigmentation of the scar
Capsular contracture
Wound dehiscence
Nerve injury (permanent or temporary; motor or sensory)
Compartment syndrome

Seroma

Seromas are statistically the most common complication occurring in implant surgery. They

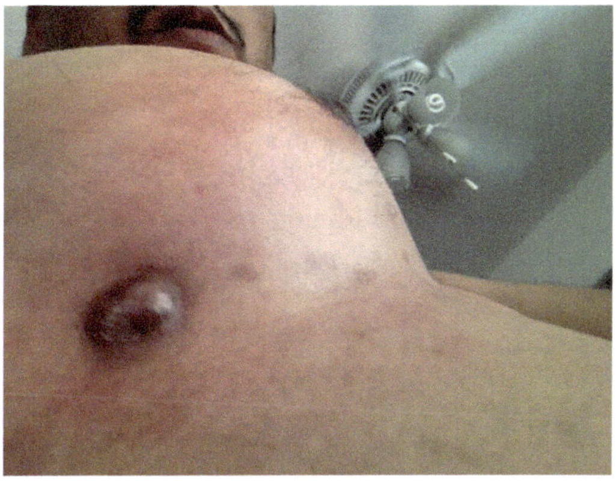

Fig. 5.17 Right pectoralis region with obvious swelling consistent with seroma at physical examination. There is evidence of blistering at the inferior pole of the right pectoralis region consistent with thinning of the skin in the area which did eventually lead to an exposed implant necessitating removal

typically present as new onset pain, swelling, or asymmetry. Patients who have had persistent seromas may also show signs of skin blistering or a thinning of the skin. This may be the precursor to an exposed implant (Fig. 5.17). The treatment of choice remains percutaneous aspiration. This complication is best prevented with patient compliance with compression vests and proper implant placement at the time of surgery, thereby minimizing dead space. In the senior author's experience, it is noncompliance with compression garments and postoperative early return to vigorous activity that result in seroma formation rather than technical issues. Sorensen's early work with silicone implants for pectus excavatum revealed a seroma rate of 52.9 % (9/17) [14]. In their long-term review of pectus excavatum reconstructions with silicone implants, Snel et al. noted a seroma rate of 31 % (5/16) [28]. Hodgkinson [16] in his 15-year review of pectoral augmentation reports a seroma rate of 30 %, typically presenting 7–10 days postoperatively. The authors' data has demonstrated a seroma rate of 4.2 % (11/259). The seroma rate is very low likely due to strict compression of the chest for 1 month postoperatively and our emphasis on not returning to full activity for 4–6 weeks after surgery.

Primarily treatment of a seroma is aspiration; however, a seroma that is resistant to drainage warrants implant removal. Long-standing seromas that fail to resolve can at times cause a thinning of the overlying skin and have led to exposed implants. Should an implant become exposed, immediate implant removal along with closure and pocket washout is imperative. The patient may have the implant replaced 3–6 months later (Fig. 5.18).

Hematoma

To date, the authors have not experienced any hematomas in the series of patients. In the event of a hematoma, rapid evacuation, pocket irrigation, and reimplantation are the mainstays of therapy. This complication is best prevented by meticulous hemostasis at the time of surgery and good compression of the chest postoperatively to prevent potential space creation.

Asymmetry

This can occur as a product of preexisting variability in the patient's chest or variability in dissection of the pocket bilaterally. This is best minimized by good preoperative photography and noting any asymmetries preoperatively. To avoid creation of asymmetry, it is important to maintain the same pattern of dissection and pocket creation bilaterally. Ideally, the pocket created should be tight and minimize the chance of implant migration. Should a pocket be over dissected and patients note postoperative asymmetry due to a pocket's over dissection, the patient may require a return to the operating room to adjust the pocket. A revision case should be planned for no sooner than 3 months postoperatively, allowing a capsule to form around the implant. On return to the operating room (OR), the capsule can be tailored to more appropriately fit around the implant, typically requiring a lateral capsulorrhaphy to prevent lateralization of the implant. The authors had an asymmetry rate of 6.2 % (16/259). While only two of these required surgical intervention to achieve a satisfactory result, this complication occurred most frequently in patients that had

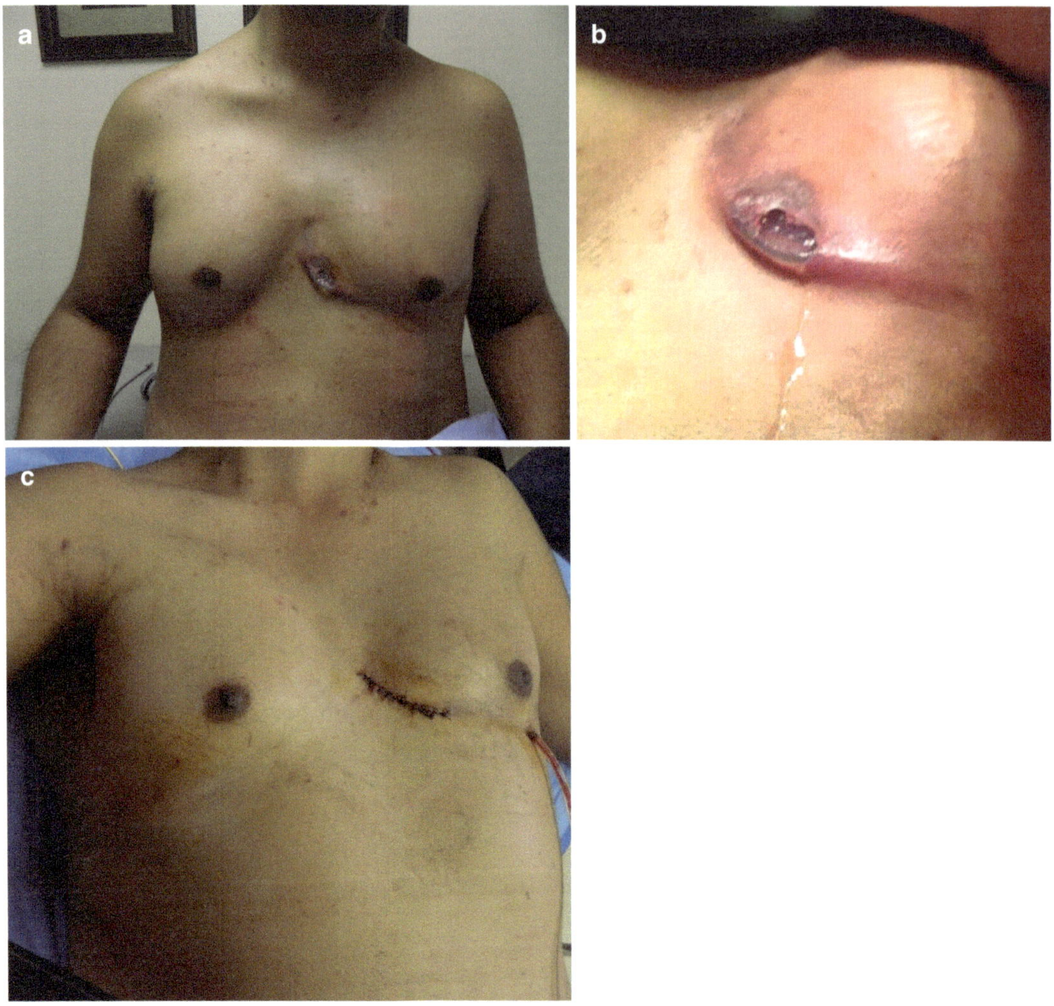

Fig. 5.18 (a–c) A 46-year-old male presented for pectoral augmentation with style 2, size 2 implants. He had recurrent seromas that were percutaneously drained over the course of 2 months. The patient presented for evaluation after he noted that he "saw" his implant along with fluid leaking from his chest. The patient was urgently taken to the OR for removal of his exposed pectoral implant. The site of implant exposure was excised elliptically and closed with interrupted silk sutures. The patient is awaiting replacement of his pectoral implant

preexisting asymmetries that were amplified by the pectoral augmentation by pushing things further forward.

Implant Visibility

Implant visibility is a rare complication of pectoral augmentation due to the deep plane of implant placement below skin, subcutaneous tissue, and muscle. However, those patients that have very thin and atrophic chests to begin with or who suffer from Poland syndrome may have implants that are palpable and visible. Patients should be counseled on this fact preoperatively if there is a feeling that the patient could be at risk. Another way to minimize implant visibility is trimming of the implant as needed to maximize muscular coverage over the implant. This is best done with a heavy mayo scissors, taking care to maintain smooth edges that would not be visible or palpable.

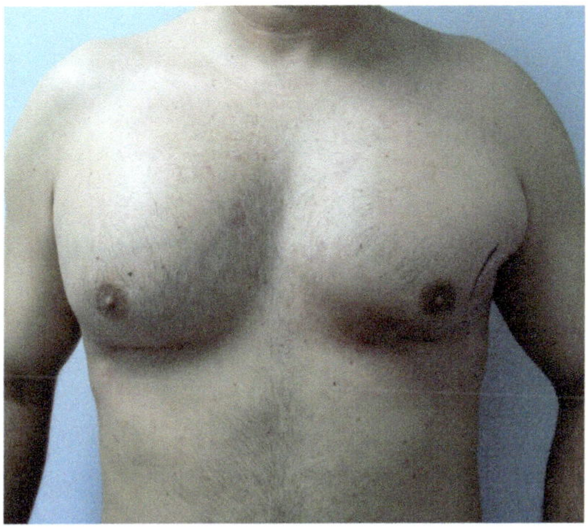

Fig. 5.19 Rotated implant. Lateral edge of implant is marked to show its degree of rotation

Implant Dislodgment/Migration (Fig. 5.19)

Sorensen [14] noted an implant migration rate of 5.8 % (1/17) in his series of pectus repairs with silicone implants. Pereira et al. [29] noted that one out of eight patients (12.5 %) treated in their 5-year study on Poland syndrome reconstructions suffered an implant displacement which presented 2 months postoperatively with rotational shift of the implant. Operative correction is the solution for implant dislodgement or migration. Oftentimes this complication can be avoided with minimal pocket dissection at the time of surgery and strict adherence to postoperative instructions concerning return to full activities (at least 4–6 weeks postop) and use of compression garments (24/7 for 1 month).

Double-Fold/Double-Bubble Deformity

This complication is a contour irregularity that forms at the inferior pole of the chest region where the lower edge of the implant and the lower edge of the existing breast tissue are seen as two separate creases. This is best prevented with good dissection at the primary surgery avoiding excessive caudal dissection.

Scar Hyperpigmentation and Hypertrophy

To date, the authors have not noted any significant issues with scar hyperpigmentation in the axilla. The key to reduction of these problems is careful layered closure as previously described.

Capsular Contracture

This is a possible late sequelae of any implant placement, most frequently described in the breast augmentation literature. To date, the authors have had three cases of capsular contracture after pectoral augmentation (1.2 %). Patients were initially started on Accolate 10 mg orally BID for 3 months in the hope of softening the capsule. This was successful in two cases. In one case, a return to the OR was necessary to perform capsulotomies. By lengthening the axillary incision by 2 cm in the anterior aspect, a lighted retractor was advanced and radial capsulotomies were performed under direct visualization. A capsulectomy would be difficult to perform in pectoral augmentation cases unless a periareolar incision was made or a significant lengthening of the axillary incision was undertaken.

Wound Dehiscence

Wound dehiscence is a product of poor wound closure under too much tension typically. In order to prevent this, meticulous closure in three layers is paramount: fascia, deep dermis, and skin. To date, we have seen three cases of wound dehiscence, none greater than 2 cm (1.2 %). These dehiscences occurred in patients that began more vigorous activity than recommended before the 1 month mark. All wounds healed by secondary intention with minor local wound care.

Nerve Injury

Permanent nerve injury is rarely a problem with this procedure as the majority of dissection is performed in a blunt, atraumatic fashion. It is quite common for patients to complain of some numbness over the area of the axilla; however, this returns within 1–3 months postoperatively without sequelae. Major motor and sensory deficits can accompany compartment syndrome, and this must be ruled out immediately if any significant deficits are appreciated.

Compartment Pressure Problems/ Compartment Syndrome

Although rarely described as an isolated compartment syndrome of the pectoral region, Tarkin et al. [30] described their experience with an exercise-induced compartment syndrome of the chest and deltoid region. As with compartment syndrome of the extremity, nerve and muscle cells start to die within 4–8 h. Compartment syndrome typically presents as a tensely swollen compartment with extreme pain, out of proportion to examination, on palpation. This is sometimes accompanied by referred pain to the affected compartment with passive stretch of muscles. There may or may not be a neuropathy, typically described as a burning or prickling sensation, appreciated over the skin of the affected region. The patient may experience frank pulselessness or paralysis of muscles in the affected compartment or distally in the extremities. However, the patient who presents with these final findings has typically progressed beyond the point of muscle salvage.

In patients with a compatible history and a tense extremity, clinical diagnosis may be sufficient. If the diagnosis is in doubt, compartment pressures may be measured with a handheld Stryker device. An absolute pressure greater than 30 mmHg in any compartment, or a pressure within 30 mmHg of the diastolic blood pressure in hypotensive patients, or a patient with a concerning history who demonstrates the constellation of signs and symptoms of compartment syndrome are all possible indications for surgical intervention and removal of the implant immediately.

Special Cases of Pectoral Augmentation

Pectus Excavatum

Pectus excavatum, Latin for "hollowed chest," is a deformity of the sternum whereby there is a depression in this area as a result of abnormal boney and cartilaginous development [27]. It occurs in an estimated 1 in 150–1,000 births, with male predominance (male-to-female ratio of 3:1). Rarely, this depression may cause compression of internal organs such as the heart and lung; however, more than anything the depression results in a cosmetically distressing defect that brings patients to the surgeon for correction [31, 32]. Classically, the deformity is corrected with extensive thoracic procedures such as the Ravitch and Nuss procedures which introduce bars to restructure the sternum and surrounding bony and cartilaginous structures [1, 29, 31]. The modified Ravitch procedure requires exposure of the sternum and surrounding area, removal of abnormal cartilages, and fixation of the sternum in a more normal position with a metal bar. This metal bar remains in place for at least a year and then is removed with another operation. While this procedure has a good history of correcting the condition, it requires an incision (and scar) on the front of the chest to resect the abnormal cartilage – an operation that takes several hours and requires hospitalization for pain management. Physical activity is severely restricted for several months as the costal cartilages slowly grow back together. The Nuss procedure is considered a minimally invasive alternative to the Ravitch procedure. Through two small incisions in the side of the chest, an introducer is pushed along posterior to the sternum and ribs and anterior to the heart and lungs. Then a concave stainless steel bar is slipped under the sternum, through the incisions in the side of the chest. A third, smaller incision is made to insert a thoracoscope used to help guide the bar. This bar is left in place. This bar is later removed at 2–4 years after initial placement. Regardless of the procedure chosen, it requires at least two surgeries and may leave patients with scars that are not esthetically pleasing and is associated with serious complications [31].

Rather than correcting the structural deformity, some surgeons began to report success in using solid implants to camouflage the matter [13, 19]. Used in both pectus excavatum cases and soft tissue deformities of the pectoral region, these implants provided a good to excellent cosmetic result without the need for all the risks and complications associated with the surgeries typically used to correct the underlying anatomic deformity. Snel et al. [28] sought to further evaluate long-term results with the reconstruction of the chest with silicone implants and found that there was a satisfaction rate of 83 % in their population of chest wall reconstructions using silicone prostheses. They stress that implant use is best reserved for less severe cases of pectus excavatum that present at a more advanced age and are able to better participate in decision making with the surgeon.

In 1997, Hodgkinson [16] reviewed his experience of 15 years using silicone implants to correct a wide range of chest wall deformities, including pectus excavatum. Via a substernal incision, he described his technique of developing a pocket at the level of the perichondrium/periosteum with partial release of the pectoralis muscle. He explains the need to trip or thin the implant using large scissors to prevent "show" of the implant in areas covered only by skin and subcutaneous tissue. The implants used for his patients were customized using a firm moulage plastic kit, providing implants suited to the individual patient.

Case 1 (Fig. 5.20)
A 37-year-old male (MG) underwent pectoral augmentation with style 2, size 2 pectoral implants (367 mL) along with left chest liposuction for minor asymmetry secondary to lipohypertrophy. His primary complaint at consultation was a minor defect in his chest wall consistent with a mild form of pectus excavatum. He denied any associated cardiopulmonary issues. He is seen preoperatively and 8 months postoperatively.

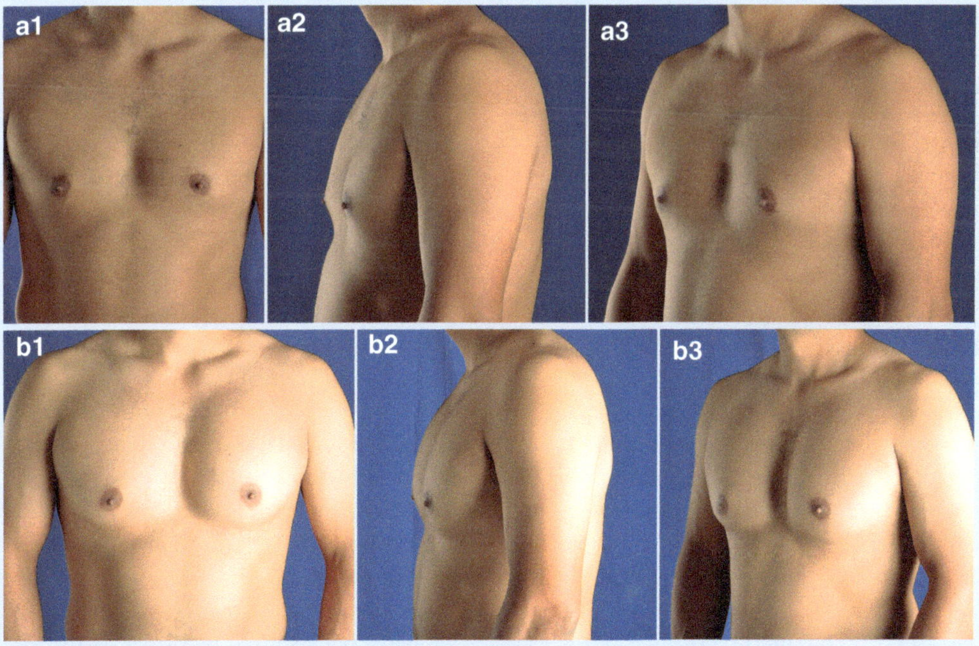

Fig. 5.20 (**a**) Preoperative. (**b**) Postoperative

Case 2 (Fig. 5.21)
A 31-year-old male (SR) underwent pectoral augmentation with style 2, size 2 pectoral implants (367 mL) for a mild case of pectus excavatum. He is seen preoperatively and 1 month postoperatively.

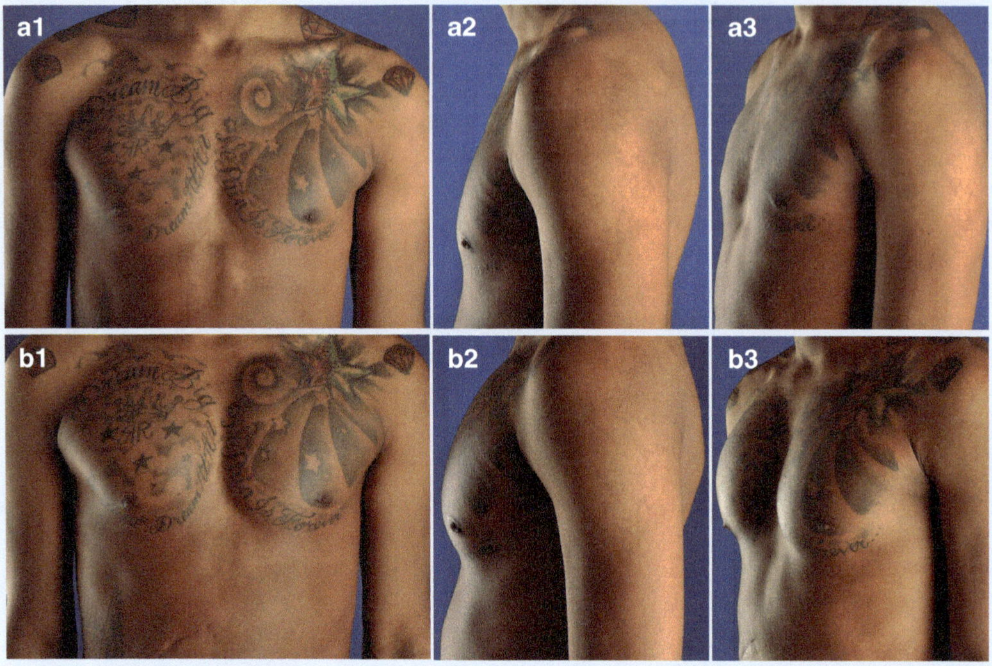

Fig. 5.21 (**a**) Preoperative. (**b**) Postoperative

Poland Syndrome

Poland syndrome is a rare deformity of the chest whereby there is an underdevelopment or absence of the pectoralis major on one side of the body [31]. It is usually associated with webbing of the fingers (syndactyly) and may also be accompanied by nipple or breast deformity. In severe cases, there may be partial agenesis of the ribs and sternum; scoliosis; absence of the latissimus dorsi, serratus anterior, and other nearby structures [33]. Poland syndrome most often affects the right side of the body (75 % of the time) and occurs more frequently in males than females (3:1 ratio). The incidence is estimated to be 1 in 7,000–1 in 100,000 live births [34]. While, little disability is noted due to this disorder, even in the most severe of cases, patients often complain of embarrassment due to a self-perceived cosmetic deformity [33]. Thoracic surgery may be a means of repairing the deformity if there is evidence of sternal rotation and very prominent, projecting costal cartilages. Also, latissimus flaps have been used to replace the void in the area of muscle agenesis or underdevelopment but have been met with unfavorable results due to muscle atrophy and contractures and unaesthetic back scars [31].

Several authors over the last two decades have suggested implant use to camouflage the deficiency in the chest region in more minor cases of Poland syndrome, helping to bring about greater symmetry between the two sides of the anterior thorax [16, 29, 33].

Case 3 (Fig. 5.22)
A 28-year-old male presented for correction of his right pectoralis region. From early childhood, he had been diagnosed with Poland syndrome. He now wished to attain greater symmetry of his chest. The patient is seen preoperatively and 1 month postoperatively. Although not exactly symmetrical (something explained to all Poland patients preoperatively), there is significant improvement in symmetry. Preoperative marking of the patient is done marking both clavicles as this is typically one of the only major landmarks that one can use. The proposed site of implant placement is marked and compared to the dimensions of the existing pectoral region. Intraoperatively, one can better appreciate the significant defect from the basilar view.

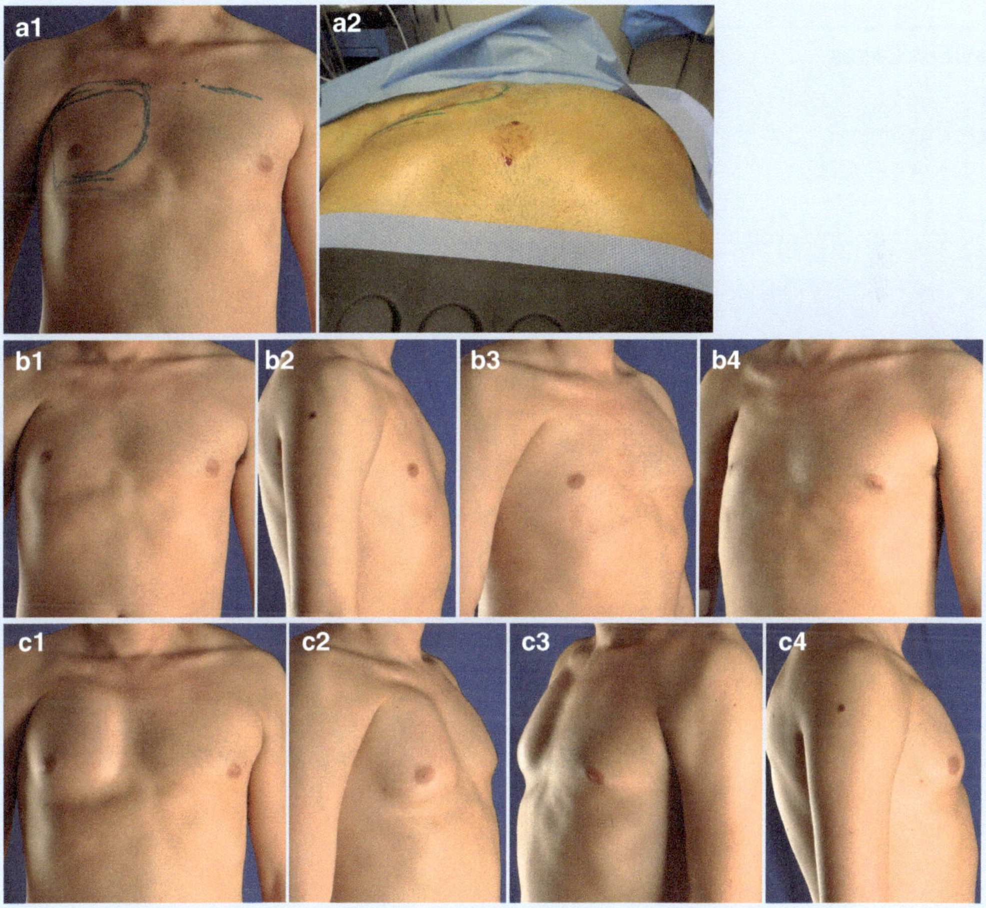

Fig. 5.22 (**a**) Preoperative marking right chest. (**b**) Preoperative. (**c**) Postoperative

Pectoral Augmentation with Fat Grafting

Work by Coleman in the field of fat grafting has accelerated the surgeon's understanding of what can be done with autologous fat packets. To date, the authors have not recommended fat grafting for pectoral augmentation as most men wish to have a more solid and chiseled appearance. Fat is inconsistent in its take but most importantly does not provide a firm, male physique.

Authors' Personal Results

In reviewing the primary author's (NVC) own experience with the procedure, there have been a total of approximately 259 pectoral augmentations performed since beginning to perform the procedure in 1995. During that time, the seroma rate has been 4.2 % (11/259). The infection rate has also been 3.0 % (8/259). Asymmetry was noted in 16 of 259 cases, giving an incidence of 6.2 % (16/259). There were three cases of capsular contracture in the 259 cases of pectoral augmentation (1.2 %). Overall satisfaction with the procedure was noted to be 95 % (246/259). Dissatisfaction arose because of the patient's complaint of inadequate augmentation.

Patient Cases

Case 4 (Fig. 5.23)
A 32-year-old male seeking pectoral augmentation. He underwent augmentation with style 2, size 2 pectoral implants (367 mL). He is seen preoperatively and 2 years postoperatively.

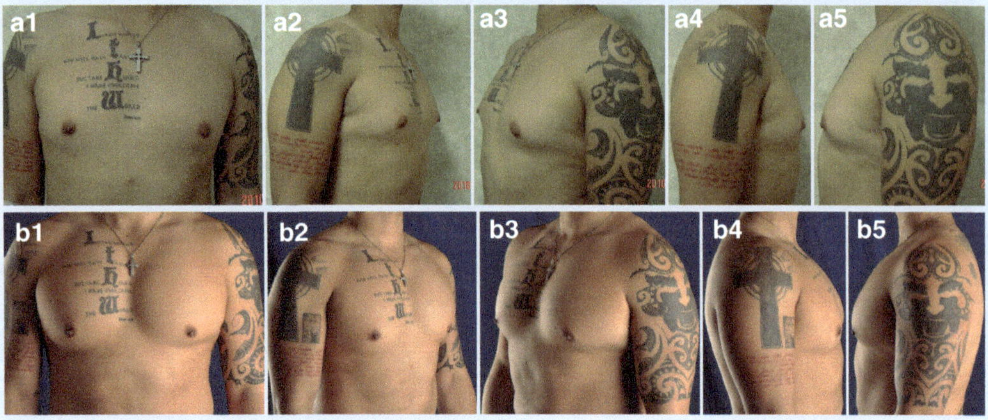

Fig. 5.23 (**a**) Preoperative. (**b**) Postoperative

Case 5 (Fig. 5.24)
A 46-year-old male seeking pectoral, biceps, and triceps augmentation. He received style 8, size 3 biceps implants. He received style 8, size 20 triceps implants. He also received style 2, size 2 pectoral implants. He had minor abdominal liposuction (300 mL fat harvested). He is seen 1 week postoperatively.

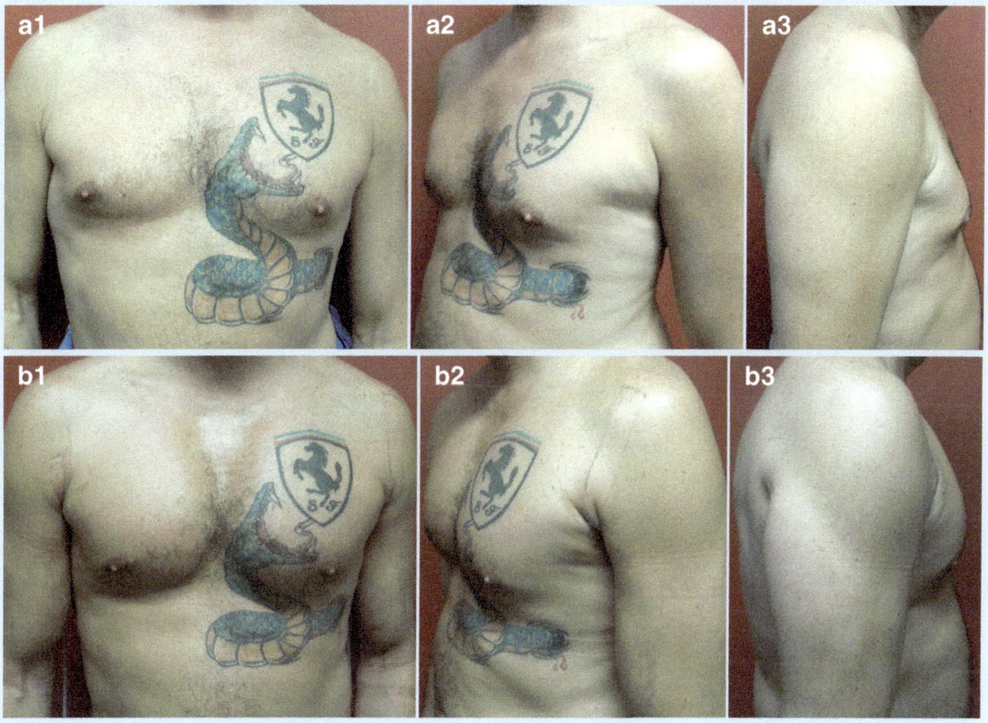

Fig. 5.24 (**a**) Preoperative. (**b**) Postoperative

Case 6 (Fig. 5.25)
A 30-year-old male seeking pectoral augmentation. He underwent augmentation with style 2, size 2 pectoral implants (367 mL). He is seen preoperatively and 8 months postoperatively.

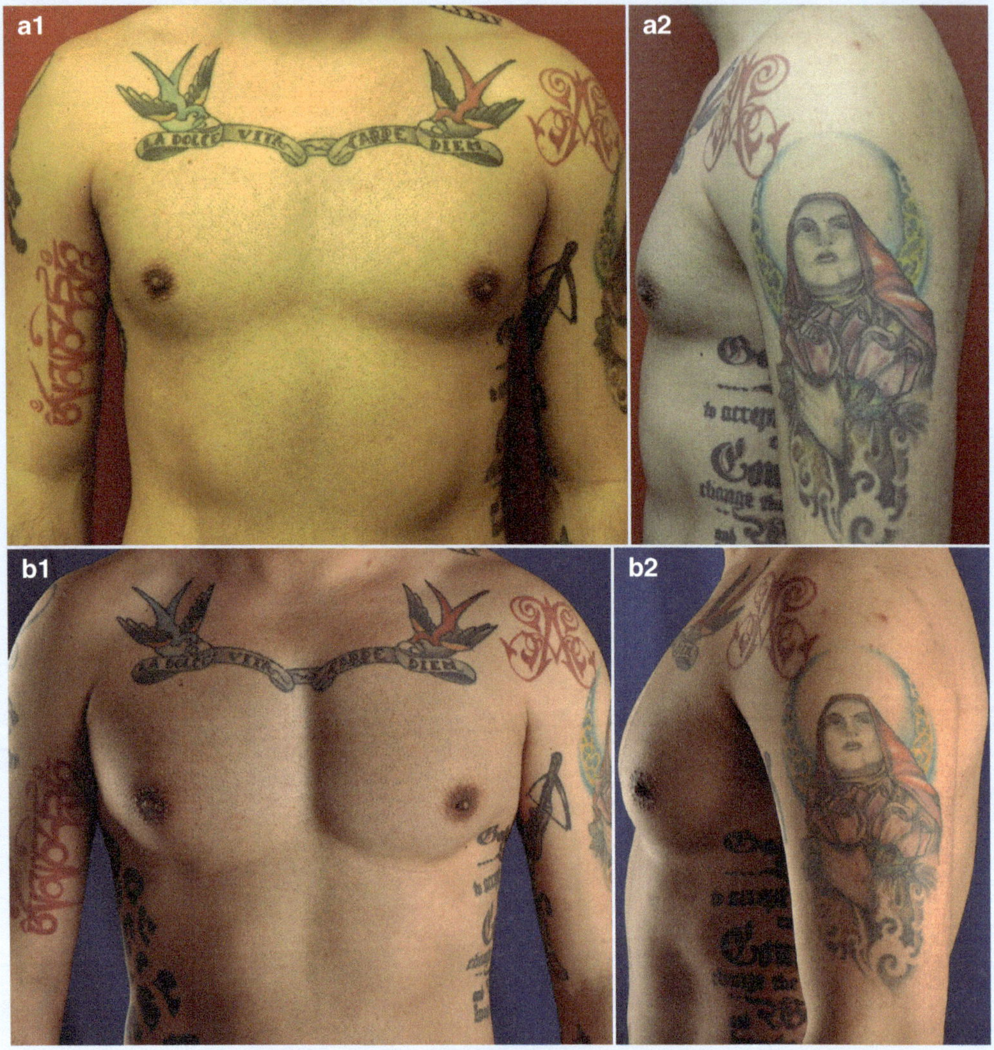

Fig. 5.25 (**a**) Preoperative. (**b**) Postoperative

Case 7 (Fig. 5.26)
A 38-year-old male seeking pectoral augmentation. He underwent augmentation with style 2, size 2 implants (367 mL). He is seen preoperatively and 5 months postoperatively.

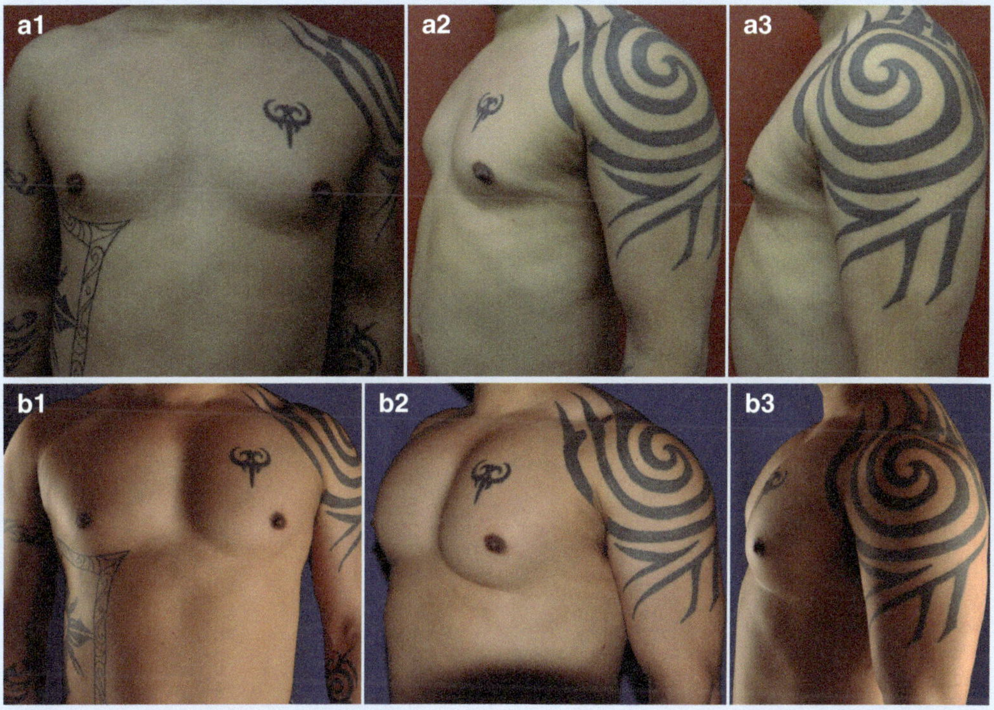

Fig. 5.26 (**a**) Preoperative. (**b**) Postoperative

Case 8 (Fig. 5.27)

A 23-year-old male underwent pectoral augmentation with style 2, size 2 pectoral implants (367 mL).

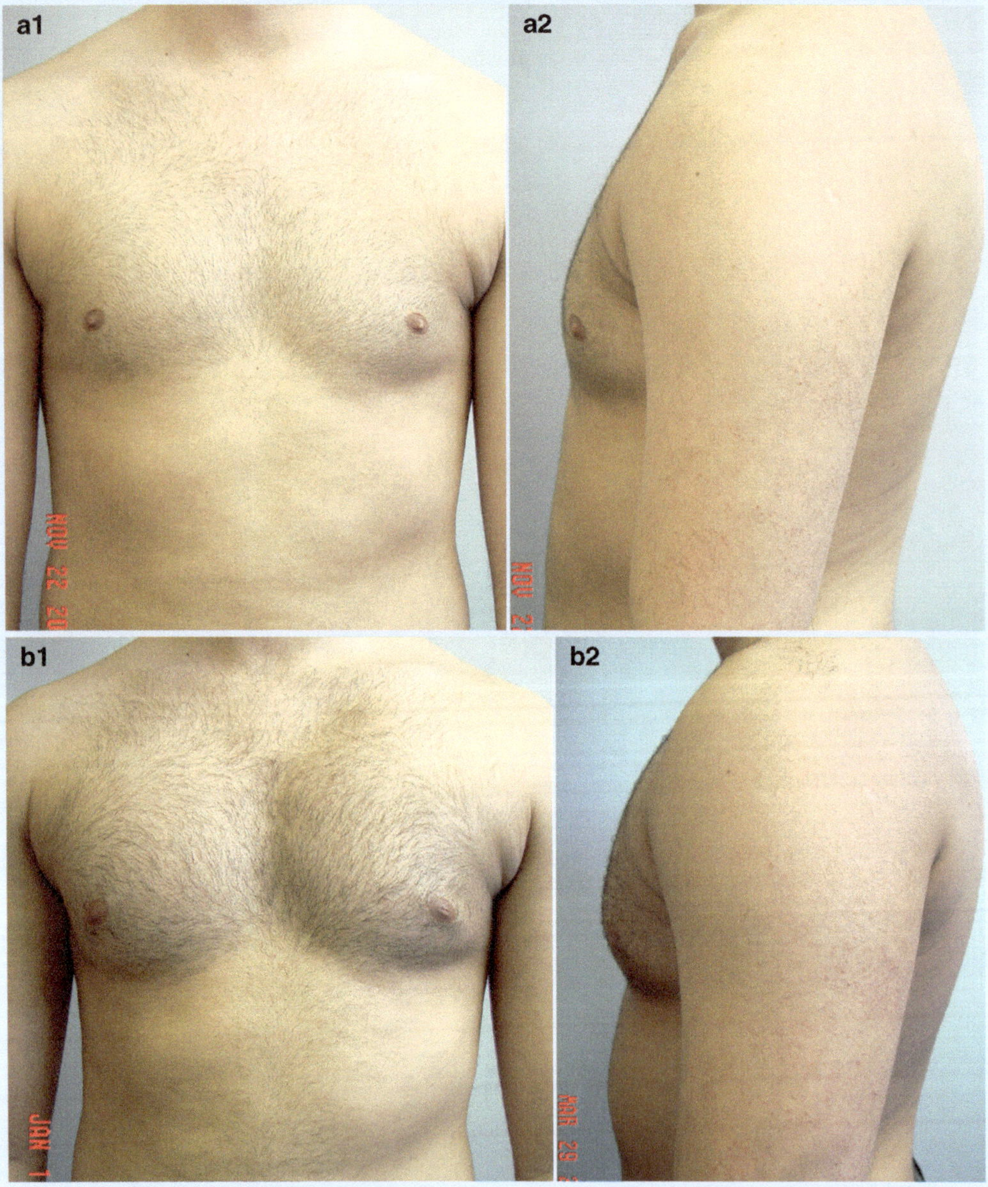

Fig. 5.27 (**a**) Preoperative. (**b**) Postoperative

Case 9 (Fig.5.28)

A 27-year-old male underwent pectoral augmentation with style 2, size 3 pectoral implants and biceps augmentation with style 8, size 1 biceps implants. He is seen preoperatively and 1 month postoperatively.

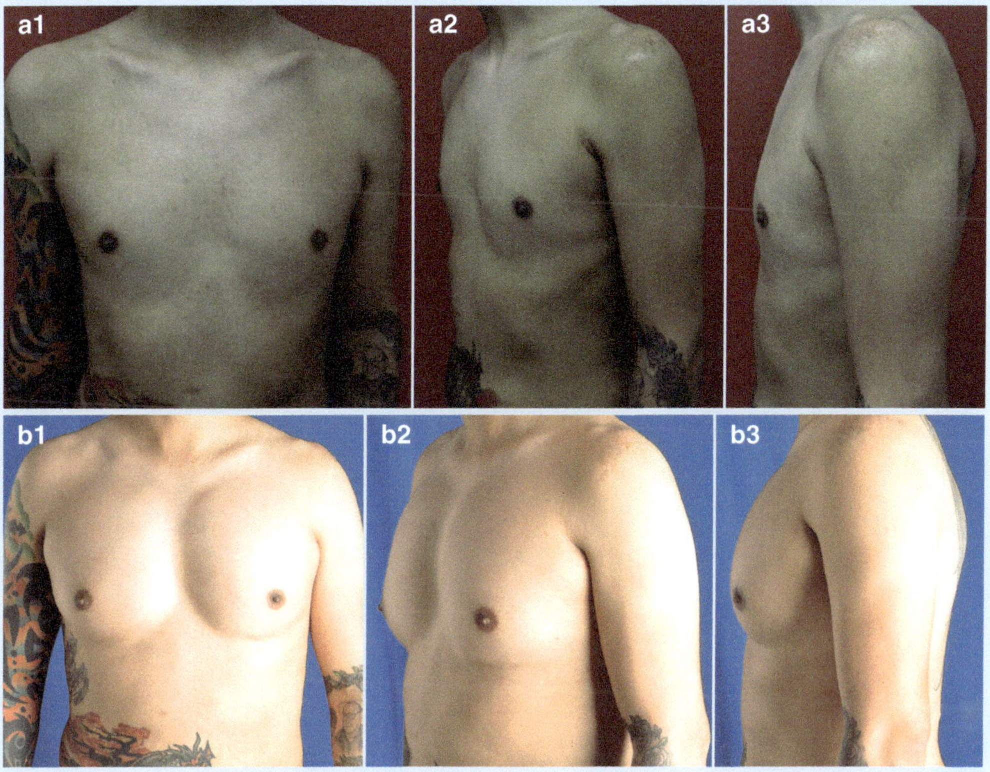

Fig. 5.28 (**a**) Preoperative. (**b**) Postoperative

Case 10 (Fig. 5.29)

A 45-year-old male underwent bilateral biceps, triceps, and pectoral augmentation with excision of breast tissue for gynecomastia and liposuction of the chest. He received a style 2, size 3 pectoral implant. He received a style 8, size 1 biceps implant and a style 8, size 20 triceps implant. Three hundred milliliter of fat was aspirated from the chest with gland excision. He complained of "hanging breasts" and wanted a more masculine figure. Due to the excessive amount of loose skin, he was offered a formal breast lift but instead he opted for the pectoral implants to fill out his chest and the loose skin envelope. He is seen preoperatively and 4 months postoperatively.

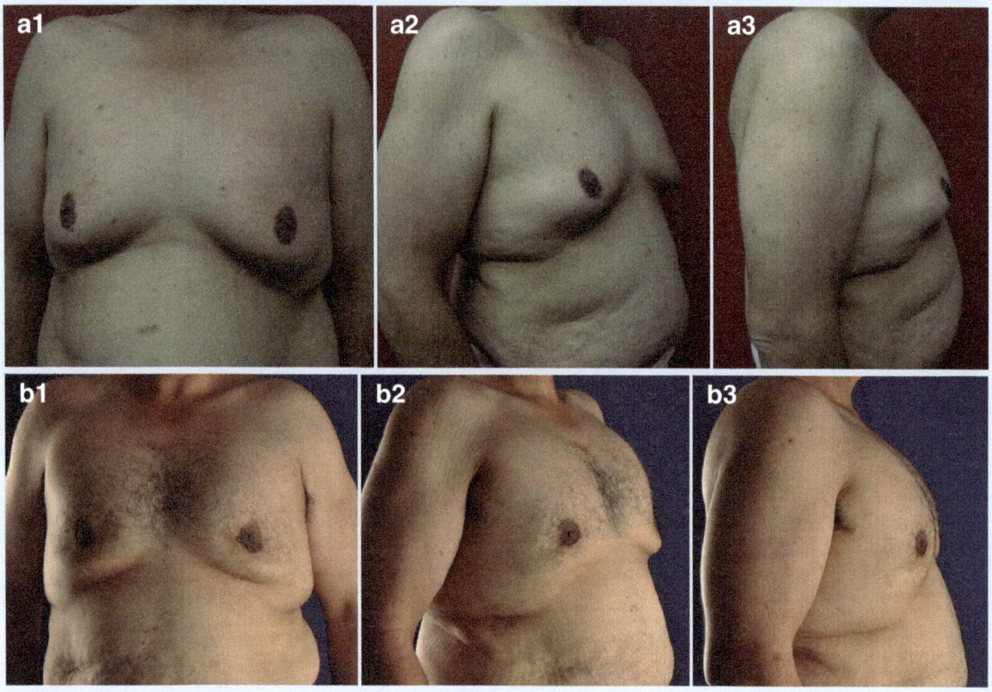

Fig. 5.29 (**a**) Preoperative. (**b**) Postoperative

Case 11 (Fig. 5.30)
A 35-year-old male underwent augmentation with style 1, size 3 (349 mL) implants. This was one of our early cases, and we have since preferred a block shaped implant as these early implants used can give a more "breast-like" appearance to the augmentation.

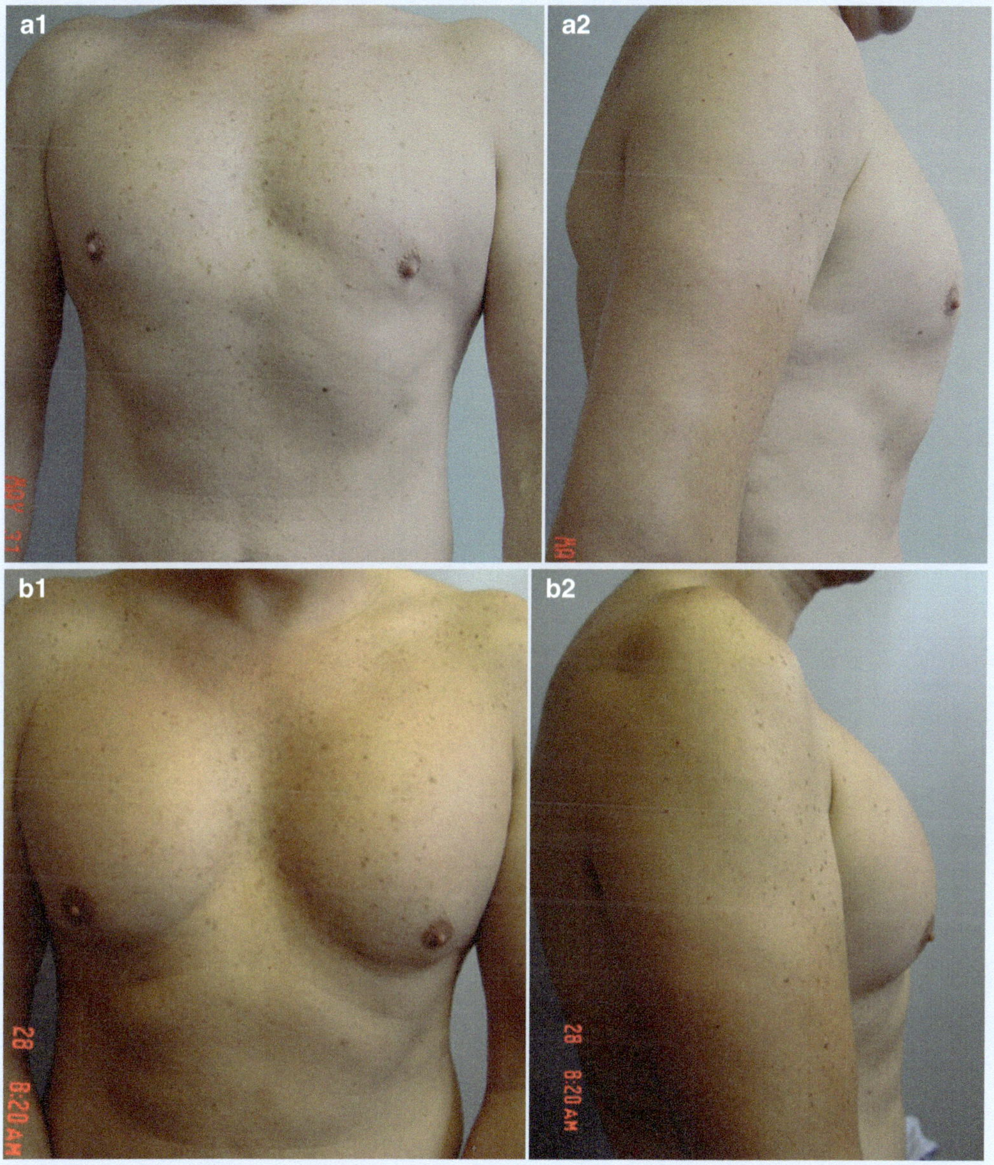

Fig. 5.30 (**a**) Preoperative. (**b**) Postoperative

Case 12 (Fig. 5.31)

A 26-year-old male underwent pectoral augmentation with style 1, size 3 (349 mL) implants. This was one of our early cases, and we have since preferred a block shaped implant as these early implants used can give a more "breast-like" appearance to the augmentation.

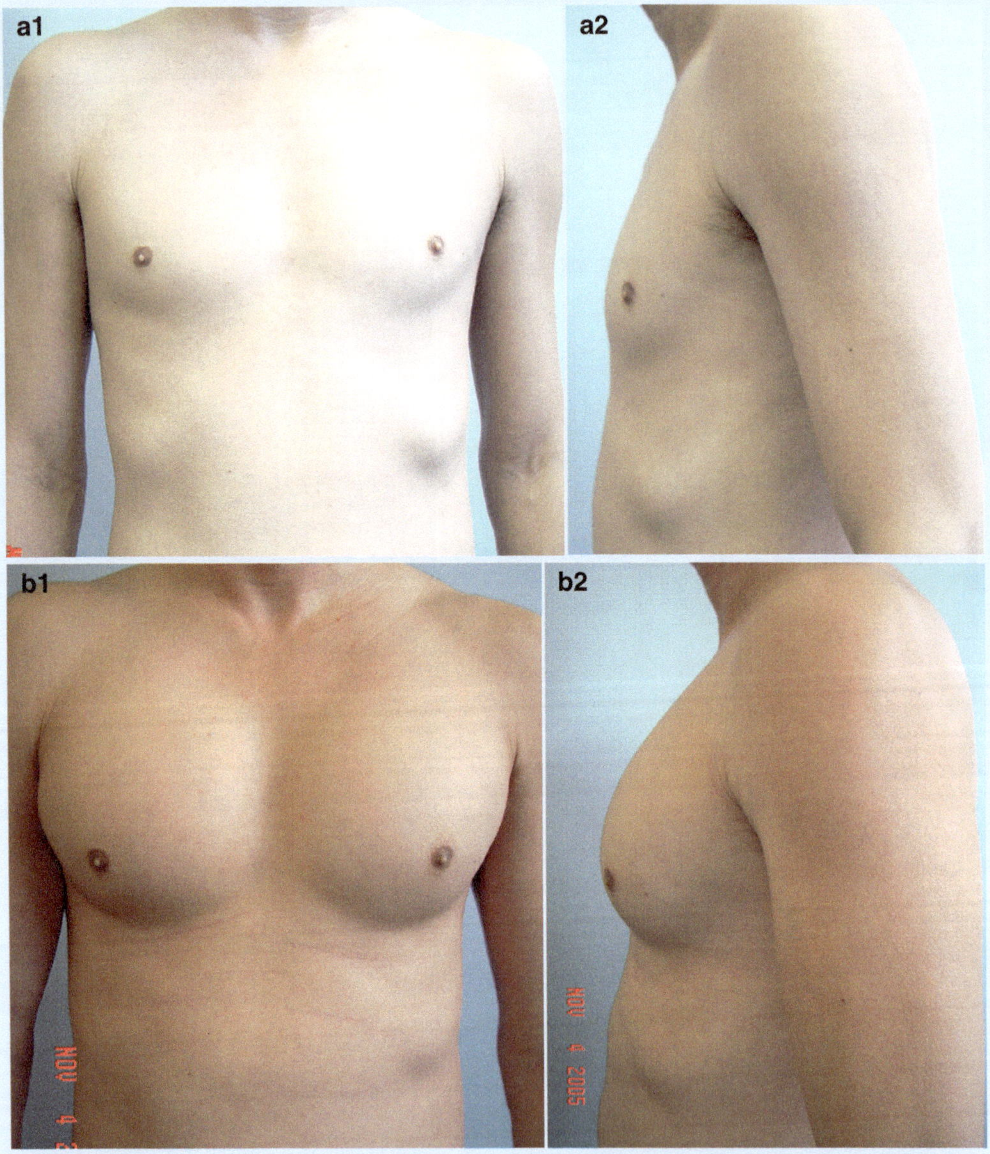

Fig. 5.31 (**a**) Preoperative. (**b**) Postoperative

Conclusions

Pectoral augmentation has long stood as an option for reconstruction of defects of the chest. Beginning in the early 1990s, multiple surgeons began to see the benefit of pectoral augmentation to meet the needs of patients who wished to augment a hypoplastic chest despite attempts to increase chest size with conventional and sometimes even aggressive exercise regimens. At this time, pectoral augmentation with silicone elastomer implants is an excellent way to help men achieve greater definition and muscularity, bringing them closer to the muscular ideals of the "manly man" currently widespread in society today.

References

1. Plastic Surgery Statistics Report. 2012. http://www.plasticsurgery.org/Documents/news-resources/statistics/2012-Plastic-Surgery-Statistics/full-plastic-surgery-statistics-report.pdf. Accessed 5 Sept 2013.
2. American Academy of Cosmetic Surgery Procedural Census. 2008. http://multivu.prnewswire.com/mnr/aacs/36867/docs/36867AACS2008ProceduralSurveyResults.pdf. Accessed 5 Sept 2013.
3. Phillips KA. Body image and body dysmorphic disorder. In: Cash T, Smolak L, editors. Body image: a handbook of science, practice, and prevention. 2nd ed. New York: The Guilford Press; 2011. p. 305–13.
4. Pope HG, Gruber AJ, Mangweth B, Bureau B, de Col C, Jouvent R, Hudson JI. Body image perception among men in three countries. Am J Psychiatry. 2000;157(8):1297–301.
5. Olivardia R, Pope HG, Borowiecki JJ, Cohane GH. Biceps and body image: the relationship between muscularity and self-esteem, depression, and eating disorder symptoms. Psychol Men Masculin. 2004;5(2):112–20.
6. Leit RA, Pope HG, Gray JJ. Cultural expectation of muscularity in men: the evolution of playgirl centerfolds. Int J Eat Disord. 2001;29(1):90–3.
7. Cafri G, Thompson JK, Ricciardelli L, McCabe M, Smolak L, Yesalis C. Pursuit of the muscular ideal: physical and psychological consequences and putative risk factors. Clin Psychol Rev. 2005;25(2):215–39.
8. Pope HG, Olivardia R, Gruber A, Borowiecki J. Evolving ideals of male body image as seen through action toys. Int J Eat Disord. 1999;26(1):65–72.
9. Chugay N, Racanelli J, Hsu J, Chugay P. Bicipital augmentation. Am J Cosmet Surg. 2006;23(1):33–6.
10. Chugay N, Chugay P. Bicipital augmentation: a retrospective review of 94 patient cases. Am J Cosmet Surg. 2009;26(4):241–5.
11. Chugay NV, Chugay PN. Triceps augmentation: early experience with the procedure. Am J Cosmet Surg. 2010;27(4):200–3.
12. Nuss D. Recent experiences with minimally invasive pectus excavatum repair "Nuss procedure". Jpn J Thorac Cardiovasc Surg. 2005;53(7):338–44.
13. Mendelson B, Masson JK. Silicone implants for contour deformities of the trunk. Plast Reconstr Surg. 1977;59(4):538–44.
14. Sorensen JL. Subcutaneous silicone implants in pectus excavatum. Scand J Plast Reconstr Surg Hand Surg. 1988;22(2):173–6.
15. Aiache AE. Male chest correction. Pectoral implants and gynecomastia. Clin Plast Surg. 1991;18(4):823–8.
16. Hodgkinson DJ. Chest wall implants: their use for pectus excavatum, pectoralis muscle tears, Poland's syndrome, and muscular insufficiency. Aesthetic Plast Surg. 1997;21(1):7–15.
17. Novack BH. Alloplastic implants for men. Clin Plast Surg. 1991;18(4):829–55.
18. Povencher MT, Handfied K, Boniquit NT, Reiff SN, Sekiya JK, Romeo AA. Injuries to the pectoralis major muscle: diagnosis and management. Am J Sports Med. 2010;38(8):1693–705.
19. Antosh IJ, Grassbaugh JA, Parada SA, Arrington ED. Pectoralis major tendon repairs in the active-duty population. Am J Orthop. 2009;38(1):26–30.
20. Lim CT, Wee J, Lee KT. Early surgical treatment of pectoralis major tendon rupture: a case report. Malays Orthop J. 2012;6(4):38–40.
21. Chugay NV, Quach Q. Pectoral augmentation. Int J Cosm Surg. 1999;7(1):43–482.
22. Horn G. A new concept in male chest reshaping: anatomical pectoral implants and liposculpture. Aesthetic Plast Surg. 2002;26(1):23–5.
23. Benito-Ruiz J. Buttock implants for male chest enhancement. Plast Reconstr Surg. 2003;112(7):1951.
24. Benito-Ruiz J, Raigosa JM, Manzano-Surroca M, Salvador L. Male chest enhancement: pectoral implants. Aesthetic Plast Surg. 2008;32(1):101–4.
25. Gray H. Anatomy of the human body. Philadelphia: Lea & Febiger; 1918.
26. David S, Balaguer T, Baque P, de Peretti F, Valla M, Lebreton E, Chignon-Sicard B. The anatomy of the pectoral nerves and its significance in breast augmentation, axillary dissection and pectoral muscle flaps. J Plast Reconstr Aesthet Surg. 2012;65:1193–8.
27. Hoffman GW, Elliott F. The anatomy of the pectoral nerves and its significance to the general and plastic surgeon. Ann Surg. 1987;205(5):504–6.
28. Snel BJ, Spronk CA, Werker PM, van der Lei B. Pectus excavatum reconstruction with silicone implants: long-term results and review of the English-language literature. Ann Plast Surg. 2009;62(2):205–9.
29. Pereira LH, Sabatovich O, Santana KP, Picanco R, Sterodimas A. Surgical correction of Poland's syndrome in males – a purposed designed implant. J Plast Reconstr Aesthet Surg. 2008;61(4):393–9.
30. Tarkin IS, Perricelli BC, Pape HC. Exercise induced compartment syndrome of the pectoralis major/

deltoid in a professional tree climber. J Shoulder Elbow Surg. 2009;18(2):e17–20.
31. Shamberger RC. Congenital chest wall deformities. Curr Probl Surg. 1996;33(6):469–542.
32. Guller B, Hable K. Cardiac findings in pectus excavatum in children: review and differential diagnosis. Chest. 1974;66(2):165–71.
33. Seyfer AE, Icochea R, Graeber GM. Poland's anomaly: natural history and long term results of chest wall reconstruction in 33 patients. Ann Surg. 1988;208(6):776–82.
34. Fokin A, Robicsek F. Poland's syndrome revisited. Ann Thorac Surg. 2002;74(6):2218–25.

6 Buttocks Augmentation

Introduction

The popular media has put a premium on particular physical attributes that are attractive, and none of these have been more prominent in the last two decades than the buttocks. Stars such as Shakira, Jennifer Lopez, and Kim Kardashian have been revered for their round, plump bottoms (Figs. 6.1 and 6.2). Cultures such as those in South America, which openly display the human form, have increasingly sought ways to contour the gluteal region as it is considered a very important secondary sexual characteristic. To that end, many patients present to aesthetic practices for augmentation of the buttocks, in the hope of making them look shapelier. In 2006, according to the American Society for Aesthetic Plastic Surgery, 2,556 gluteal augmentations were performed in the United States [1]. When considering the patients that are undergoing buttock augmentations, the vast majority of patients are in the 20–39-year age group [2, 3]. Whether fat grafting to the buttocks or implant placement is the right choice for the patient is at the discretion of the surgeon based on physical findings at the time of consultation. Herein, we will discuss the evaluation of the gluteal region, discuss the gluteal augmentation procedure, and recommend the patients that are best suited for implant surgery versus other options.

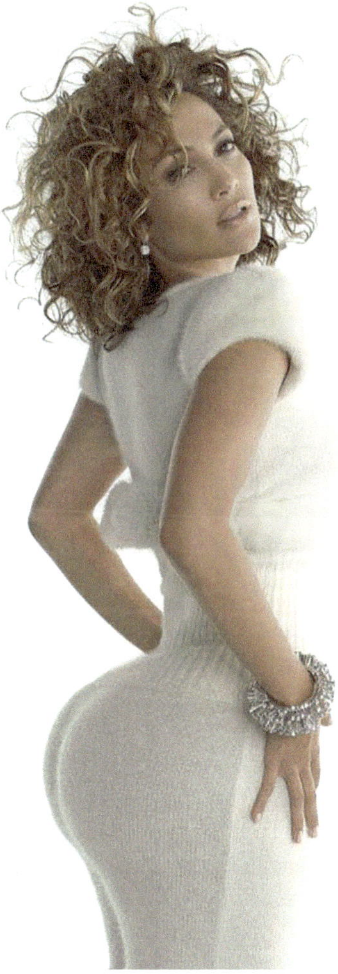

Fig. 6.1 Jennifer Lopez

N.V. Chugay et al., *Body Sculpting with Silicone Implants*,
DOI 10.1007/978-3-319-04957-1_6,

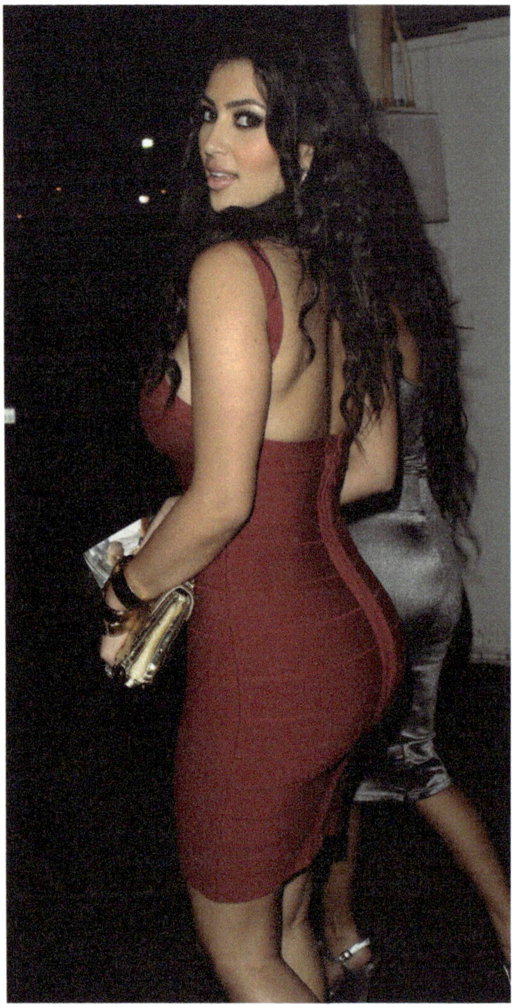

Fig. 6.2 Kim Kardashian

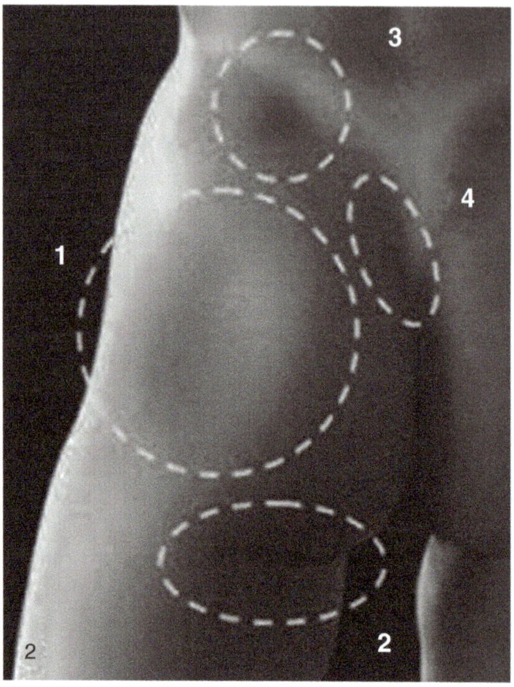

Fig. 6.3 Cuenca-Guerra Buttock Landmarks. Take note of the following: *1* A mild lateral depression that corresponds to the greater trochanter of the femur. *2* Short infragluteal folds that do not extend beyond the medial two-thirds of the posterior thigh. *3* A well-defined dimple on each side of the medial sacral crest that correspond to the posterior-superior iliac spines (PSIS). *4* A V-shaped crease (or sacral triangle) that arises from the proximal end of the gluteal crease

Gluteal Aesthetics and Classification Systems

Although the standards to define a beautiful buttock region may vary slightly from culture to culture, there is little debate about the allure of the hourglass female figure. Singh [4] proposed that there is one female body shape (full buttocks and a narrow waist) that men universally find attractive; and this is defined by an ideal female waist to hip ratio (WHR) of 0.7. The waist to hip ratio is defined as the ratio of the circumference of the waist at its narrowest point to the circumference of the thighs at the level of maximal lateral projection (level of the trochanteric depression). (See Chap. 7 for more details.) A successful gluteal augmentation procedure is therefore defined as one in which the surgeon successfully brings the woman as close to the ideal WHR of 0.7 as possible [5].

Since the advent of body contouring surgery, many different ways of evaluating the gluteal region have been proposed to help surgeons achieved optimal results in contouring of and around the buttocks. In 2004, Cuenca-Guerra et al. [6] first reported their analysis of more than 24,000 images of the gluteal area taken from various media sources. He defined four recognizable characteristics of an aesthetically pleasing gluteal region (Fig. 6.3):

1. Two well-defined dimples on each side of the medial sacral crest that correspond to the posterior-superior iliac spines (PSIS)
2. A V-shaped crease (or sacral triangle) that arises from the proximal end of the gluteal crease

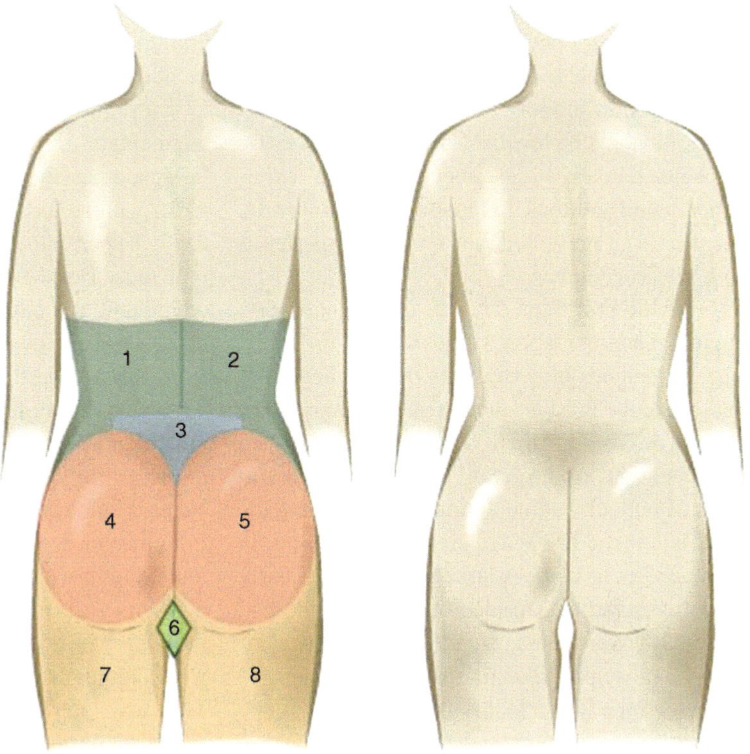

Fig. 6.4 The 8 gluteal aesthetic units of Centeno include *1*, *2* two symmetrical flank units, *3* one sacral triangle unit, *4*, *5* two symmetrical gluteal units, *7*, *8* two symmetrical thigh units, and *6* one "infragluteal diamond" unit

3. Short infragluteal folds that do not extend beyond the medial two-thirds of the posterior thigh
4. Two mild lateral depressions that correspond to the greater trochanter of the femur

Centeno in 2006 [7] described one of the other primary methods for evaluation of the buttocks to help plan body contouring procedures. From the posterior-anterior view of the patient, he defined eight gluteal aesthetic units that help form an aesthetic bottom. By his estimation, the gluteal region consists of two symmetrical "flank" units, a "sacral triangle" unit, two symmetrical gluteal units, two symmetrical thigh units, and one "infragluteal diamond" unit (Fig. 6.4). Accentuation of these units with liposculpture, buttock implants, or hip implants would aid in producing a more aesthetically pleasing contour to the buttock region. When considering procedures that involve incisions, Centeno recommended careful incision placement to respect the junctions of these aesthetic units.

Mendietta in 2006 [8] described a gluteal evaluation system where he analyzed the underlying bony framework of the buttocks, the skin, and the subcutaneous fat distribution, in addition to the musculature of the region. First, he recommended an evaluation of the pelvic frame. Next, the gluteus muscle is evaluated in its height and width. He divided the buttock into four quadrants: upper inner, lower inner, upper outer, and lower outer. Determination of volume addition should be based on analysis of these four quadrants of the buttock. Any additional procedures that need to be performed (e.g., buttock lift or liposculpture) can then be determined by the analysis of these defined criteria.

History of the Procedure

Many surgeons on many continents have added to the knowledge base and growing amount of literature on gluteal augmentation procedures. Gluteal augmentation surgery began in 1965 when Bartels first used a mammary prosthesis (Cronin prosthesis) in the gluteal region to produce a more round and supple bottom side [9]. Subsequently, Cocke in 1973 [10], Douglas in

1975 [11], and Buchuk in 1980 [12] described their early experiences with aesthetic gluteal augmentation. Robles in 1984 [13] reported on his placement of a submuscular gluteal implant with an incision in the medial sacral line. In 1991, Gonzalez Ulloa [14] described his 10-year experience with buttock augmentation. Recently, Vergara [15] presented his 15-year experience with the procedure.

Over the past three decades of advancements in gluteal augmentation, surgeons have proposed various methods of performing the augmentation to achieve the most aesthetic result with minimal complications. Gonzalez Ulloa [16] is regarded by most as one of the great pioneers and grandfathers of buttock augmentation, having begun his work late in the 1970s and presenting his work in Mexico City in 1977. A large portion of his early procedures were performed on patients who had suffered severe damage and/or deformation of the gluteal region due to silicone, collagen, or guaiacol injections. In his early reports of the procedure, he recommended placement of the implant above the gluteus maximus muscle with an incision in the subgluteal sulcus. This subcutaneous plane has largely been abandoned by many surgeons as it can produce an unnatural look and has a large risk of implant migration. Robles in 1984 [13] reported on placement of implants in the submuscular plane with an incision along the medial sacral line. In 1995, the primary author evaluated Robles' work and felt that the potential for injury to the sciatic nerve was too great and began working to place gluteal implants in a more superficial submuscular space, which would later be termed the "intermuscular" space. His initial work on 22 gluteal augmentations performed in the intermuscular space was published in early 1997 as a "modification of buttock augmentation" [17]. The intermuscular space was defined as the potential space that was visualized between the gluteus maximus above and the medius and minimus below during surgical dissection. An implant could easily be placed into this position, thereby minimizing trauma to the gluteus maximus muscle and avoiding injury to deeper muscles and neurovascular structures. Vergara and Marcos [15] later described their use of the "intramuscular" plane for gluteal implant placement based on cadaver dissections which showed an intramuscular anatomic space available for augmentation, larger in size than the submuscular space previously noted by Robles [13]. This paper validated the placement of a silicone prosthesis between the fasciculi of the gluteus maximus muscle and avoided the deeper plane which would put the patient at greater risk of sciatic nerve injury. However, this description differed from that of the primary author in that Vergara attempted placement of the implant within the gluteus maximus muscle rather than placing the implant fully under the maximus muscle. Vergara, along with other authors that use the intramuscular plane, emphasizes the need for maintaining a superior muscle flap covering the implant that is at least 3 cm thick [17–19]. Later in 1997 Peren et al. [20] described their work with augmentations done in the subfascial plane. This was then revisited in 2004 by de la Pena [21]. The limitation of the subfascial plane is that large volume implants with significant projection increase cannot be used due to the tightness of the pocket. Additionally, because of its more superficial position, there is a greater chance of implant palpability. Most recently, Gonzalez [22] introduced the XYZ method for gluteal augmentation. Gonzalez uses the same intramuscular plane as described by Vergara but introduces a means of orienting the gluteal implants to maximize symmetry and aesthetic results. He defines a point X as representing the center of the gluteus maximus muscular mass at the site of access to the submuscular plane. He performs dissection cephalically up to a point Y which is just past the lower iliac spine. Then along a vector named line G, he dissects caudally down to a point Z which is at the level of the trochanter and still beneath the gluteus muscle. Gonzalez asserts that his technique is important in gluteal augmentation as natural and reliable pelvic landmarks are used for dissection as preoperative cutaneous markings often provided a distorted view of the anatomy when the patient is in the prone position for surgery, helping to produce more reliably aesthetic outcomes [22].

In considering incision placement for the procedure, early surgeons worked through bilateral infragluteal sulcus incisions [9–12, 14]. This was then followed by bilateral coccygeal incisions as used by Gonzalez Ulloa [9]. Later surgeons felt that less incisions could lead to less postoperative morbidity. For this reason, incision placement turned to use of a single 5–7 cm incision hidden in the intergluteal cleft [13–15, 17, 18]. Mendietta in 2005 [23] presented his approach to gluteal augmentation, suggesting two paramedian incisions in order to decrease the risk of wound dehiscence. By placing two incisions, there was less trauma to the incision and tension was minimized. Most recently, in 2007, Badin and Vieira [24] discussed their experience with a small intergluteal crease incision with pocket dissection using endoscopic technology aimed at minimizing the risks of sciatic nerve injury and maximizing aesthetic gain.

Implants Used (Table 6.1)

In 2006, De la Pena [25] described the history of gluteal augmentation and briefly discusses the differences in implants used for buttock augmentation between the United States and countries outside it. He notes that there are two primary types of buttock implants available commercially: semisolid elastomer implants and cohesive gel implants. In 2012, Bortoluzzi Daniel [19] sought to evaluate the durability of gluteal prostheses and noted that cohesive gel implants, as used in his native Brazil, had a high failure rate and risk of rupture when compared to the semisolid elastomer-type implants used by surgeons in the United States. Cohesive gel implants have a shortened useful lifespan due to the fact that creases can sometimes fold in the implant itself combined with the significant force of compression produced by sitting on the implants. Studies performed on breast augmentation patients suggest that cohesive gel implants may need replacement in 20–40 % of patients at 8–10 years. Based on the research of Bortoluzzi Daniel, this half lift is considerably shorter for gluteal implants because of the constant tension that they are subjected to. Although the search for the ideal implant continues, the semisolid elastomer implant and cohesive gel implant have underscored the major developments in buttock augmentation surgery.

Table 6.1 Types of buttock implants used

Implant type	Advantages	Disadvantages
Semisolid elastomer	Does not rupture	Firmer buttocks
Cohesive gel	Soft and natural feel	Possibility of rupture
	Less palpable	Not available in the United States

The large majority of the US companies are making implants that are semisolid and rigid. Implantation of these types of implants does have the advantage of not rupturing; however, it can lead to a more firm buttock region. This is in contrast to the implants frequently used in Latin American countries that are often made of a cohesive gel within a thick and resilient silicone shell (Fig. 6.5). These implants are softer and have a more natural feel according to physicians that use them. The major downside of these implants, however, is the risk of rupture. In our own practice, it is our feeling that implants made by AART (Aesthetic and Reconstructive Technologies, Inc., Reno, NV) not only provide rigidity needed to provide a solid augmentation but are pliable enough to make them natural in their look and feel when implanted.

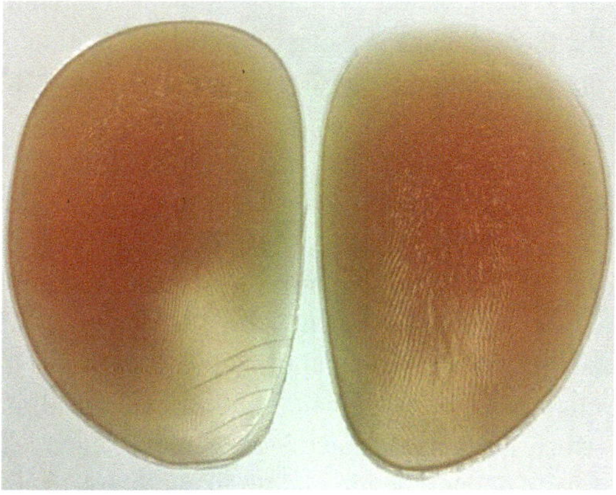

Fig. 6.5 Cohesive gel implants used for gluteal augmentation

Relevant Anatomy

In Centeno's [7] work, there are four superficial landmarks that should be identified and potentially accentuated in buttock augmentation/contouring. These four areas are the sacral dimples (overlying the PSIS), the sacral triangle (formed by the two PSIS and the coccyx inferiorly), the lateral depression correlating to the greater trochanters of the femur, and the short infragluteal fold. When performing buttock augmentation, one should be careful not to obliterate these landmarks and may even consider the adjunctive use of liposculpture to further enhance these landmarks in addition to performing the buttock augmentation.

The buttock region has investing fascia that helps prevent gluteal ptosis and provide structural support to the gluteal area. The superficial fascia as described by Lockwood [6] fuses with the deep gluteal fascia at the level of the infragluteal fold to create a tight adherence which needs to be respected in augmentation and liposculpture procedures [26]. A violation of this tight adherence can lead to significant gluteal ptosis which is difficult to reconstruct if lost. In addition to helping to create the infragluteal fold, the superficial fascial system along with the deep investing fascia of the gluteus muscle is key to providing a sound closure at the end of the procedure and should be employed in a layered closure of the midline buttock incision.

The muscles that comprise the buttock region are several, but the primary volume is formed by the three gluteus muscles (Fig. 6.6). The gluteus maximus muscle originates on the fascia of the gluteus medius muscle, the external ilium, the fascia of the erector spinae, the dorsum of the lower sacrum, the lateral coccyx, and the sacrotuberous ligament [27]. It inserts on the iliotibial tract and proximal femur. The muscle is a powerful extensor of the flexed femur and provides lateral stabilization of the hip. The gluteus medius originates on the external ilium and inserts on the lateral greater trochanters. It acts to abduct the hip and thigh and helps to stabilize the pelvis during standing and walking. During dissection, it can be differentiated from the gluteus maximus because of its vertically oriented fibers. The gluteus minimus originates on the external surface of the ilium and inserts on the anterior-lateral greater trochanter. This muscle abducts the femur and also serves as a pelvic stabilizer.

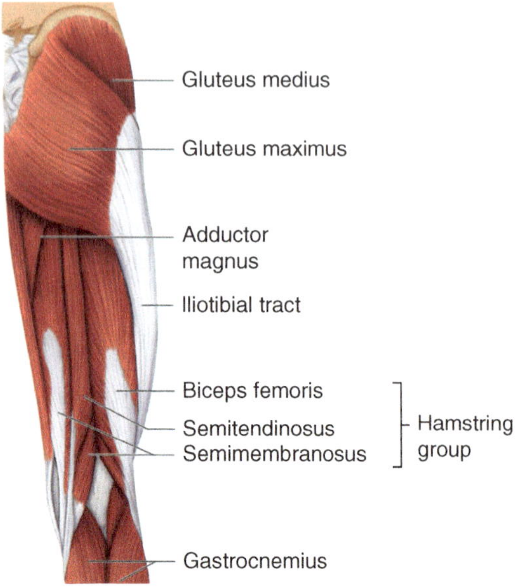

Fig. 6.6 Gluteal muscles (maximus, medius) depicted and their relationship to key muscular structures in the lateral hip/thigh and lower extremity. Gluteus minimus is not depicted

Blood supply in the gluteal region is rich and reliable. The musculocutaneous structures in the gluteal region are largely supplied by the perforating branches of the superior and inferior gluteal arteries, which are terminal branches of the internal iliac artery [28]. Accessory blood supply comes from the deep circumflex iliac, lumbar, lateral sacral, obturator, and internal pudendal arteries. The superior and inferior gluteal veins provide venous drainage of the region. When considering dissection of the gluteus muscle, one must be careful to avoid sharp dissection very close to the sacrum and sacrotuberous ligament as injury to the gluteal arteries can occur [22].

There is a rich complex of nerves that innervate the muscles of the buttock region and provide sensation to the overlying skin. They largely originate from the lumbosacral plexus. The gluteus maximus is innervated by the inferior gluteal nerve. This nerve comes from the pelvis to the gluteal area, crossing the great sciatic foramen posteriorly and in a way medial to the sciatic nerve. It divides into three collateral branches: the gluteus (motor nerve of the gluteus maximus), the perineal, and the femoral (sensory nerve). The branches of the inferior gluteal nerve are like a crow's foot when dividing into its branches. These branches then course between the gluteus muscle and its anterior fascia, with the largest segments (fillets) of this nerve being close to the sacrum and sacrotuberous ligament. It is for this reason that undermining inside the gluteus muscle must never be performed to close to the sacrum, the sacrotuberous ligament, or the sciatic tuberosity [22].

The gluteus medius and minimus are innervated by the superior gluteal nerve. Sensation to the gluteal region and lateral trunk comes from several sources: the dorsal rami of the sacral nerve roots 3 and 4, the cutaneous branches of the iliohypogastric nerve, and the superior cluneal nerves that originate from the L1, L2, and L3 roots. The iliohypogastric and ilioinguinal nerves, branches of the L1 nerve root, supply the skin overlying the lateral gluteal region and can be injured with aggressive lipocontouring of the lateral buttock region. Lastly, the sciatic nerve is the largest nerve of the body and originates from the nerve roots of L4 through S3 (Fig. 6.7). It exits the gluteal region through the greater sciatic foramen below the piriformis muscle and above the superior gemellus muscle to enter the posterior compartment of the thigh. Compression or injury of the sciatic nerve may cause loss of function of the posterior thigh compartment muscles and all muscles of the leg and foot and loss of sensation in the lateral leg and foot as well as the sole and dorsum of the foot [29].

Indications

Gluteal augmentation with implants is indicated in patients who suffer from insufficiency of the gluteal region. These patients are typically young and have good muscle and skin tone but lack volume or definition to the gluteal region. Gluteal implants are also indicated in patients who suffer from

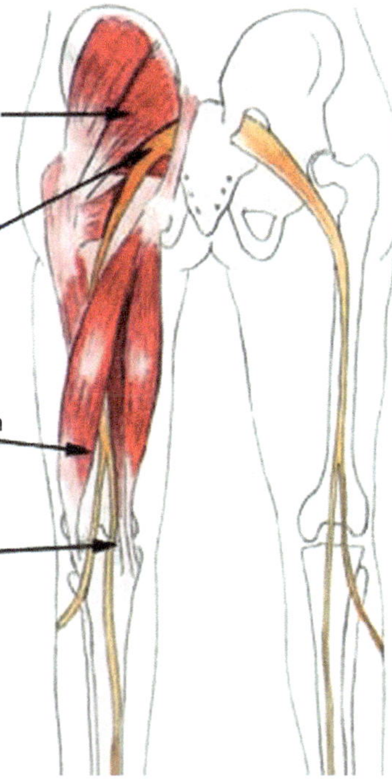

Fig. 6.7 Course of the sciatic nerve with its exit at the inferior pole of the gluteus muscle. Because of its course, this nerve is at risk for injury during submuscular placement of a gluteal prosthesis either by traction injury or by direct compression by the implant

ptosis of the gluteal region and wish to have a perkier appearance to the buttocks. Another set of patients that benefit from gluteal augmentation with implants are those who have a congenital gluteal deformity or acquired asymmetry (due to trauma, postoperatively, or post-oncologic resection).

Contraindications/Limitations

Relative contraindications to the procedure are few and typically deal with tissue irregularities in the area to be augmented. One such limitation is a depressed scar in the buttock area which may require adjunctive procedures to cause a release of the scar. Patients who have suffered from radiation to the area have a relative contraindication to surgery as their tissues may be indurated and healing may not be optimal postoperatively. Another patient who may have a relative or absolute contraindication to implant surgery is the patient who presents with deficiency of the lateral and inferior portions of the buttocks. When performing buttock augmentation with implants, the inferior pole remains largely unchanged as too caudal a dissection can put the sciatic nerve at risk of injury. For that reason patients who have a significant deficiency at the lower pole should be counseled to consider fat grafting and implant augmentation. Similarly, deficits in the lateral aspect of the butt are largely unchanged with implant augmentation. Although there will be a slight improvement in the lateral curvature of the buttocks, significant deficits may best be treated with fat grafting or possibly a hip implant. Patients who suffer from autoimmune diseases may be at increased risk postoperatively and should be counseled appropriately prior to pursuing any implant surgery. A patient who presents with unrealistic expectations or suffers from major psychological illness is not an appropriate candidate for buttock augmentation surgery.

Consultation/Implant Selection

A thorough history and physical are paramount to preventing complications at the time of buttock augmentation. Questions are posed regarding the patient's reasonable attempts to build the muscle with conventional means. During the consultation, patient's expectations are managed and assessment of the patient's mental state is undertaken. It is made clear to the patient the expected augmentation that can be achieved, and limitations of the procedure are also explained.

After completion of the history portion of the consultation, an evaluation of the patient's buttocks is made. Any asymmetries or defects are pointed out to the patient. The patient's muscles are then evaluated. The skin and fat content are similarly assessed at this time as a patient with minimal adipose and thin skin is more at risk for implant palpability. Measurements of the patient's buttocks in the transverse axis are then taken in the midportion of the gluteal region beginning 1 cm lateral to the intergluteal crease and ending at the lateral palpable edge of the buttock muscle. This measurement allows the physician to choose an implant that will adequately fill out the gluteal region and is analogous to determining the base width in breast augmentation. Measurement of the vertical height of the buttock is taken from its most cranial portion to its most caudal portion 2 cm short of the infragluteal crease.

Available Implants (Tables 6.1, 6.2, 6.3, and 6.4)

The authors' preference is the style 3, round implant.

Table 6.2 Style 1 buttock implants (Aesthetic and Reconstructive Technologies, Inc., Reno, NV)

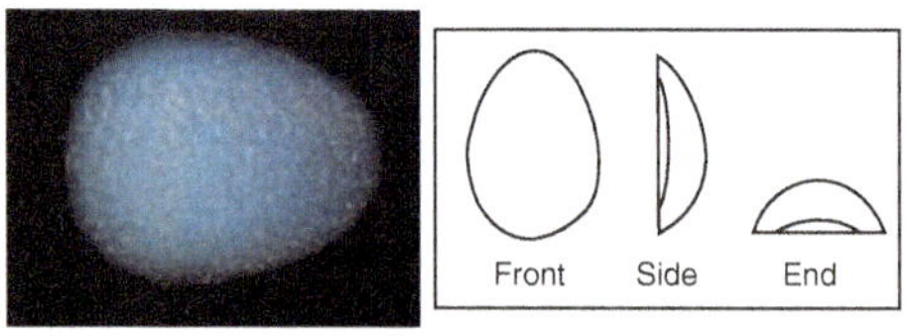

Size	Catalog #	Width	Length	Projection	Volume (cc)
1	501–101	10.4	15.0	2.5	207
4	501–102	11.0	15.6	3.1	250
3	501–103	13.5	18.0	4.6	545
4	501–104	11.1	16.2	3.2	303
5	501–105	11.5	16.6	3.6	328
6	501–106	12.9	18.0	4.2	435

Table 6.3 Style 2 buttock implants (Aesthetic and Reconstructive Technologies, Inc., Reno, NV)

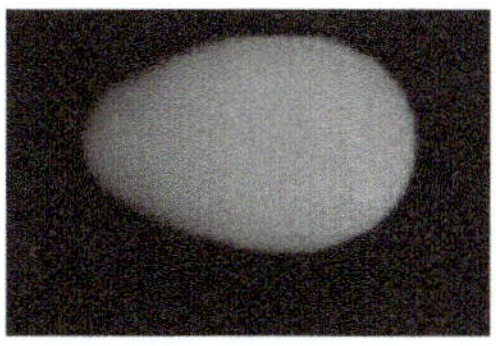

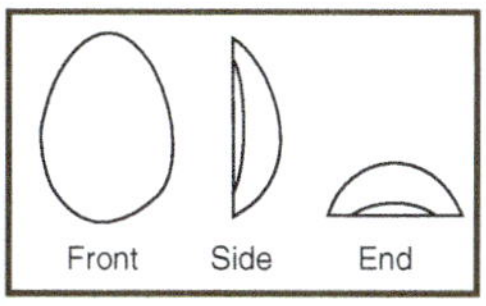

Size	Catalog #	Width	Length	Projection	Volume (cc)
1	501–201	12.4	14.5	2.5	194
2	501–202	12.7	15.4	2.9	234
3	501–203	12.8	16.5	3.3	292
4	501–204	13.4	18.0	3.8	375
5	501–205	14.6	19.3	4.8	575
6	501–206	12.5	16.4	4.6	430

Table 6.4 Style 3 buttock implants (Aesthetic and Reconstructive Technologies, Inc., Reno, NV)

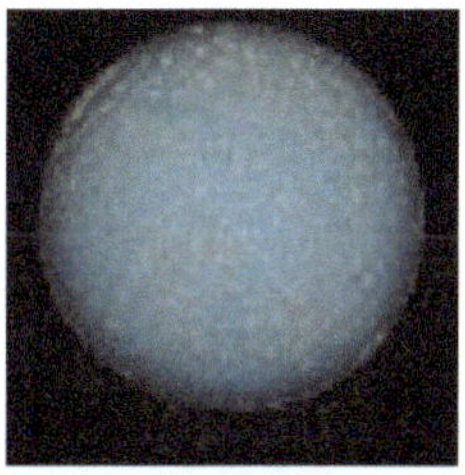

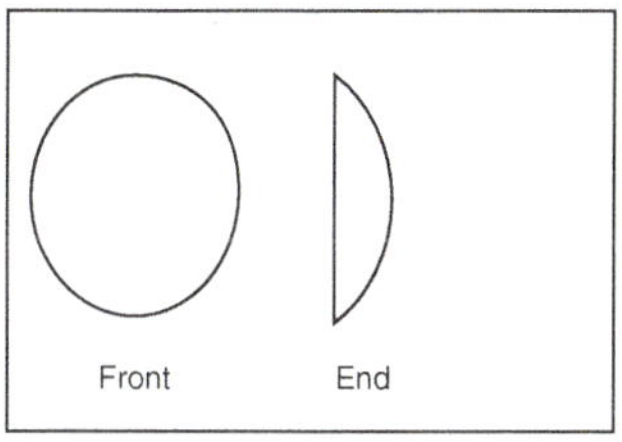

Size	Catalog #	Diameter	Projection	Volume (cc)
0	501–300	10.5	2.5	117
1	501–301	12.5	2.8	189
2	501–302	13.4	3.6	276
3	501–303	14.5	3.8	379
4	501–304	13.4	4.9	434
5	501–305	13.5	3.7	301
6	501–306	15.0	5.5	713
6	501–307	12.5	4.0	296
8	501–308	12.0	3.5	215
9	501–309	15.0	4.5	485
10	501–310	15.0	5.0	550

Preoperative Planning and Marking

On the day of the surgery, the patient is met in the preoperative holding area. It is here that the patient's consent is verified and again risks, benefits, and alternatives are reviewed with the patient. With the patient in the erect position, the proposed site of incision is marked, measuring approximately 5–7 cm. The site of incision should be in the intergluteal cleft, starting at the apex of the cleft and proceeding caudally. This line of incision must be marked in the upright position preoperatively as the intergluteal sulcus loses its definition when the patient is in the prone position during surgery. The area around the anus should be respected, and incisions should not exceed a 5 cm boundary around the anus to avoid injury to the sphincter complex. Once the site of the incision is marked, the site of the proposed implant is marked taking into account the patient's anatomy and existing deficit along with the desires of the patient (Fig. 6.8).

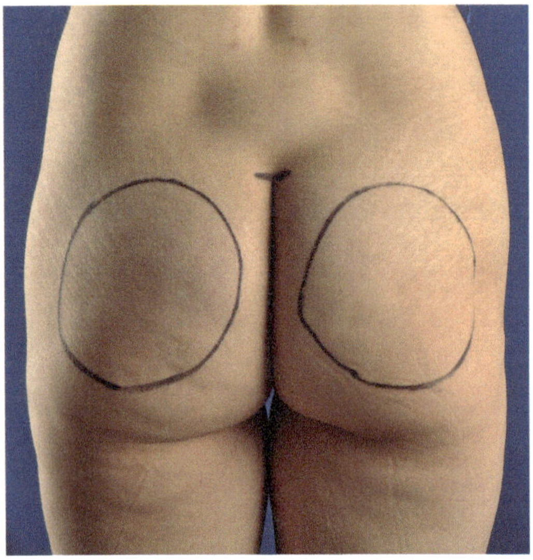

Fig. 6.8 Preoperative markings. Note the superior most *horizontal marking* indicating the beginning of the natural intergluteal fold. Just below this line is the starting point for the intergluteal fold incision. The site of the proposed implants is marked preoperatively, taking care to ensure that they are evenly placed away from midline (ruler used to ensure symmetric placement). The outline of the implant helps to control dissection intraoperatively

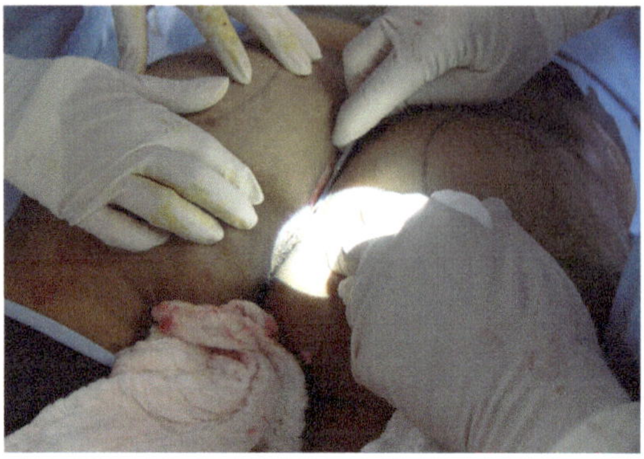

Fig. 6.9 Incision in the intergluteal fold

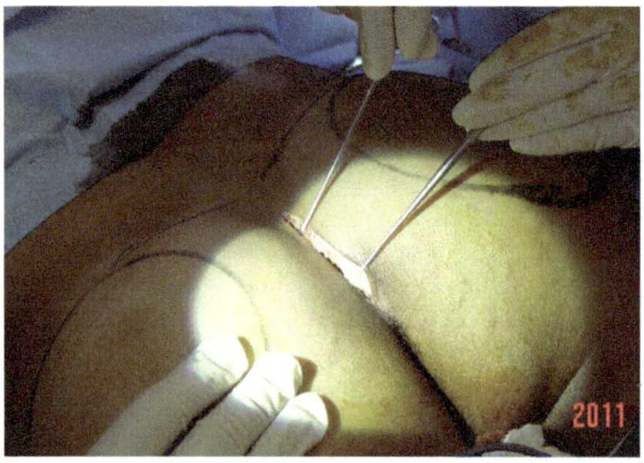

Fig. 6.10 Hooks placed in the skin to aid in dissection of the subcutaneous plane, taking care to preserve the presacral fascia which will be used at closure

The superior excursion of the buttock is marked with manual manipulation of the buttock in the cephalic direction if liposuction of the hips is to be done. The sacral triangle is marked for reference if liposuction of the sacrum/flanks is to be performed at the same time.

Operative Technique

The patient is brought to the operative suite. Anesthesia is administered. The patient is then placed in the prone position. The buttocks and perianal region are prepped and draped in sterile fashion. The previously marked incision site in the intergluteal cleft is incised with a #15 blade scalpel, taking care not to violate the 5-cm safe zone proximal to the anus (Fig. 6.9). Dissection is carried through the subcutaneous tissues using electrocautery, using hooks in the skin to provide adequate visualization (Figs. 6.10 and 6.11). The incision is carried down to the level of the presacral fascia, making sure to maintain the presacral

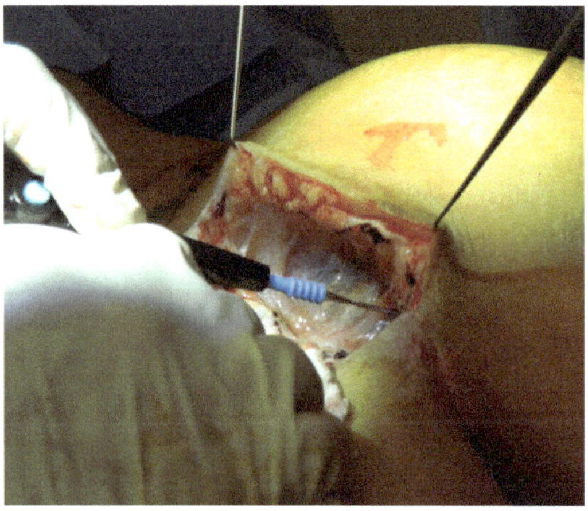

Fig. 6.11 Dissection through the subcutaneous tissue using electrocautery

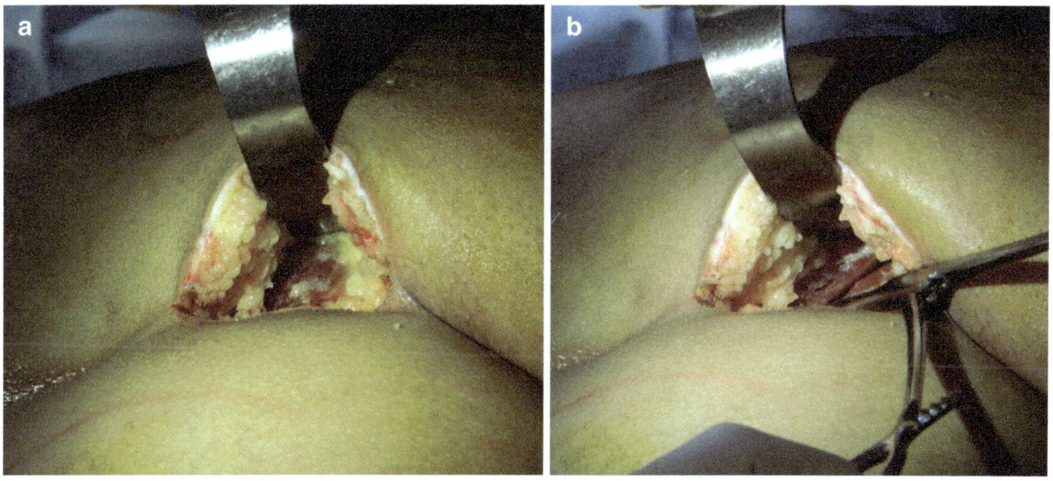

Fig. 6.12 (**a**) Subcutaneous tissue has been dissected away from underlying muscle, exposing the gluteus muscle. (**b**) Gluteus maximus muscle is split in its midportion in line with its fibers using a Kelly clamp

fascia intact as the closure will utilize this fascia as an anchor to recreate the intergluteal sulcus. Dissection is carried laterally to the gluteal fascia (Fig. 6.12). Dissection is carried laterally for approximately 3–4 cm to better expose the gluteal fascia. At a point found to be in the midsection of the gluteus maximus muscle, the gluteus is split in line with its fibers using a large Kelly clamp to achieve a plane below the gluteus maximus muscle (Fig. 6.12). The opening in the gluteus maximus muscle is then extended using electrocautery to create a 6–7 cm defect in the muscle. A spatula dissector and hockey stick dissector, along with finger dissection, are used to further develop this plane, in line with the proposed site of implant placement (Figs. 6.13 and 6.14). The pocket is created in such a way that the gluteus maximus adequately covers the position of the implant in the medial, lateral, and superficial levels. The gluteus medius and minimus then create the floor of the implant pocket (Fig. 6.15). When considering dissection of a buttock augmentation procedure, the medial extent of dissection should respect the sacral triangle. Care is also taken to minimize dissection in the lower third of the buttock which is the support zone of the buttock and supports the weight of the body when sitting. A key point for the novice surgeon at this stage is that one should err on the side of a tight pocket to minimize the risk of over-dissection and increased potential for implant migration that comes with too loose a pocket for the implant. The pocket is then packed with peroxide-soaked sponges, and attention is turned to the contralateral side for similar dissection (Fig. 6.16). Once all dissection has been completed, implant pockets are evaluated for hemostasis. Hemostasis is achieved as necessary with electrocautery. Next, the pocket is irrigated with an antibiotic solution containing Betadine, normal saline, 80 mg gentamicin, and 1 g of Ancef (if the patient is not penicillin allergic). The irrigant is then suctioned out. Ten milliliters of

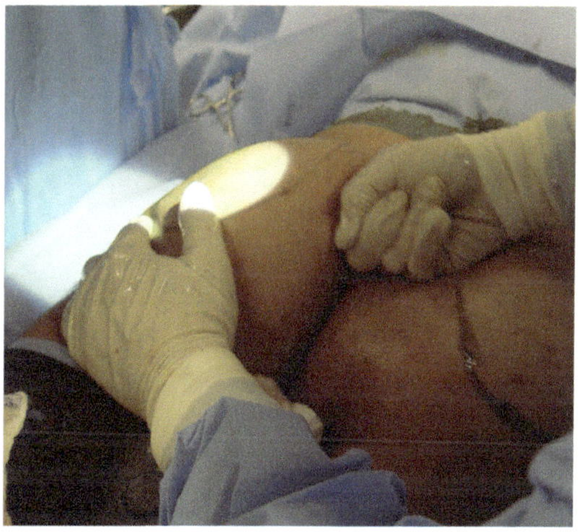

Fig. 6.13 Initial dissection of the intermuscular plane using blunt finger dissection

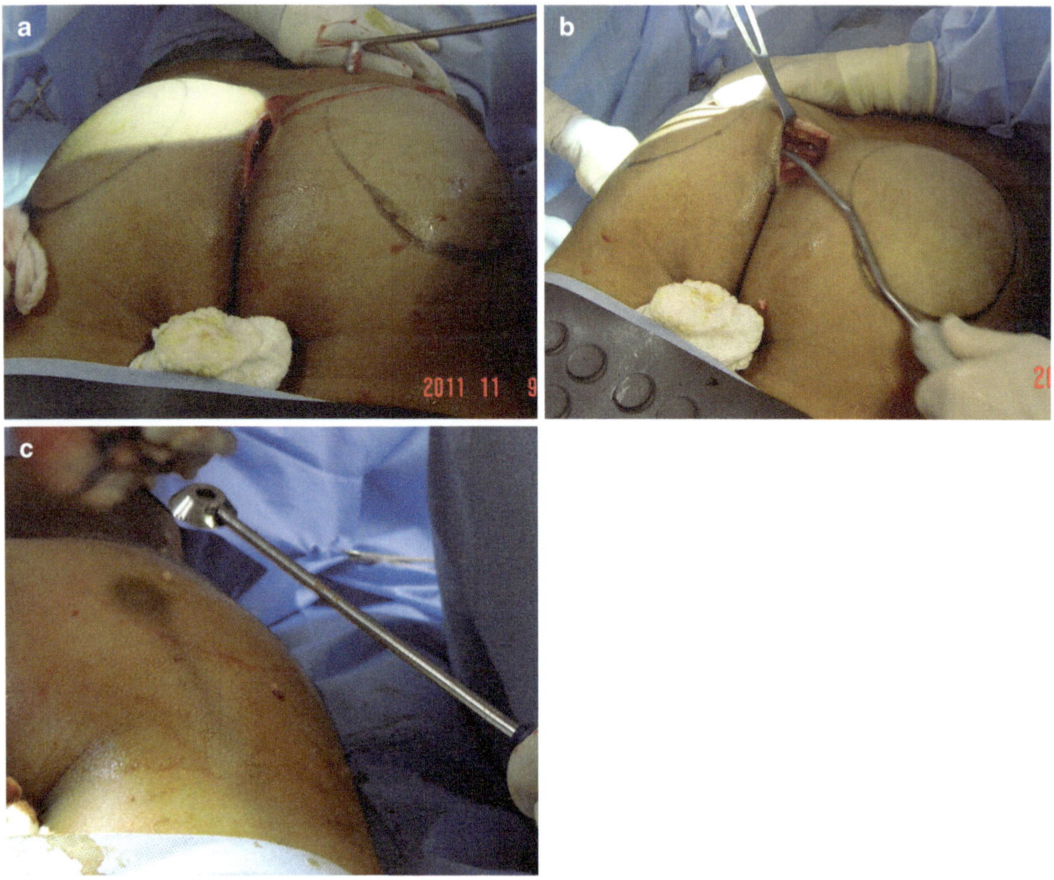

Fig. 6.14 (**a**) Dissection of the intermuscular plane using a hockey stick dissector. (**b**) Dissection of the pocket using a spatula dissector. (**c**) A serrated dissector may be used if there are resistant strands of gluteus muscle that need to be freed to accommodate the implant

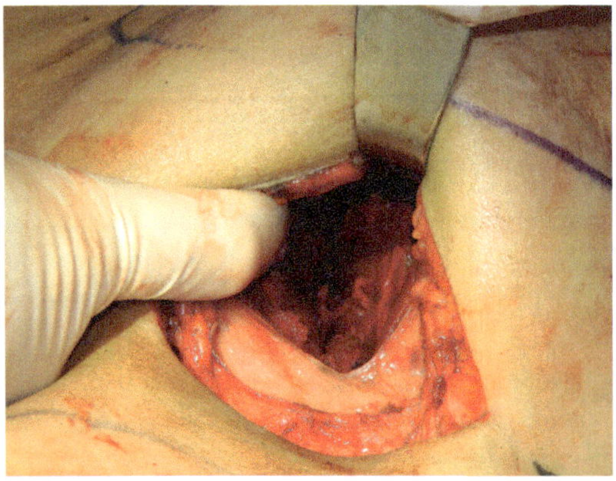

Fig. 6.15 Dissection of the intergluteal plane has been completed. The subcutaneous tissues and gluteus maximus are elevated demonstrating the underlying gluteus medius muscle with transversely directed fibers

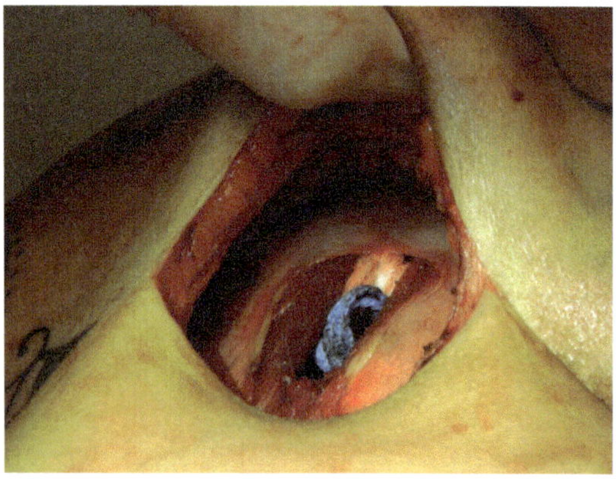

Fig. 6.16 Lap sponges in position in the intermuscular plane

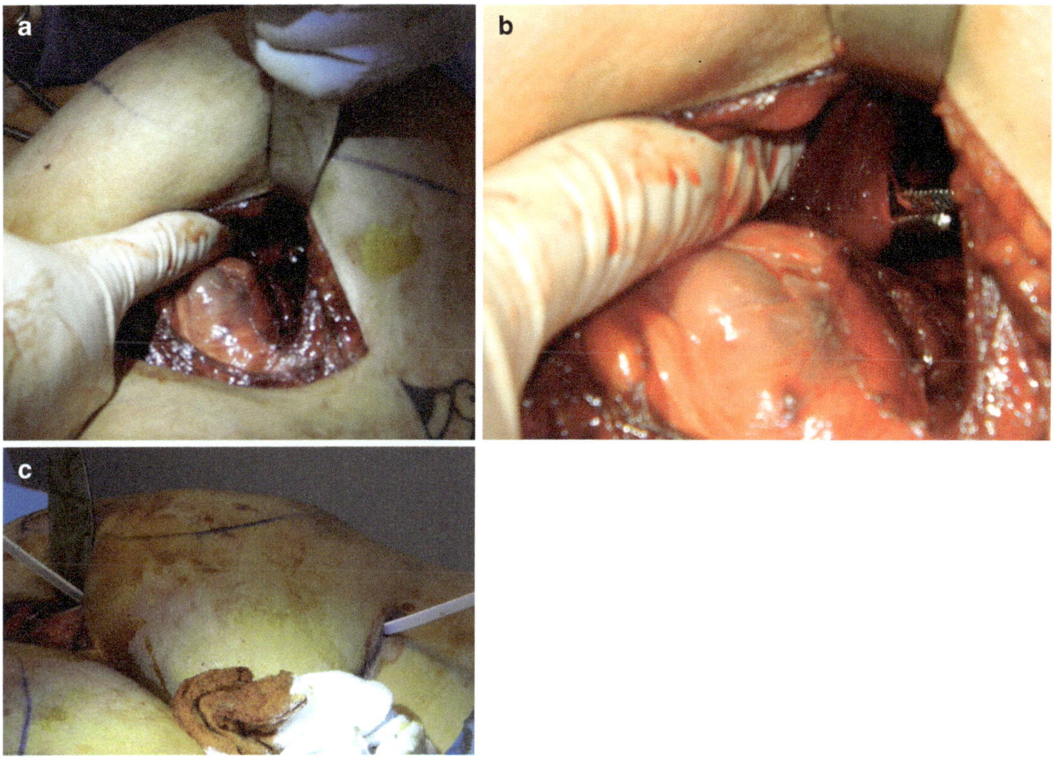

Fig. 6.17 (**a**) Drain placement via a stab incision in the infragluteal fold. (**b**) Close-up view of Kelly clamp being extended into the intermuscular pocket with the tip of the Kelly spread to accept the drain. (**c**) Drain in position with exit in the infragluteal fold

0.5 % Marcaine is instilled into the pocket to allow for postoperative pain control. Drains are placed via stab incisions in the infragluteal fold using a #15 blade scalpel. Jackson-Pratt drains are then introduced into the pocket and laid into the base of the pocket and secured with 3-0 Nylon suture (Fig. 6.17). The appropriately selected gluteal implant is folded in half (like a taco) and introduced through the incision in the gluteus maximus (Fig. 6.18). The implant is placed in the contralateral side in the similar fashion. Symmetry is then assessed. Once this is deemed to be satisfactory, closure is begun. A 0-Prolene suture (or permanent suture of surgeon's preference) is then used in interrupted fashion to close the gluteus muscle and fascia over the implant (Fig. 6.19). Once the implant has been fully covered, the intergluteal incision is closed in layers. First, 2-0 Vicryl suture is used to reapproximate the deep subcutaneous tissues and deep dermis to the presacral fascia to recreate the gluteal cleft. 3-0 Vicryl is used as necessary to fully approximate the dermis. 3-0 silk sutures in interrupted fashion are used to close the skin. The patient's wound is dressed with Neosporin and absorbent pads. The patient is then placed in a compression garment. Anesthesia is discontinued and the patient is taken to the postanesthesia care unit (PACU).

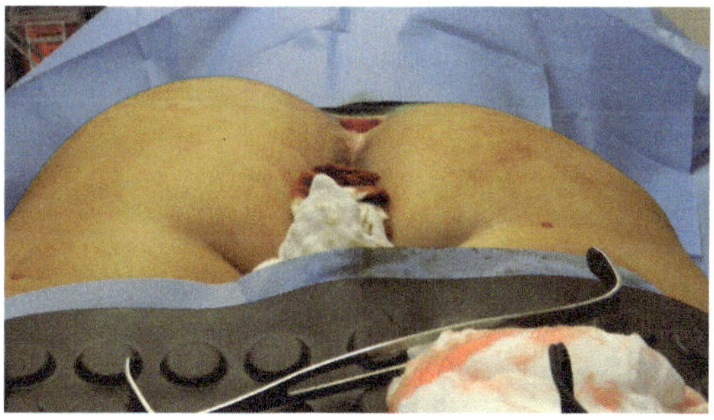

Fig. 6.18 *Left side* augmented with surgeon now returning to the *right side* for removal of packs and placement of right gluteal implant

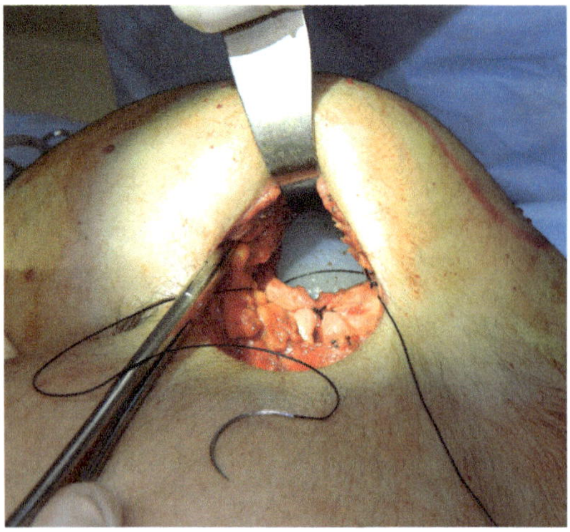

Fig. 6.19 Closure of gluteus maximus muscle over the underlying implant using permanent suture

Postoperative Care/Instructions

Postoperatively the patient may begin ambulating starting on the evening of the procedure. They may shower POD 2, making sure to keep the dressings clean. The buttock region is dried and antibiotic ointment is applied in a thin layer. Patients are then allowed to begin light activity at week 2 and full unrestricted activity at weeks 4–6. Patients are asked to wear an elastic compression garment for 4 weeks postoperatively to prevent dead space, thereby helping to reduce the risk of seroma formation. The legs are to be elevated as much as possible to allow for better lymphatic/venous drainage. Narcotic analgesics are prescribed along with muscle relaxants (diazepam 5 mg every 8 h as needed for spasm) to assist with postoperative pain. Patients are placed on broad-spectrum antibiotics for 7 days. The authors' preference is to use ciprofloxacin 500 mg BID for its broad coverage, both gram positive and gram negative. For 2 weeks postoperatively, the patient is asked to sleep on their abdomen or side and avoid direct pressure to the buttocks. After 2 weeks, the patient is cleared to sleep on their buttocks and sit on their new bottom side with the intention of slowly stretching the newly forming scar capsule. In the early postoperative period, patients may sit on their bottom side but favoring a "bird on a perch" position with the majority of bodily weight being focused on the posterior thigh region rather than directly on the midportion of the buttocks.

Table 6.5 Potential complications of buttock augmentation

Potential complications of buttock augmentation surgery
Infection
Seroma
Hematoma
Asymmetry
Implant visibility
Implant bottoming out/double-bubble deformity
Implant rupture
Hypertrophic scarring
Hyperpigmentation of the scar
Capsular contracture
Wound dehiscence
Nerve injury (permanent or temporary, motor or sensory)
Pulmonary embolism
Compartment syndrome

Complications

In performing buttock augmentation, there is a host of complications that can arise (Table 6.5).

Infection

Infection, either superficial or deep, is a possibility in hip/lateral thigh augmentation surgery. There is a reported infection rate of between 1.4 and 5 % in gluteal augmentation surgery, including both superficial and deep infections [15, 30, 31]. The most likely culprits would be *Staphylococcus aureus* and *Staphylococcus epidermidis*, relatively common skin flora. However, gram-negative infections are also possible secondary to the close proximity to the anal canal. Prior to making incision, standard practice should be the administration of 2 g of Ancef IV (or 300 mg IV clindamycin in a penicillin- or cephalosporin-allergic patient). During the procedure, irrigation of the pocket with a standard antibiotic solution containing normal saline, Betadine, Ancef, and gentamicin should be performed. During surgery, a Betadine-soaked gauze is secured over the anus to prevent contamination. Postoperatively, a 7–10-day regimen of oral antibiotics covering normal skin flora along with gram-negative organisms should be administered. The authors' standard practice is administration of ciprofloxacin 500 mg orally twice daily for 7 days postoperatively. If a deep infection occurs, the standard of practice is removal of the implant, closure, and possible reimplantation in 3–6 months. There are reports in other forms of implant surgery (breast surgery) that conservative management and implant salvage are possible. This should be left to the discretion of the surgeon and performed with careful counseling of the patient. There are reports of late postoperative gluteal infections after augmentation gluteoplasty, but these are quite rare and typically relate to some trauma to the area [32–34]. These delayed infections are typically managed with drainage of the abscess, implant removal, and antibiotics.

Seroma

Seromas are statistically the most common complication occurring in implant surgeries. They typically present as new onset pain, swelling, or asymmetry. The treatment of choice remains percutaneous aspiration. This complication is best prevented with patient compliance with compression garments for 1 month and proper implant placement at the time of surgery, thereby minimizing dead space. In larger studies, such as those by Vergara and Gonzalez Ulloa, the seroma rate for intramuscular augmentations is reported to be between 4 and 10 % [14, 15, 20, 30]. Other large volume studies such as those by Senderoff [30], evaluating 200 consecutive augmentation cases, report seroma rates as high as 28 %. Seromas are best prevented with drain use in the implant pocket. The authors' standard practice is to leave Jackson-Pratt drains in place until drainage is less than 30 mL/24 h period for 48 consecutive hours.

Occasionally, patients will present with recurrent seromas that are recalcitrant to drainage. If this is the case, a discussion must be had with the patient regarding possible implant removal. Some

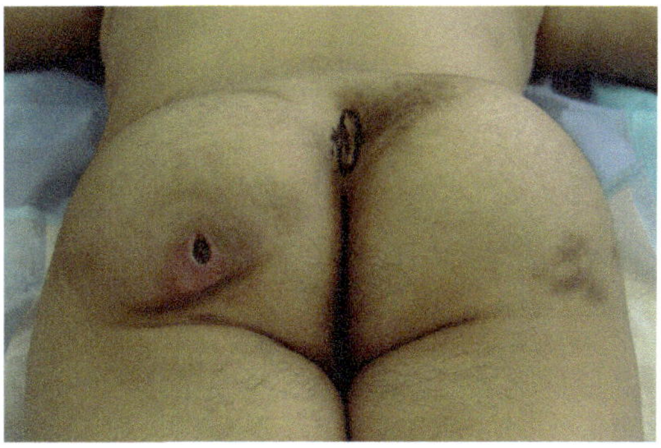

Fig. 6.20 A 26-year-old female underwent buttock augmentation with style 3, size 7 implants and suffered from persistent seromas for 1.5 months that were aspirated in sterile fashion using an 18-gauge needle. After 1.5–2 months, she was noted to have skin thinning in the lower pole of the buttock (dependent) and presented with an exposed implant on the *left side*. Note opening in caudal portion of left buttock with exposed implant

patients, however, wish to do everything they can to maintain their implant. In this case, the patient does run the risk of having tissue thinning of the buttock due to the constant pressure of the underlying fluid and implant. In one such case, a 26-year-old female underwent buttock augmentation with style 3, size 7 implants and suffered from persistent seromas for 1.5 months that were aspirated in sterile fashion using an 18-gauge needle. After 1.5–2 months, she was noted to have skin thinning in the lower pole of the buttock (dependent) and presented with an exposed implant on the left side (Fig. 6.20). She was taken to the operating room for implant removal, pocket washout, and closure of the defect in the skin. She is awaiting replacement of the left buttock implant to re-achieve symmetry of the buttocks.

Hematoma

Although a rare occurrence due to the relatively avascular plane of dissection for the hip augmentation procedure, a hematoma is always a possibility in surgical procedures. There is a reported incidence of 2 % in buttock augmentation surgery [30]. Small branches of the lateral circumflex femoral artery, a branch of the profunda femoris, can be injured during the dissection for hip augmentation.

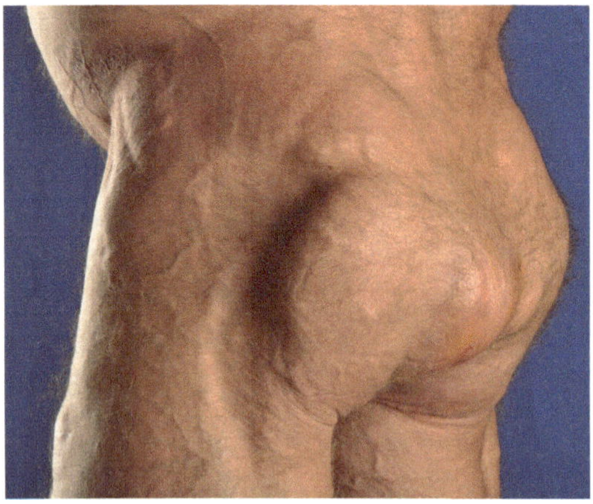

Fig. 6.21 A 46-year-old male, who was HIV positive, suffered a delayed hematoma years after his initial augmentation

In the event of a hematoma, rapid evacuation, pocket irrigation, and reimplantation are the mainstays of therapy. This complication is best prevented by meticulous hemostasis at the time of surgery and good compression of the buttock postoperatively to prevent potential space creation.

In the authors' series, there was one case of a delayed hematoma. A 46-year-old male, who was HIV positive, suffered a delayed hematoma years after his initial augmentation (Fig. 6.21). He had previously undergone buttock augmentation 11 years ago and then noted in the last several months prior to presentation that he had increased volume in the buttocks region that was soft to touch. He was subsequently taken to the operating room (OR) for drainage. Four hundred milliliters of serosanguinous matter was suctioned and likely was the result of a capsular tear (Fig. 6.22). No active bleeding was noted on evaluation of the region.

Asymmetry

This can occur as a product of preexisting variability in the patient's legs or variability in dissection of the pocket bilaterally. This is best minimized by good preoperative photography and noting any asymmetries preoperatively (Fig. 6.23). To avoid creation of asymmetry intraoperatively, it is important to maintain the same pattern of dissection and pocket creation bilaterally. Vergara

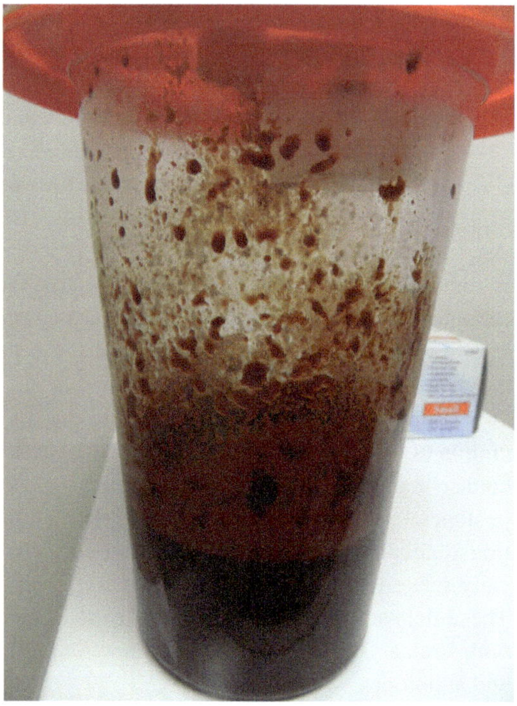

Fig. 6.22 Evacuated hematoma in patient with delayed hematoma

[15], in his 15-year experience with intramuscular placement of gluteal implants, reports an incidence of 2.6 % of asymmetry. Mendieta [31] reports an incidence of 5 %.

Implant Visibility/Palpability

Due to the intermuscular placement of the implant, in our practice, this is indeed a rare complication. For surgeons that perform the augmentation in the subfascial plane, there is a greater risk of implant palpability just by virtue of less tissue covering the implant [20, 21, 25]. Mendieta [31] in the first large volume US study on buttock augmentation with implants noted a rate of implant exposure of 2.7 % (2/73). However, those patients that have very thin and atrophic buttocks to begin with may suffer from implant palpability and visibility. Patients should be counseled on this fact preoperatively if there is a feeling that the patient could be at risk. Several authors who espouse the intramuscular approach to gluteal augmentation do warn

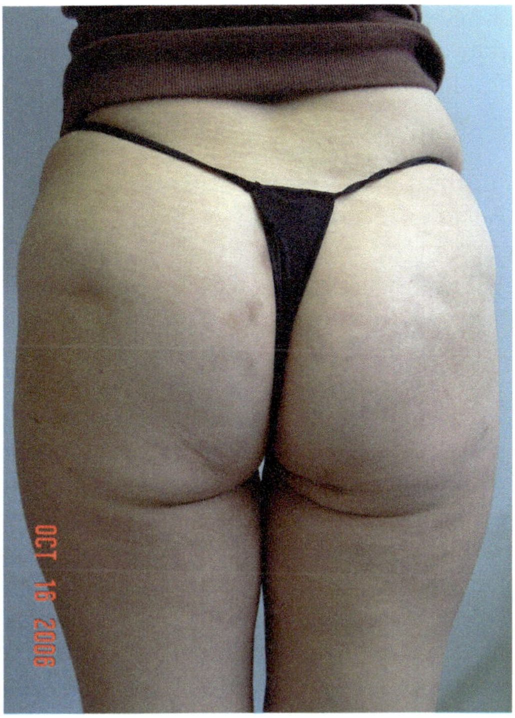

Fig. 6.23 Patient who presented for buttock augmentation and had preexisting asymmetry of the buttocks. There is a wider buttock on the *left side* with much more shapely buttock on the *right side*. The patient has a small indentation of the left buttock. The creases inferiorly are also asymmetric with two creases noted in the right gluteal area when compared to the single crease on the left. Cellulite is also evident in the buttocks. All of these existing irregularities should be pointed out to a patient prior to augmentation as there will still be asymmetry postoperatively

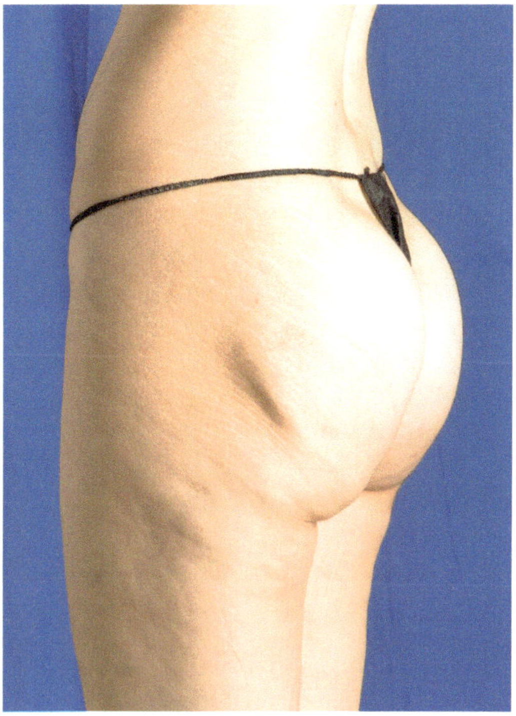

Fig. 6.24 Lateral exposed implant in a patient that was thin and had dissection in the superficial plane laterally causing exposure of the implant. This was corrected at subsequent surgery with placement of the implant below the existing capsule to better hide the implant edge

about the risk of becoming too superficial in the lateral dissection of the implant pocket, which could leave the implant exposed, due to the tapering of the gluteus maximus muscle in the lateral buttock region. For that reason, care must be taken in the dissection of the lateral aspect of the pocket, making sure to drive the dissector into a deeper plane to avoid leaving the implant covered only by subcutaneous tissues in the lateral aspect [15, 22, 23]. It is for this reason that Gonzalez [22] strongly recommends the XYZ approach to intragluteal gluteoplasty, as reliable anatomic points of reference may be used to guide pocket dissection. In the authors' practice, patients did at times present with implants that were palpable in the lateral aspect due to overly superficial dissection in the lateral aspect, leaving the implant not fully covered by muscle laterally (Fig. 6.24). This can be corrected with a reoperation no sooner than 3 months after the initial surgery. At the time of the second surgery, the surgeon will find a capsule formed and will then place the implant below the formed capsule, camouflaging any lateral implant palpability. A partial anterior capsulectomy should also be considered at this time to minimize the risk of a seroma formation postoperatively in the previously created pocket which will now be devoid of implant. Also, patients have presented to the practice with flipped implants (Fig. 6.25). This has been seen in patients that are thin to begin with and have minimal surrounding tissue around the implant and experience a flipping of their implant with movement. An in-office procedure or manual manipulation at home will typically correct this problem. Should this continue to repeat itself, the surgeon may consider a submuscular placement of the implant, but this

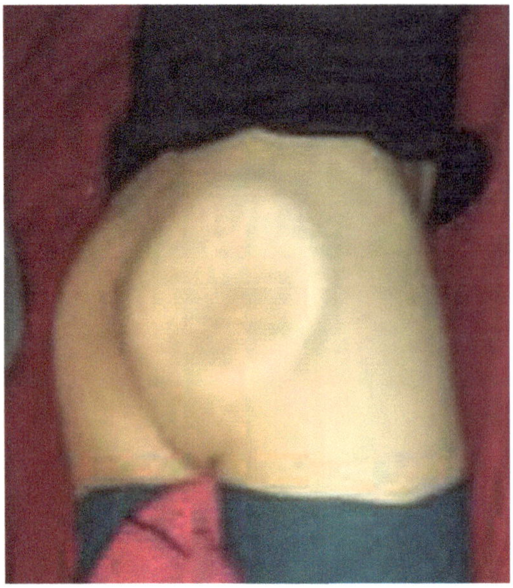

Fig. 6.25 Flipped right implant in a patient who was 120 lb at the time of her buttock augmentation and then lost 20 lb secondary to illness, creating very thin and loose tissues. She was able to easily manipulate the implant into position. She is slated for surgery to place the implant in a deeper submuscular position

increased risk of neurovascular injury must be fully discussed with the patient prior to proceeding down this route.

Implant Bottoming Out/Double-Bubble Deformity

With implants placed in the subcutaneous plane, there is a risk of implant bottoming out. This occurs as there is insufficient support around the implant to maintain its position. The skin and subcutaneous tissues are left to fight gravity and are unable to sustain the implant (Fig. 6.26). In the worst case scenario, the implant can move so far inferiorly as to create a double-bubble deformity, where the edge of the implant is noted as well as the natural crease of the buttock (Fig. 6.27). These complications are best corrected with implant placement in a deeper, intermuscular, intramuscular, or submuscular position.

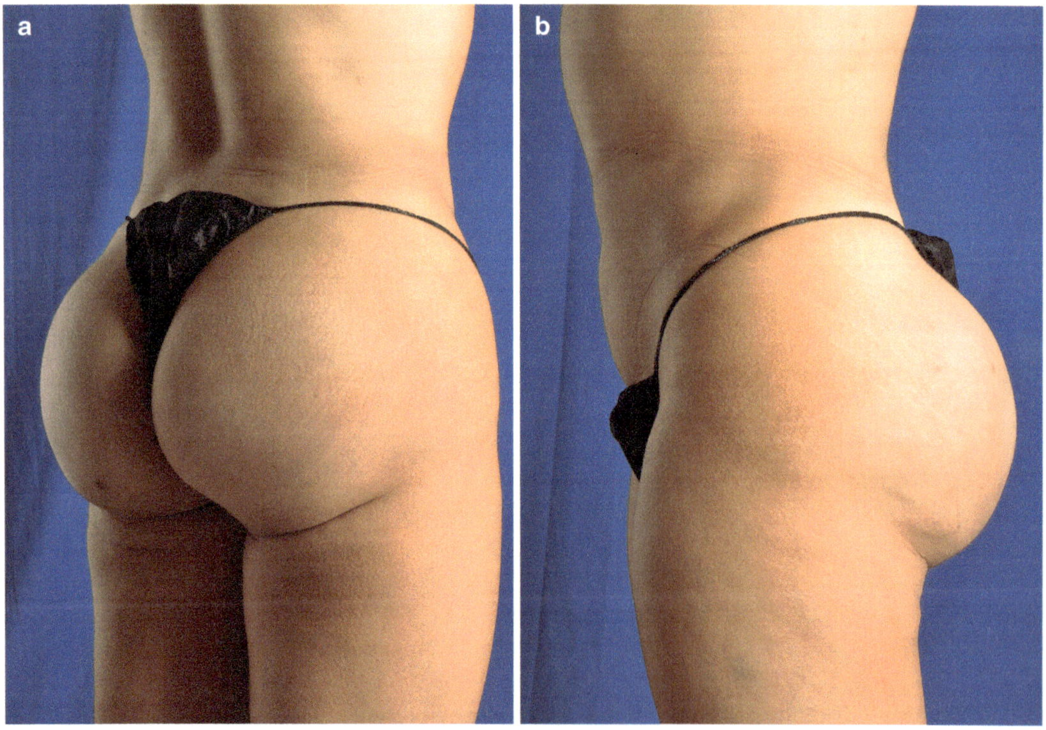

Fig. 6.26 (**a**, **b**) A 33-year-old female had undergone buttock augmentation in 2004 with another physician in the subcutaneous plane. Over time, she noted a bottoming out of her implants

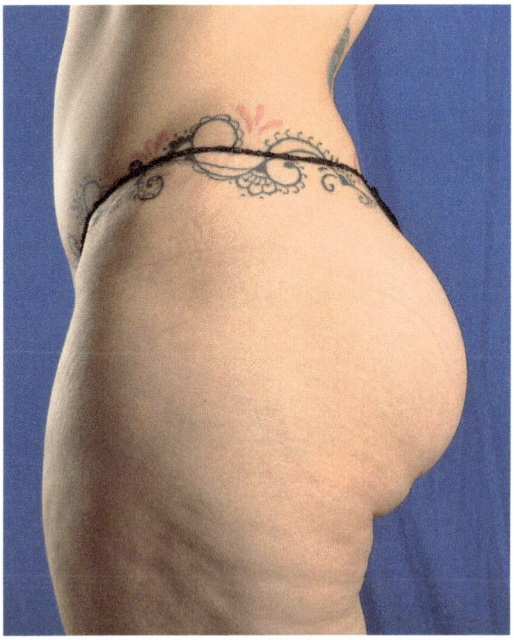

Fig. 6.27 A 32-year-old female had undergone buttock augmentation in 2006 with another physician in the subcutaneous plane. Over time, she noted drooping in the buttock to the point of creating a double-bubble deformity in the inferior aspect of her butt

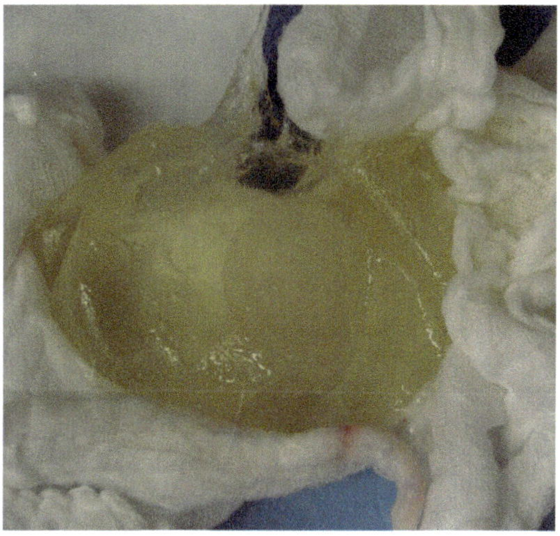

Fig. 6.28 Ruptured cohesive gel implant after removal from the patient's buttocks. She had undergone augmentation in South America and presented because of significant hardening of the buttocks with the left being harder than the right. The left buttock implant was noted to be ruptured

Implant Rupture

Implants used in the early days of buttock augmentation, typically breast implants, were filled with liquid silicone and were subject to rupture (Fig. 6.28) [32]. Since that time, the majority of US surgeons have begun performing buttock augmentation with semisolid elastomer implants which do not have a gel component. While the implants used in our practice cannot be ruptured, fractures of the implant are possible.

Scar Hyperpigmentation and Hypertrophy

The key to reduction of these problems is careful layered closure. Patients with a history of keloid or hypertrophic scar formation may require the use of steroid injected at the site of incision. Careful layered closure can produce very aesthetically pleasing scars that are difficult to notice. In addition, the use of silicone gels and silicone sheeting may help patients achieve nearly "invisible" postoperative scars (Fig. 6.29).

Capsular Contracture

This is a possible late sequela of any implant placement, most frequently described in the breast augmentation literature. In the buttock augmentation literature, the rate is typically noted to be about 1–2 % [15, 30]. In the event that a patient presents with signs/symptoms of capsular contracture (e.g., induration of the implant site, tightness in the leg, new onset pain, new onset swelling), ultrasound or CT evaluation of the affected extremity is warranted. If a capsule is identified, typically characterized by calcifications, then a partial or complete capsulectomy is warranted (Fig. 6.30). Capsular contracture is best prevented by meticulous hemostasis, good sterile technique, and avoidance of bleeding in the postoperative period. In 2012, the primary author defined a staging system for capsular contracture to better define the entity (Table 6.6).

In 2012, the authors sought to evaluate the results with buttock augmentation and the incidence of capsular contracture. It was noted that with respect to capsular contracture, there

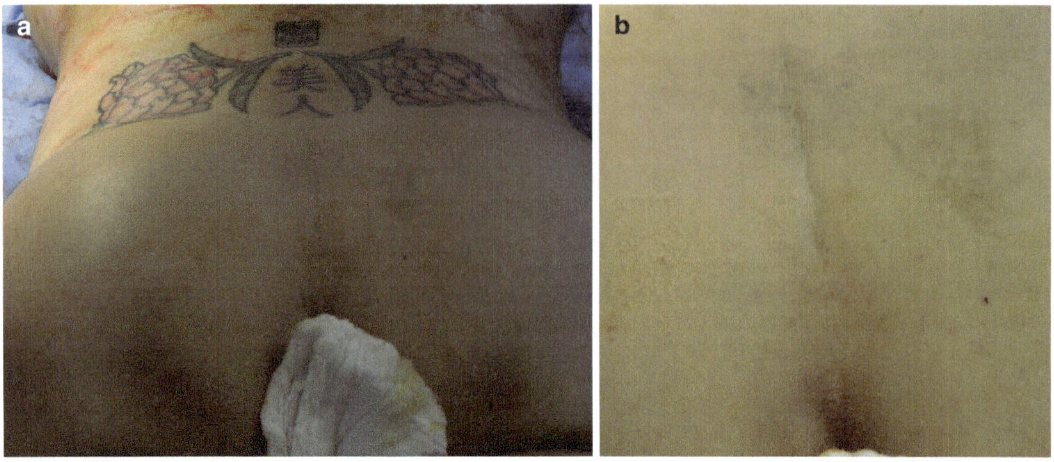

Fig. 6.29 (**a**, **b**) A 34-year-old patient 1 year post-gluteal augmentation. Closure was performed in a subcuticular fashion with the use of silicone on the incision for months 2–4 to improve scar quality

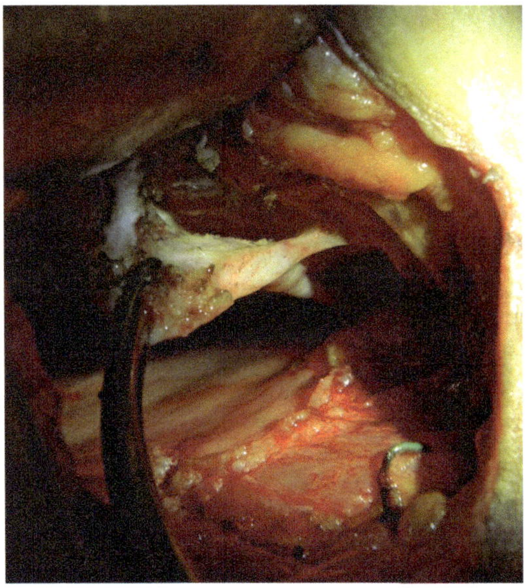

Fig. 6.30 Capsulectomy being performed in a patient who developed significant capsular contracture. The Kelly is grasping the capsule and electrocautery is used to free it from surrounding tissue

Table 6.6 Chugay staging system for capsular contracture with buttock implants

Grade of contracture	External deformity	Implant displacement
I	Firmer buttock but no deformity	None
II	Palpable hardening of buttock	Minimal or none
III	Minor external deformity	Moderate
IV	Marked external deformity	Severe

Table 6.7 Incidence of capsular contracture as noted in the authors' series from 2008 to 2011. There is note of decreased incidence of capsular contracture with time

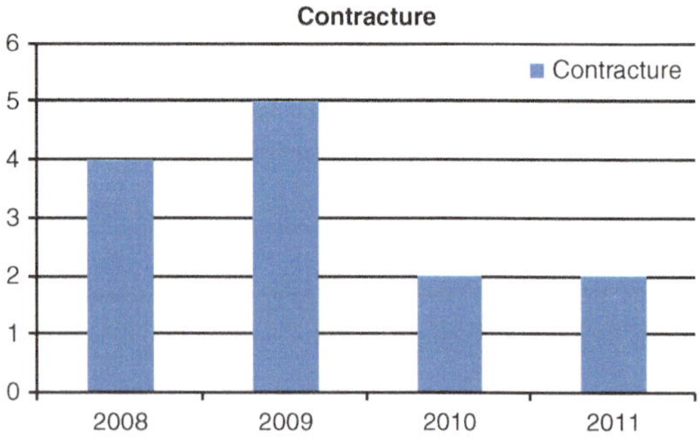

was an overall rate of 13.5 % (13/96) over the 4-year period [35]. However, over that period, there was a drop in the rate of capsular contracture from an average of 4.5 contractures/year in 2008 and 2009 versus 2 contractures/year in 2010 and 2011 (Table 6.7). To minimize capsular contracture, a much stricter and more regimented postoperative care plan was utilized for the patients that began in late 2009. Patients were asked to sleep on their back 2 h/night for 6 months beginning at week 2. This helps keep the implant pocket soft and allows the pocket to be stretched out adequately. In addition, a 7–10-day course of postoperative antibiotics is prescribed, and the pocket is irrigated with antibiotic solution to take the bacterial load as low as possible, which has been suggested as a possible source of capsules. JP drain suction is maintained until drainage is less than 30 mL/24-h period for 48 h. While these measures do not eliminate the possibility of having a capsular contracture, the authors believe that the results demonstrate a decreased incidence.

Case 1

A 35-year-old female underwent buttock augmentation with a previous physician. She presented with significant capsule formation in the left buttock with noted asymmetry. She underwent removal of old implants, left-sided capsulectomy, with placement of new style 3, size 3 implants. During the operation, she was noted to have significantly thickened capsule below the muscle. There was some residual serous fluid in the pocket which leads one to believe that seromas and hematomas may play a large role in capsule formation. Using a combination of sharp dissection with electrocautery and blunt dissection with a Lareux tissue dissector, the capsulectomy was completed (Figs. 6.31 and 6.32). The capsule was noted to be significantly thickened, measuring approximately 1 cm (Fig. 6.33).

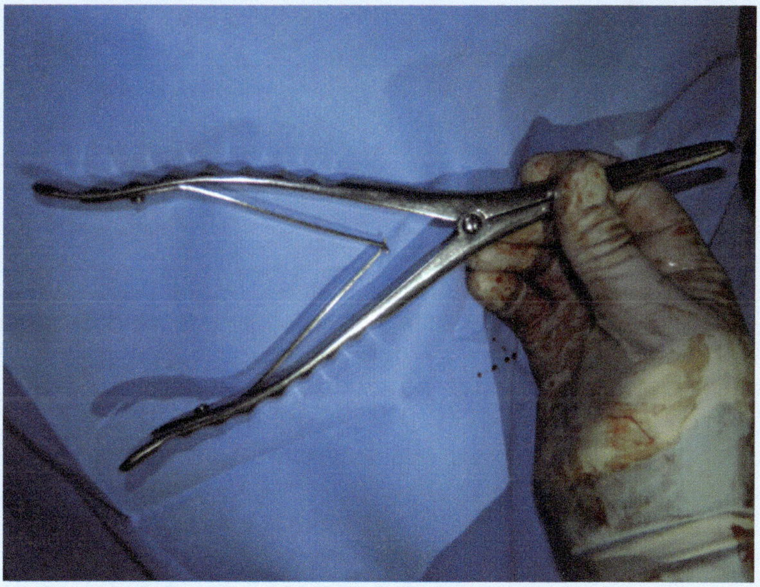

Fig. 6.31 Lareux tissue dissector

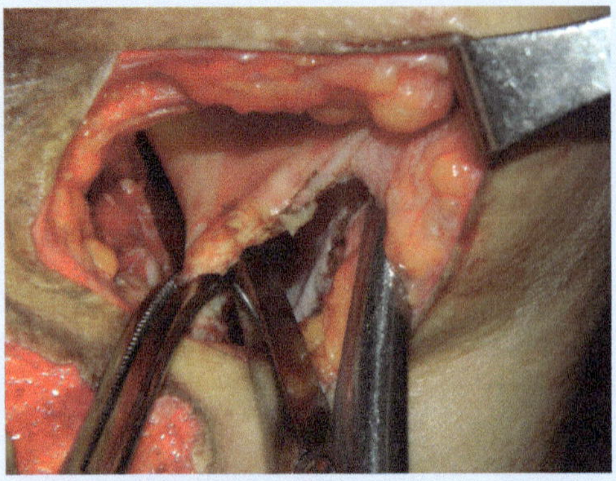

Fig. 6.32 Dissection of capsule away from surrounding muscle using sharp dissection with electrocautery and Lareux tissue dissector

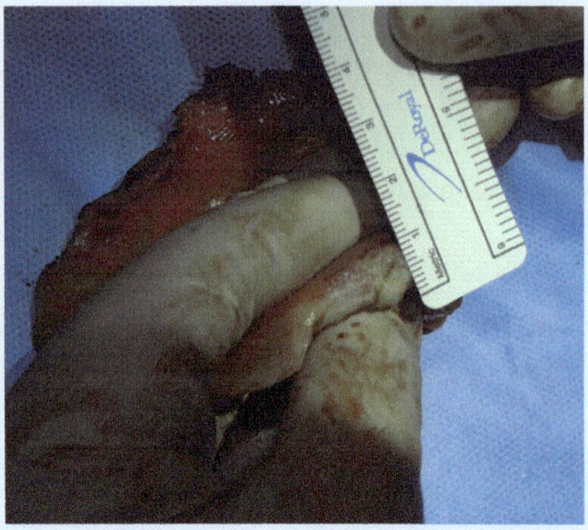

Fig. 6.33 Capsule from patient undergoing buttock capsulectomy for capsular contracture. The capsule measures approximately 1 cm in thickness

Wound Dehiscence

In the field of surgery, wound dehiscence is typically a product of surgeon error and poor attention to wound closure. It may also be produced by inadequate blood supply or due to excessive tension at the site of the incision. In the case of buttock augmentation, the cause is likely an amalgam of these. Bruner et al. [36] proposed that the cause of dehiscence in buttock augmentation is that the site of the incision is a "watershed" area with no perforating vessels in the area overlying the sacrum. The blood supply to the healing wound is entirely based on small capillaries that approach the midline from the lateral aspect. He then recommends that to minimize the risk of dehiscence, one must be delicate with the tissues at the site of the incision, avoiding desiccation and excessive traction. There is little that the physician can do to combat the marginal blood supply to the healing wound. Therefore, in the authors' estimation, the best way to prevent this complication is meticulous closure in three layers: fascia, deep dermis, and skin. Mendietta [23] also noted that dehiscences are significantly increased in overweight patients and also in patients in which an implant of more than 350 cc or more than 3.5 cm projection is used. His data demonstrates an 80 % dehiscence rate in this population. For this reason, he uses intraoperative tissue expansion while dissecting the contralateral side. If the muscle still cannot be closed with minimal tension, a smaller implant must be used. This means that it is incumbent on the surgeon to properly select the appropriate patient for buttock augmentation and to choose the implant that best suits the patient without being overly large and risking wound dehiscence.

It is very common in buttock augmentation to have small segments of dehiscence due to the significant tension on the incision in the gluteal region (Fig. 6.34). The first large volume studies on buttock augmentation by Mendietta [31] and Gonzalez [22] reported wound dehiscence rates of between 14 and 30 %. The authors' work in buttock augmentation, noting a dehiscence rate of 14.5 % (14/96) over a 4-year study period, coincides with the work of Mendietta and Gonzalez and relates solely to intermuscular placement of the gluteal prosthesis [35]. Dehiscences in the study were defined as any break in the gluteal incision, ranging from 1 to 5 cm in size. A recent study of 200 gluteal augmentations by Senderoff [30] reports a dehiscence rate of 1.5 %. However, the surgeon admits that the vast majority of his cases were performed

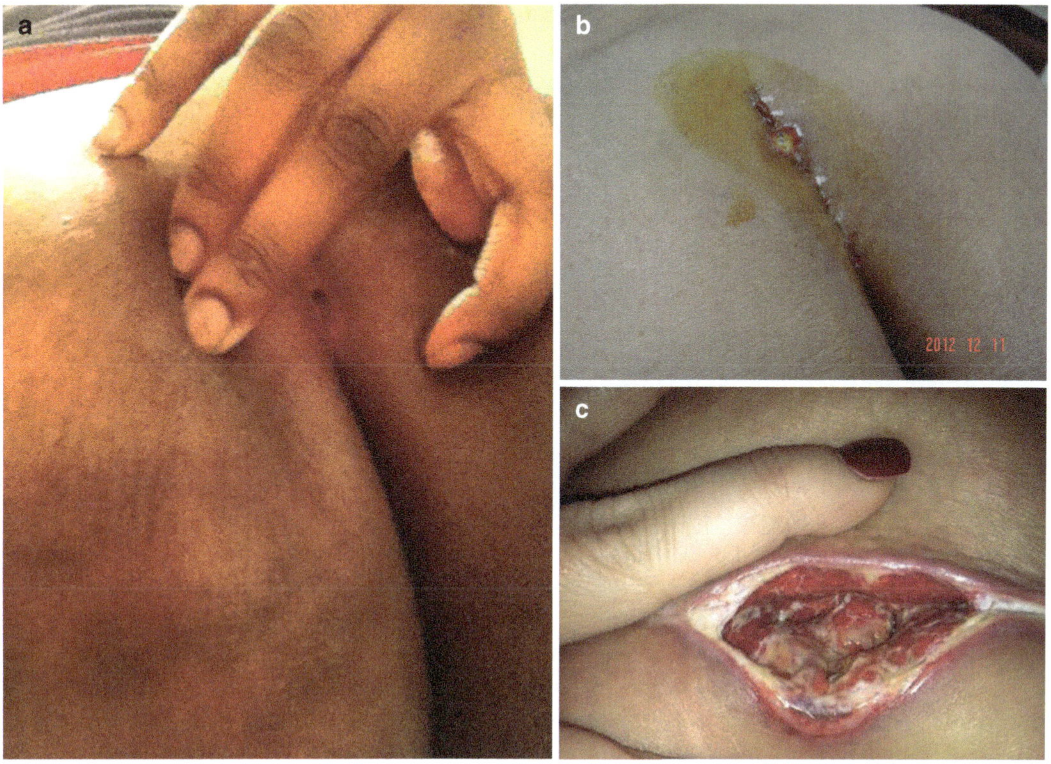

Fig. 6.34 Wound dehiscence. (**a**) Small (<2 cm). (**b**) Medium (2 cm). (**c**) Large (>2 cm)

in the subfascial plane, putting less tension on the intergluteal fold incision due to small implant sizes and potentially skewing his dehiscence rate. Therefore, depending on the plane of dissection, implant size used, and method of closure, there is a wide variability in dehiscence rates noted for gluteal augmentation.

Nerve Injury

Although frank paresis has yet to be described in the literature, there is no doubt that there is always a potential for injury either to the gluteal nerves due to their close proximity to the sacrum at the site of entry into the subgluteal plane or to the sciatic nerve in dissection of the submuscular pocket. Mendieta [31] reported a 20 % risk of transient sciatic paresthesias postoperatively, likely due to traction injury on the sciatic caused by significant pocket manipulation. If a patient has persistent discomfort, gabapentin (Neurontin) or pregabalin (Lyrica) may be considered to treat neuropathic pain. Gabapentin works by blocking voltage-dependent calcium channels, modulating excitatory neurotransmitter release. Pregabalin works by binding alpha 2-delta subunits of calcium channels and thus reduces neurotransmitter release. Treatment on either of these medications is typically continued for 1 month and patient results are evaluated at that time. Prior to discontinuation of the medication, the dosage should be tapered over the course of a week.

Pulmonary Embolism

Although this is a potential risk with any surgery performed due to the increase in stasis of the blood and the increased inflammation due to surgery, it has been a rarely reported phenomenon. In addition, patients undergoing liposculpture and fat-grafting procedures are at risk of fat emboli. These phenomena may have a low incidence that may just be due to the fact that most cases are subclinical and do not present to the attention of the surgeon. Cardenas-Camarena in 1999 [37] reported 1.5 % (1/66) incidence of fat embolism. Most large volume studies on fat emboli reveal an incidence of less than 1 % in retrospective studies and a mortality of 10–15 % in fulminant cases [38, 39].

Compartment Pressure Problems/Compartment Syndrome

Compartment syndromes, typically seen in trauma, involve an acute increase in pressure inside a closed space, thereby impairing blood flow to the affected space and potentially putting the limb at risk for loss. Clinical signs of compartment syndrome include the six Ps: pain, poikilothermia, pallor, paresthesias, paralysis, and pulseless. In conscious patients, pain out of proportion to examination is the prominent symptom. Pain with passive range of motion is particularly troubling. Although rare, gluteal compartment syndrome has been reported in the literature and has been attributed to trauma, vascular surgery, intramuscular drug abuse, altered level of consciousness from alcohol ingestion or drug overdose, prolonged immobilization, epidural analgesia after join arthroplasty, and infection [40]. In a meta-analysis of 28 cases, Henson et al. [9] note that 46.4 % of cases were diagnosed based on measuring compartmental pressures in addition to the constellation of physical findings, while 54 % were diagnosed purely based on clinical findings. This points to the fact that a physician who is aware of the potential complication can diagnose the matter without resorting to advanced testing or diagnostic assays, especially considering that there is no known pressure threshold to definitively diagnose gluteal compartment syndrome. In the cases of compartment syndrome noted in the medical literature, when compartment pressures were obtained, a compartment pressure above 30 mmHg measured with a Stryker monitor was felt to be indicative of compartment syndrome. Nonoperative treatment was used in 28.6 % of cases reviewed. The treatment of gluteal compartment syndrome is at the discretion of the treating surgeon making nonoperative management a viable option as long as close follow-up can be performed; but expeditious removal of the implant is the treatment of choice.

Discussion

Over the course of the authors' time working with gluteal implants, there are several recommendations that seem to be useful in standard practice:

1. Use of the subgluteal plane (intermuscular plane) for implant placement [17]. Authors have suggested various planes for implant placement and each has its own disadvantages. Surgeons who use the subcutaneous space are bound to have bigger problems with implant migration, implant palpability, and capsular contracture [14, 15]. The submuscular plane, as described by Robles [13], carries significant risks for damage to the sciatic that are unnecessary in gluteal augmentation surgery. The intramuscular plane, as espoused by Vergara [18], allows for complete coverage of the implant with less chance of palpability, giving a much more natural and long lasting result for gluteal augmentation. However, the intermuscular plane, in the authors' experience, avoids unnecessary injury to the gluteus maximus muscle that may occur with the creation of the intramuscular plane.
2. Use of the intergluteal fold incision. While some surgeons have suggested use of infragluteal cleft incisions, others have recommended incisions to each side of the midline. It is the authors' feeling that a single incision in the intergluteal fold is not only the most aesthetically pleasing but one that lends itself to less morbidity and disruption of the natural anatomy.
3. Placement of a bulb suction drain and maintenance until drainage is less than 30 mL/24-h period for 48 h consecutively. While this typically only remains in place for 1 week, there have been some patients who had longstanding drainage and would otherwise have developed seromas in all likelihood with early

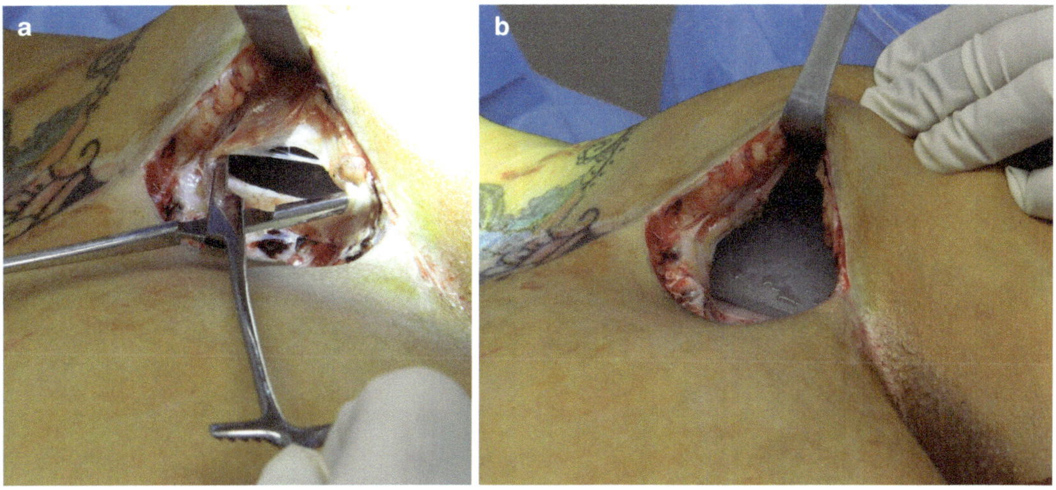

Fig. 6.35 (**a**) The implant pocket is identified and opened using a Kelly clamp to permit full visualization of the implant and facilitate removal. (**b**) The implant in its subcutaneous pocket

drain removal. We ask patients to record drain outputs twice a day and instruct patients and caregivers on proper drain care (e.g., stripping of the tubing and maintaining the bulb to suction) and recording of outputs.

Transitioning from a Subcutaneous Implant Position to Intermuscular Implant Position

The authors have seen many patients that present after having had a buttock augmentation in the subcutaneous plane and note a sagging of their buttocks within 10 years of their previous surgery. They present wanting to have their buttocks lifted and wish to regain their more youthful appearance. In managing these patients, one must be very meticulous in the operation to achieve good results that improve the patient's presenting condition.

The operation is begun by excising the existing scar in the patient's intergluteal fold. Next, subcutaneous dissection is carried to the existing implant capsule using electrocautery. The pocket is then entered and the old implant removed (Fig. 6.35). Any serous fluid that may be in the pocket is evacuated with suction. At this point, one can clearly see nothing but skin, subcutaneous tissue, and anterior capsule wall as being the only support for the implant and one begins to better understand why implant descent and drooping may occur (Fig. 6.36). An anterior capsulectomy is performed to remove the capsule as leaving it may result in a seroma in that space (Fig. 6.37). An alternative option, for those who do not feel comfortable performing a capsulectomy, may be scarification of the capsule in the hope of creating a raw surface that will better collapse postoperatively (Fig. 6.38).

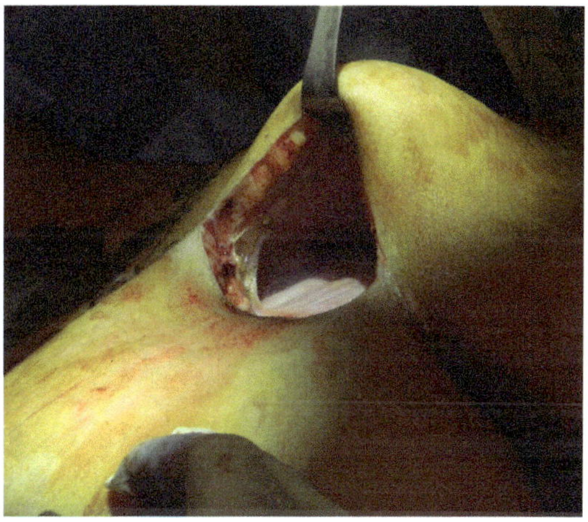

Fig. 6.36 The subcutaneous implant pocket with nothing but skin, subcutaneous tissue, and anterior capsule wall supporting the implant explaining why drooping can frequently occur with subcutaneous implant placement

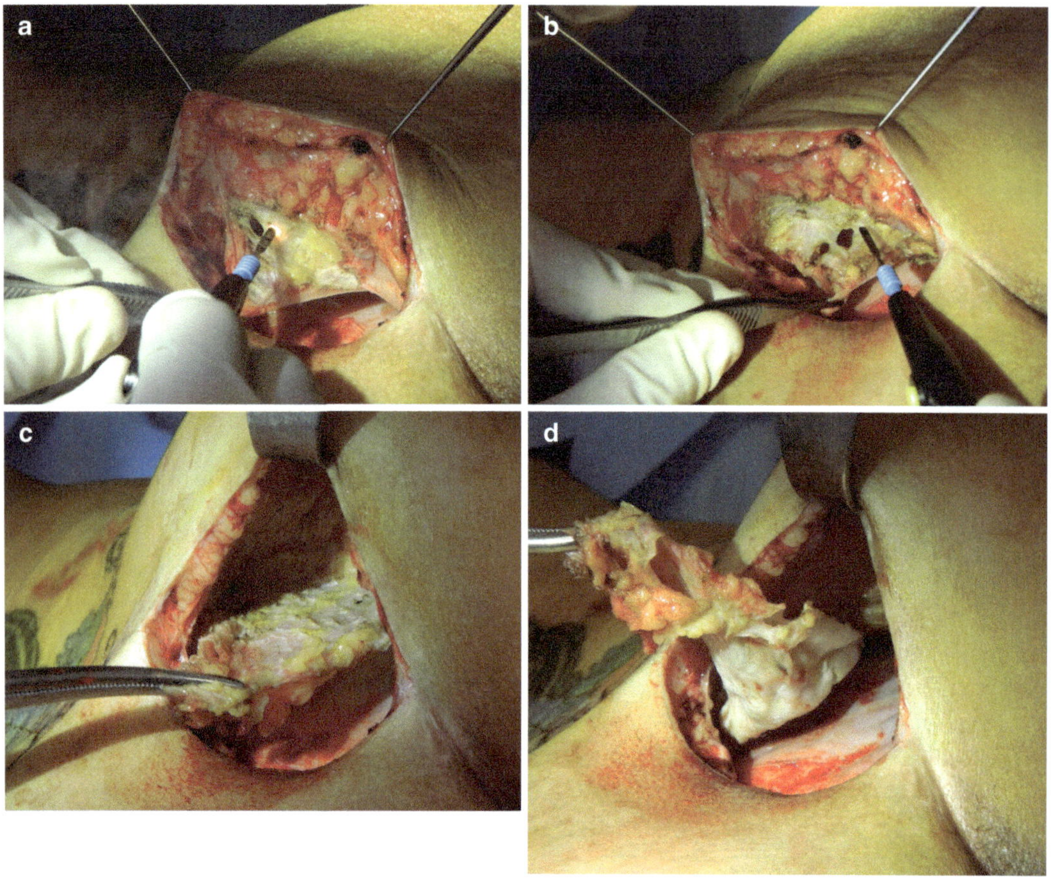

Fig. 6.37 (**a**) Beginning of capsulectomy with forceps grasping the capsule, placing traction on it and allowing for a better definition of the plane between the capsule and subcutaneous tissues. (**b**) Further dissection along the capsule using electrocautery. Small tears in the capsule may occur in trying to maintain a close dissection along the capsule wall. The surgeon should take care to minimize excess tissue removal as this may predispose the patient to a more palpable implant. (**c**) Near-complete dissection of capsule. At this point using a Kelly clamp to grasp the capsule is of great help. (**d**) Anterior capsule just prior to excision

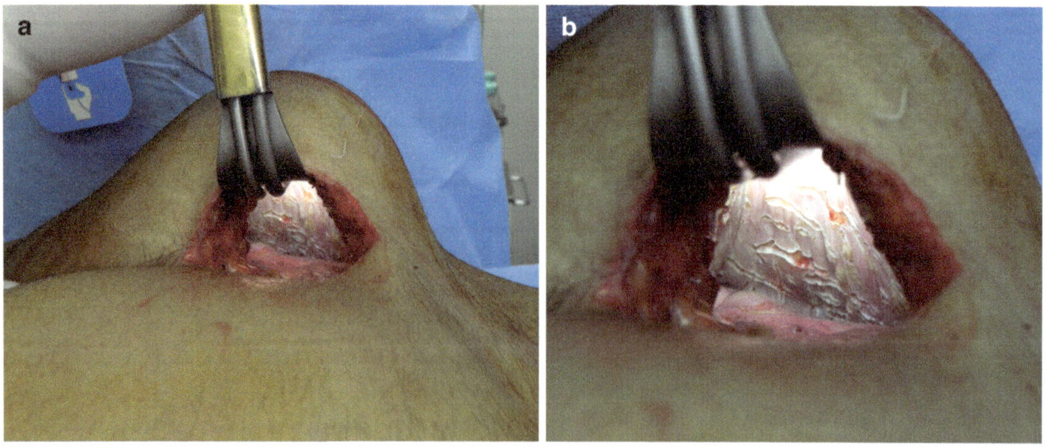

Fig. 6.38 (**a**) Scarification of the anterior capsule wall rather than capsulectomy. This may be a preferred means of capsule management in the already thin patient with thin tissues. (**b**) Close-up of the anterior capsule wall that has been scarified with electrocautery

After the management of the anterior portion of the capsule is complete, the posterior wall of the capsule is entered. Dissection through the capsule and muscle is then continued with a curved hemostat to achieve an intermuscular position (Fig. 6.39). This pocket is then dissected as done in a routing gluteal augmentation (intermuscular position). Prior to placement of the implant, a drain is placed into the newly created intermuscular plane with the tip of the drain extending through the old posterior capsule wall and into the old capsule space (Fig. 6.40). By placing the drain in this manner, one can decrease the risk of seroma formation not only around the implant but also in the old capsule space. The gluteus maximus muscle and posterior capsule wall are approximated as much as possible over the newly placed implant. Due to tension and tearing of the capsule, it may not be possible to completely incorporate all of the old posterior capsule wall. However, one should take care to create a secure and complete closure overtop the implant (Fig. 6.41). Closure of the remainder of the wound is as described in a routine gluteal augmentation.

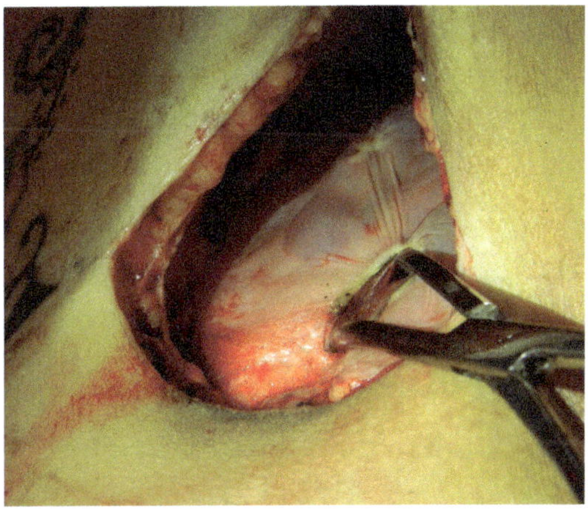

Fig. 6.39 Small incision in the posterior capsule wall was made with electrocautery, and now a hemostat is used to spread the capsule and underlying gluteus maximus to achieve an intermuscular position for implant placement

Adjunct Procedures for Gluteal Augmentation

When considering the patient for gluteal augmentation, the surgeon should evaluate the areas surrounding the buttocks for possible liposculpture or other adjunct procedures. Patients seeking augmentation of the buttocks frequently have lipohypertrophy of the flanks, sacrum, and thighs that may need attention to better define the contour of the buttocks and achieve a more aesthetic appearance [41]. Liposculpture to these areas frequently can help to better define the gluteal aesthetic units. This is especially true when performing liposuction of the flank and lower back region, which can provide a gentle “S curve” to the lower back along

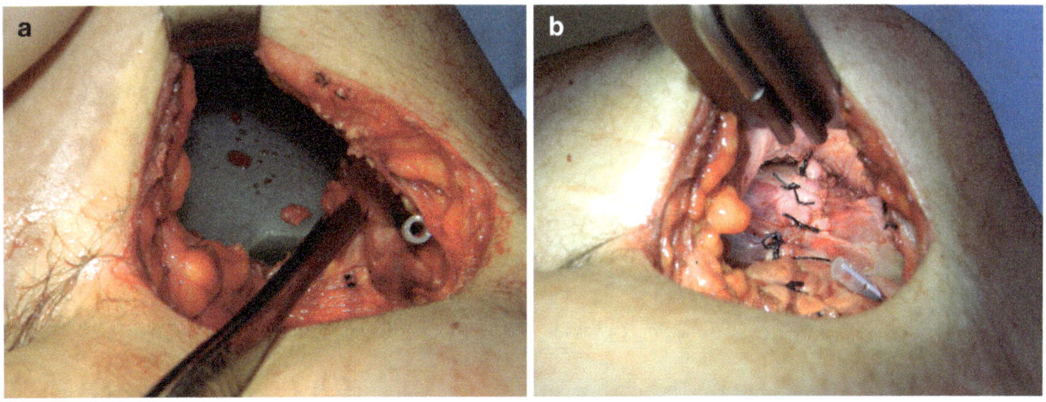

Fig. 6.40 (**a**) Drain beneath the newly placed implant and extending into the subcutaneous space and site of previous capsule. (**b**) With the capsule and muscle approximated, one can now see the tip of the drain in the subcutaneous space preventing seroma formation in the site of the previously excised capsule

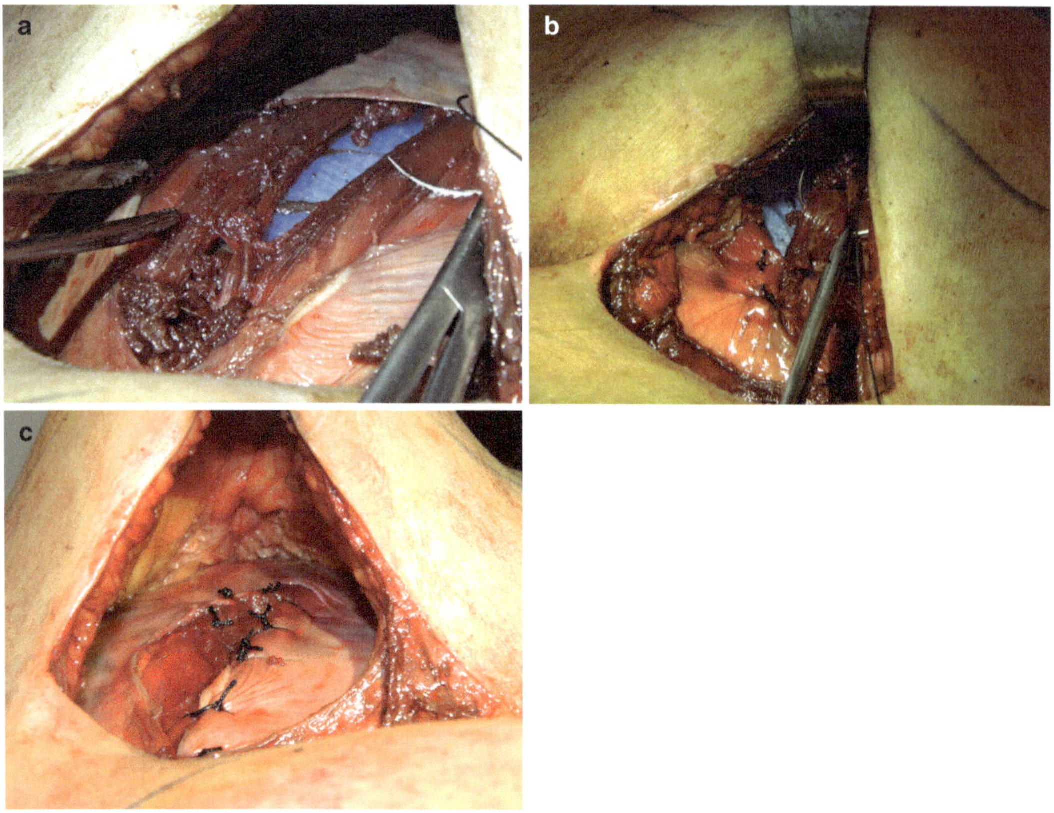

Fig. 6.41 (**a**) This demonstrates the first stitch being placed to approximate the gluteus maximus muscle and posterior capsule wall over the newly placed intermuscular implant. (**b**) Further closure of the muscle and capsule over the implant. (**c**) Final closure over the implant. Note that there are sections of the capsule that are not incorporated as attempts to bring them into the closure produced tearing of the capsule

with a narrowed waist, hence accentuating the new fullness of the buttocks. One caveat to this is that the surgeon must be careful to minimize aggressive liposuction in the area of the banana roll, as the tissues at the level of the infragluteal crease are the insertion for the fascia that surrounds the buttock muscle. Disruption of this fascia can in essence destroy the "pillars" of the buttocks and place the patient at increased risk of buttock ptosis over the crease. Another caveat is that the surgeon cannot be overly aggressive in liposuction of the presacral area at the time of simultaneous implant augmentation as there may be excessive trauma to the area which could compromise the vascular supply and significantly increase the chance of postoperative wound dehiscence.

Another adjunct procedure to consider is fat grafting to the lateral hip region overlying the trochanters to help produce a more aesthetic "S curve" in the lateral hip region. While the trochanteric depression is a natural anatomic entity, some people find it unsightly and wish to achieve a more rounded appearance to the lateral hip area [42]. Fat is an excellent means of correcting this deformity if it is available. Another option, if there is a lack of fat, would be consideration of a hip implant. While it is possible to place a hip implant over a significantly depressed trochanteric region, we recommend performing this at a separate sitting from the buttock augmentation to minimize the risk of creating one large open space between the buttocks and lateral hip region (Fig. 6.42).

One may consider a buttock lift in the gluteal region if there is a significant ptosis. Ptosis will not be corrected with a buttock implant. However, a patient who has buttock hypoplasia and ptosis may be a good candidate for both an implant and a buttock lift to eliminate a sagging bottom side.

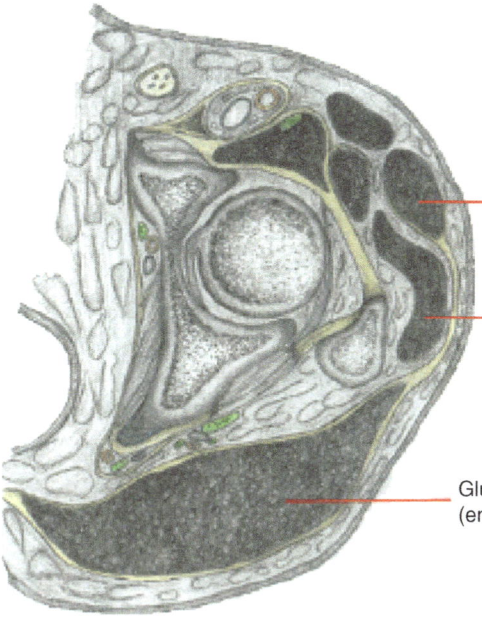

Fig. 6.42 Axial section displaying the gluteus maximus and medius muscles and their relationship to the tensor fascia lata. All of these muscles are in close proximity, and for this reason, dissection for a simultaneous hip and buttock augmentation may leave one large open space, potentially leaving the patient at risk for seromas, implant migration, and a larger chance for infection. Because of these anatomic relationships, the authors rarely perform simultaneous buttock and hip augmentations

Buttock Augmentation with Fat Grafting Compared to Implant Augmentation

The topic of the "Brazilian butt lift" and using patient's own fat to augment their bottom side has been a hot one in aesthetic surgery within the past decade (Fig. 6.43). Since the advent of liposuction, surgeons have been working to contour the body with removal of localized adiposities. The work of Sydney Coleman in the field of fat grafting has helped to propel the use of fat to augment everything from the face and hands to the butt [41, 43, 44]. Coleman's work with fat and long-term studies on permanence of the effect of grafting then pushed other surgeons to start grafting more frequently to the buttocks with significant improvement in gluteal contour [37, 45–51]. Cardenas-Camarena [37] was one of the first to report on his work. He evaluated his work with lumbosacral liposuction and fat grafting to the buttocks and found that with a mean fill of 210 mL (range 120–280 mL), it had significant improvement with excellent patient satisfaction.

Some patients who present to consultation have fat excess or lipohypertrophy in the flanks, hips, thighs, back, and/or abdomen and would benefit from liposuction. This fat can then be used to augment a hypoplastic or deflated gluteal area as opposed to using a prosthesis (Fig. 6.44). When considering a patient for augmentation gluteoplasty with fat grafting, there are several factors that must be considered by the surgeon:

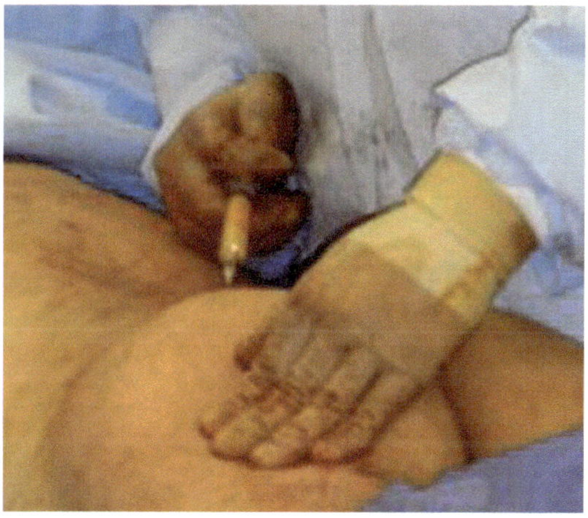

Fig. 6.43 Injection of fat into the gluteal region for an improved volume using a 3-mm cannula. Injection directly into the muscle proper will produce an increase in overall volume, while more superficial and peripheral injection will help to define the gluteal region and provide better shape

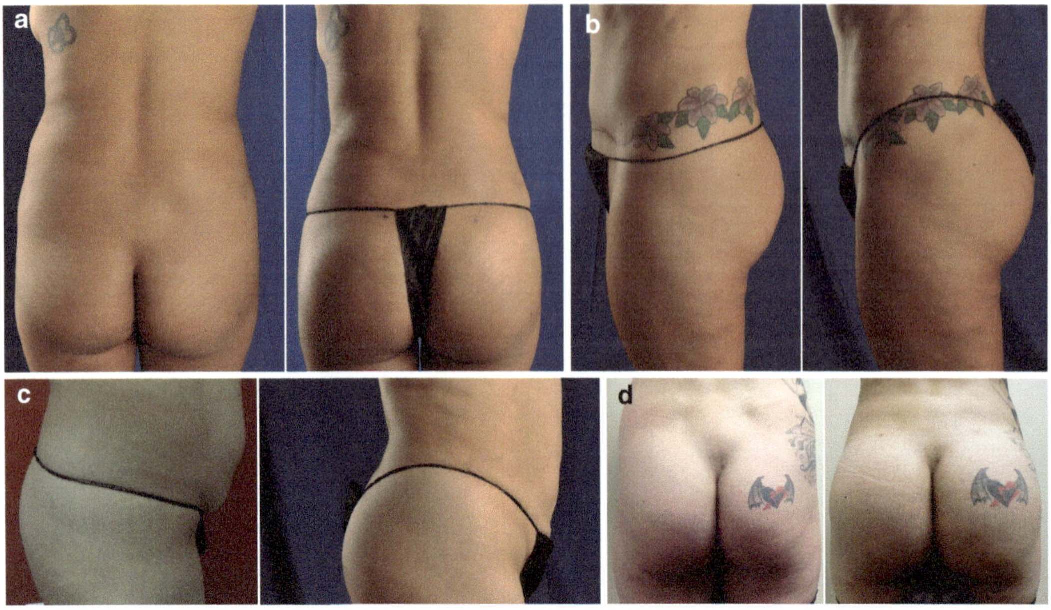

Fig. 6.44 Examples of patients undergoing buttock augmentation with fat grafting. (**a**) Patient 1 month after liposuction of the hips and back and fat transfer to butt (270 mL per buttock). (**b**) Patient 3 months after liposuction of the hips and fat transfer to the butt (235 mL per buttock). (**c**) Patient 1 month after liposuction of the abdomen and hips with fat transfer to butt (290 mL to left buttock and 270 mL to right buttock). (**d**) Patient 1 month after liposuction of the abdomen and hips and fat transfer to buttocks (410 mL to left buttock and 420 mL to right buttock)

1. First, a patient who has very little fat and cannot at least provide 300 mL of clean fat per buttock for augmentation should be dissuaded from using fat as a means of performing gluteal augmentation. In a comparative study performed at our institution, we found that patients had a mean of 280 mL grafted to each buttock (range of 30–600 mL per buttock) and achieved satisfactory results in 69.7 % of cases (23/33) [35]. Those patients who were not satisfied postoperatively were largely dissatisfied with the amount of augmentation produced; and, of those patients who were dissatisfied, it was noted that they had smaller volumes (typically less than 250 mL) grafted. Bruner and others with large volumes of buttock augmentations with autologous fat support the use of larger volumes in order to achieve aesthetically pleasing outcomes, recommending volumes of 500–900 mL of grafted fat per buttock in some cases [20, 36, 51]. While some might feel that 300 mL is an inadequate volume for augmentation, the authors feel that it maximizes aesthetic result and minimizes the risk of complications that can be seen with larger volume augmentations in the range of 500–900 mL. Some surgeons have even achieved grafts over 1,000 mL per buttock; however, it is clear that this is associated with a much higher risk of infection at the graft site and seroma formation at the harvested sites [36, 51]. For this reason, the authors discourage this practice.
2. This then brings up the second point of consideration which is the unpredictable nature of "fat take" in grafting procedures. To date, only one study has truly sought to quantify fat that was resorbed after buttock augmentation with autologous fat grafting by performing serial MRI examinations of the buttocks [51]. Unfortunately, only six patients were studied making actual quantification of fat survival near impossible. In studies performed by Coleman and others, there is an estimated typical take of fat between 50 and 70 % when stem cell therapy is not employed [36, 41, 43–45, 51]. Despite efforts to minimize trauma to the buttocks by direct pressure and the use of loose buttock compression garments, there is still no way to reliably produce a 100 % take of fat that is injected. For that reason, in order to increase the chance of "take" after fat grafting, the authors do

recommend the use of stem cell therapy for all fat-grafting patients. The authors employ Invitrx Therapeutics from Irvine, California. This is an independent laboratory that sends a technician to the office to process and purify the fat in a procedure that takes approximately 45–60 min. The physician can continue performing liposuction while the stem cell technician is processing the adipose tissue submitted to them at the onset of the case (at least 30 mL). After liposuction fat/aspirated adipose tissue and tumescent fluid is given to the technician, the adipose tissue is isolated from the tumescent fluid by centrifugation. Adipose tissue is treated with the enzyme collagenase and placed in incubation for 20 min to release adipose-derived stem cells. After incubation, to separate the enzyme from the adipose tissue and stem cells, the mixture is centrifuged again. The adipose tissue, enzyme, and stem cell pellet are separated in layers. To ensure the enzyme is fully removed from the fat, the fat and pellet are washed and rinsed with phosphate buffer saline and recentrifuged. The patient's own blood serum is added to the pellet to neutralize the enzyme. The processed fat along with the stem cell pellet is returned to the physician for implantation. After liposuction has been completed, the fat to be grafted is washed and then mixed with the harvested stem cells. While this does not ensure a 100 % take, it does increase the take of fat from the conventional 50–70 % up to 80 %, in the authors' practice [35].

3. A third point to consider is the level of vacuum applied by the suction apparatus. There has been some evidence to suggest that high vacuum levels may damage the fat cells and decrease their survival [45, 52]. For that reason, the authors do not exceed 25 mmHg on the suction apparatus. This use of aspiration at lower vacuum pressures is supported by Coleman [41, 43, 44], Pedroza [49], Bruner [36], and Murillo [51].
4. Grafting in small amounts and in variable layers. Coleman [27–29], Guerrerosantos [53], and Bruner [36] all agree that grafting in small quantities (<0.3 mL in each tunnel) improves the graft survival as there is more contact with adjacent blood supply. In addition to considering the quantity of the graft, the surgeon should aim to augment both the deeper muscular structures and the superficial structures. Addition of volume to the region is done at the level of the gluteus muscles, whereas shaping can be done with injection into the subcutaneous level. Injection in various layers also helps to spread out the grafted fat and increase the blood supply available to the grafted fat cells.
5. Postoperatively, the patient must be able to commit to 2 weeks without pressure on the buttocks. There is never an ability to achieve a 100 % fat take, but everything must be done to minimize trauma to the grafted fat. For that reason, it is recommended that the patients avoid sitting or sleeping on their back side for 2 weeks after surgery to minimize shear and compression forces.

In reviewing the authors' experiences with fat grafting and those of other physicians, the most commonly reported complications after fat grafting include infection, seromas, transient sciatic paresthesias, and tissue irregularities [33, 36, 50, 51]. Infection rates range between 7 and 18 % [36, 37]. Infection rates as high as 18 % are to be expected as every stage of harvesting, preparing, and grafting the fat has a potential for contamination [36]. This, when combined with a warm, moist, traumatized grafting environment, can help to explain why infections are a serious risk with fat-grafting procedures. Seromas are noted in areas of liposuction. Greater volumes of aspirate are more likely to result in a greater chance for seroma formation. Seroma rates vary from 6 % in Cardenas-Camarenas' work with fat grafts between 100 and 240 mL per buttock up to 40 % in Murillo's study that had average fat graft of 700 mL/buttock [20, 36, 37, 51]. In their most recent evaluation of seroma rates in their practice, Bruner [36] notes that he has seen a drop in seroma rates from approximately 40 % down to 2 % with the use of better compression in the sacral region along with closed suction drains (2) in the sacral region. Another complication often seen in fat-grafting patients is transient sciatic paresthesia. This tends to be described as minor discomfort associated with tingling and slight numbness along the course of the sciatic nerve, lasting less than 2 weeks in most cases [36]. The incidence is reported to be between 1 and 4 % [23, 51]. Bruner

[44] has made 12 mg of IV dexamethasone a routine at the beginning of the surgical procedure, hoping to minimize perioperative inflammation. As with neuralgia produced with implant augmentation, neuromodulators such as gabapentin and pregabalin are options in the recalcitrant patient.

In the only comparative study of gluteal augmentation (Table 6.8) that is available in the literature, the authors evaluated the results with implant augmentation against those with fat augmentation [35]. Over a 4-year study period, 129 patients underwent gluteal augmentation with either fat (33 patients) or implants (96 patients). The overall satisfaction of the patients receiving buttock augmentation was 76.0 % (73/96) for augmentation with implants and 69.7 % (23/33) for augmentation with fat, which was statistically significant ($P<0.001$; 95 % confidence interval [CI], 67.93–71.47). Seroma formation was more prevalent in the implant group (3.0 % versus 17.7 %; $P=0.02$; 95 % CI, 0.070–15.7). Lumps or dents were more prevalent in the fat-grafting group (33.3 % versus 2.1 %; $P<0.0001$; 95 % CI, 17.9–51.8). Complications isolated to those undergoing implant augmentation included dehiscence (14.6 %) and contracture (13.5 %). Ultimately, it was determined that although fat grafting for buttock augmentation is rising in popularity among surgeons, the results are not as consistent as those seen with buttock augmentation via implant. On the other hand, the consistency of results for implant augmentation is offset by the risk of capsular contracture and dehiscence, which are seen only in implant surgery. Regardless of the method of buttock augmentation chosen, surgeons can be confident that the results will be pleasing to the eye and to their patients as long as good surgical technique is used and the aforementioned perioperative risks are kept in mind.

Table 6.8 Summary data for 2012 buttock augmentation comparative study

Complications	Fat grafting ($n=33$)	Implant ($n=96$)	P value (CI 95 %)
Infection	1	12	0.09
Seroma	1	17	0.02
Rejection	N/A	1	N/A
Hematoma	1	0	<0.0001 (0.07–15.7)
Asymmetry	2	12	0.1
Scarring	2	1	0.003 (0.75–20.3)
Contracture	N/A	13	N/A
Post-op pain 8–10	9	20	0.37
Dehiscence	N/A	14	N/A
Lumps/dents	11	2	<0.0001 (17.9–51.8)
Satisfaction	23	33	<0.001 (67.9–71.8)

Table 6.9 Observed complications in buttock augmentation

Complication	Number ($n=450$)	Percent (%)
Seroma	74	16.44
Infection	52	11.56
Asymmetry	46	10.22
Wound dehiscence	74	16.44
Capsular contracture	51	11.33

Authors' Personal Experience

Since starting to perform buttock augmentation in 1995, the lead author (NVC) has performed approximately 450 buttock augmentation procedures, averaging approximately 25 augmentations per year. The overall satisfaction rate is 92.0 % (414/450). Patients who were dissatisfied primarily complained of an inadequate augmentation. Based on retrospective chart review, the most frequently encountered complications included seroma formation, infection, asymmetry, wound dehiscence, and capsular contracture. A patient was considered to have an infection if there was evidence of erythema around the wound or cellulitis requiring the physician to prescribe antimicrobial treatment or perform some surgical intervention. Wound dehiscence was broadly defined as any separation of the midline wound, with a maximal dehiscence of 5-cm, complete opening of the midline wound (Table 6.9).

Patient Cases

Case 2 (Fig. 6.45)
A 35-year-old female underwent buttock augmentation with a previous physician. She presented with significant capsule formation in the left buttock with noted asymmetry. She underwent removal of old implants, left-sided capsulectomy, with placement of new style 3, size 3 implants. The patient is seen preoperatively and 4 months postoperatively.

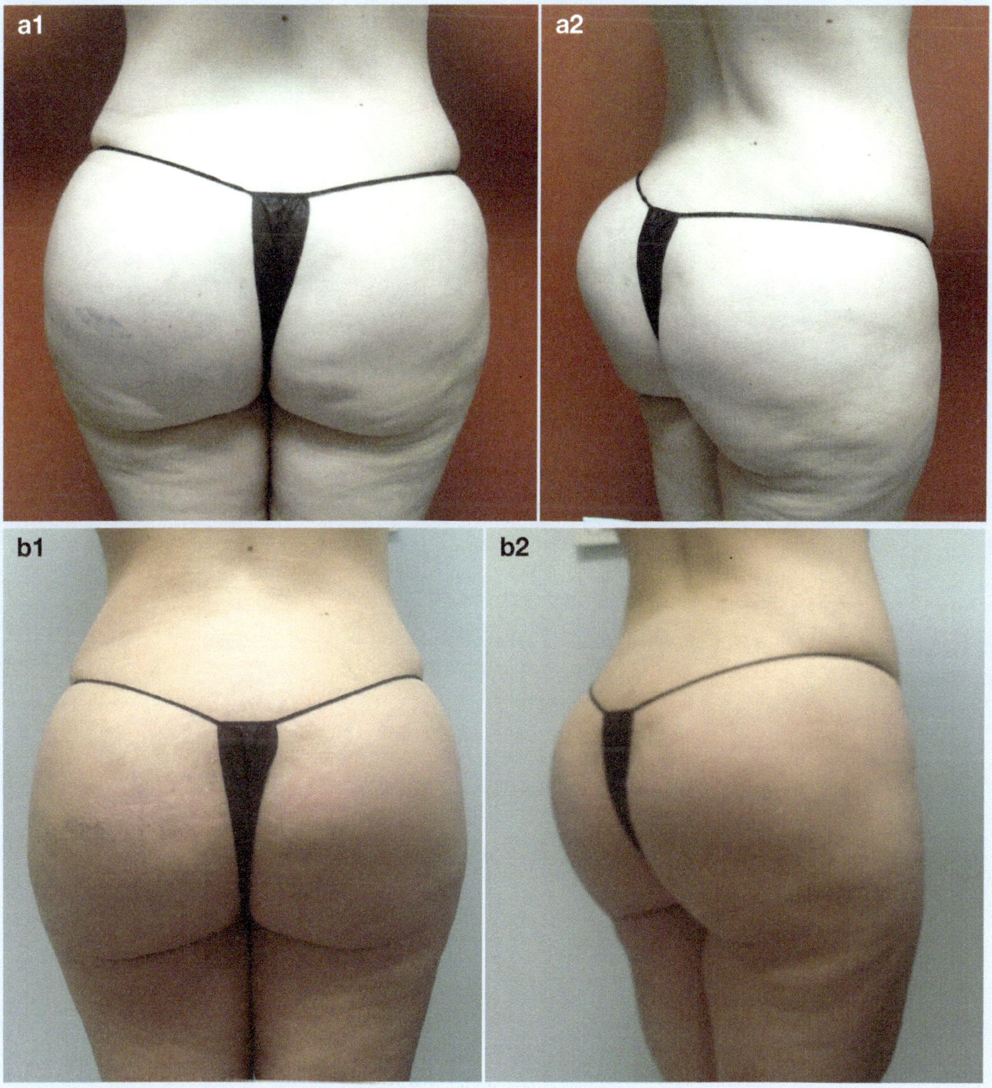

Fig. 6.45 (**a**) Preoperative. (**b**) Postoperative

Case 3 (Fig. 6.46)

A 44-year-old female underwent buttock augmentation with style 3, size 2 implants. The patient is seen preoperatively and 4 months postoperatively.

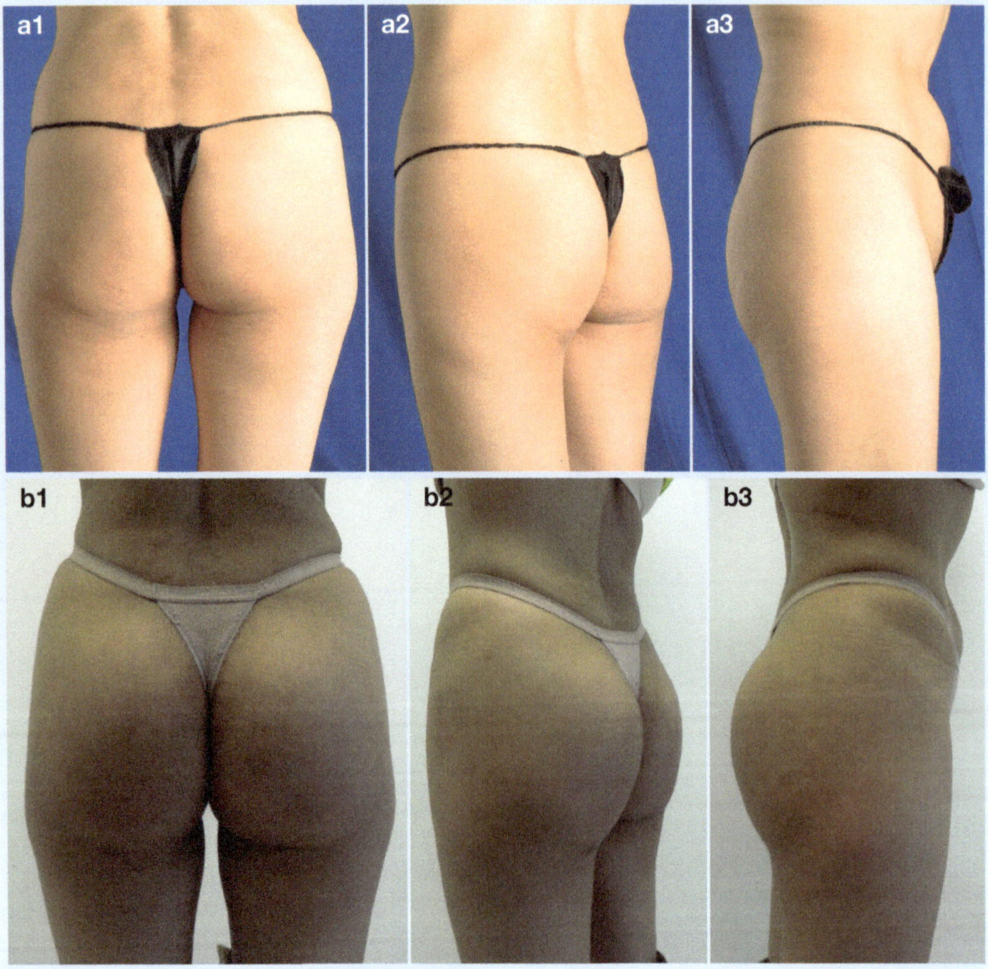

Fig. 6.46 (**a**) Preoperative. (**b**) Postoperative

Case 4 (Fig. 6.47)
A 61-year-old female underwent buttock augmentation with style 3, size 7 implants secondary to buttock hypoplasia. Patient seen preoperative and 1.5 months postoperative.

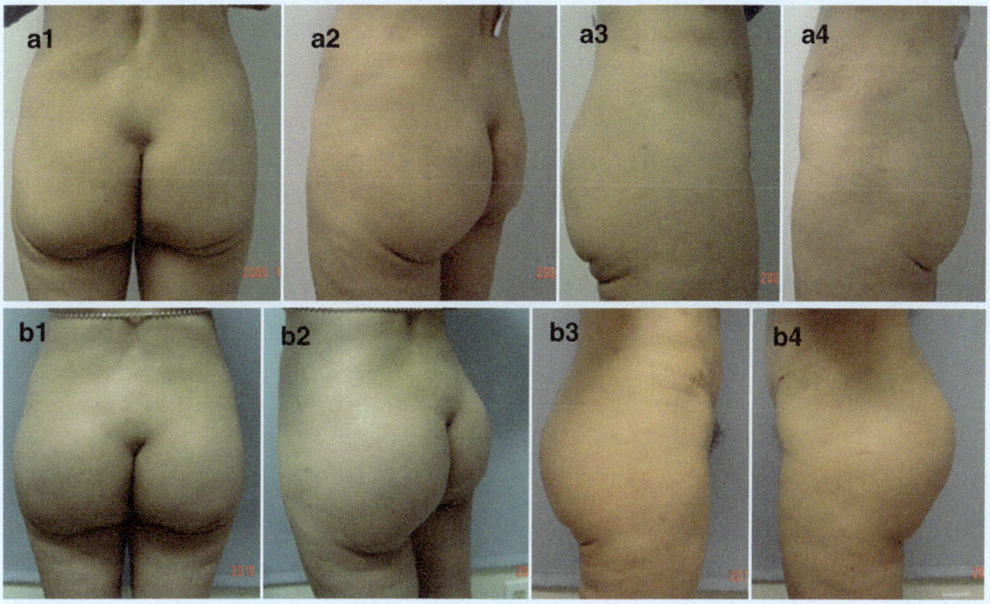

Fig. 6.47 (**a**) Preoperative. (**b**) Postoperative

Case 5 (Fig. 6.48)
A 45-year-old female underwent buttock augmentation with style 3, size 7 implants secondary to buttock hypoplasia.

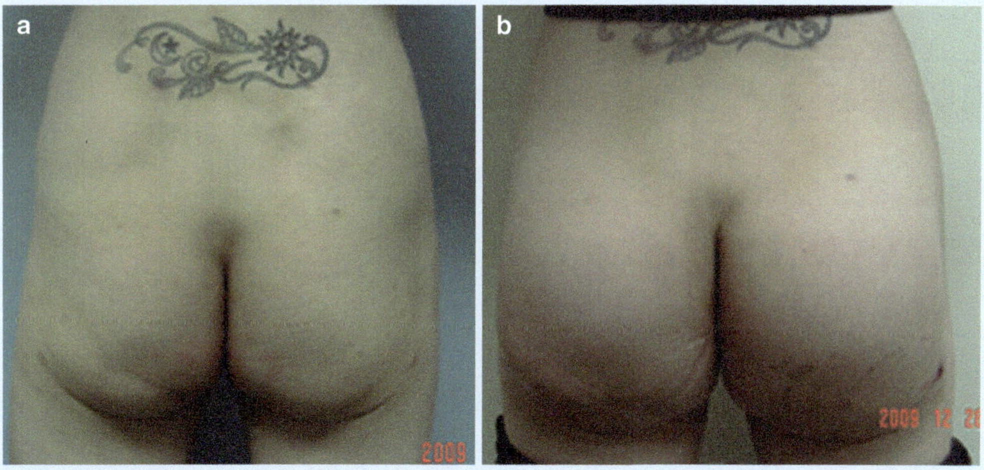

Fig. 6.48 (**a**) Preoperative. (**b**) Postoperative

Case 6 (Fig. 6.49)

A 31-year-old female underwent buttock augmentation with style 3, size 7 implants to achieve a more lifted and slightly more projected bottom side. She is seen preoperative and 3 months postoperative.

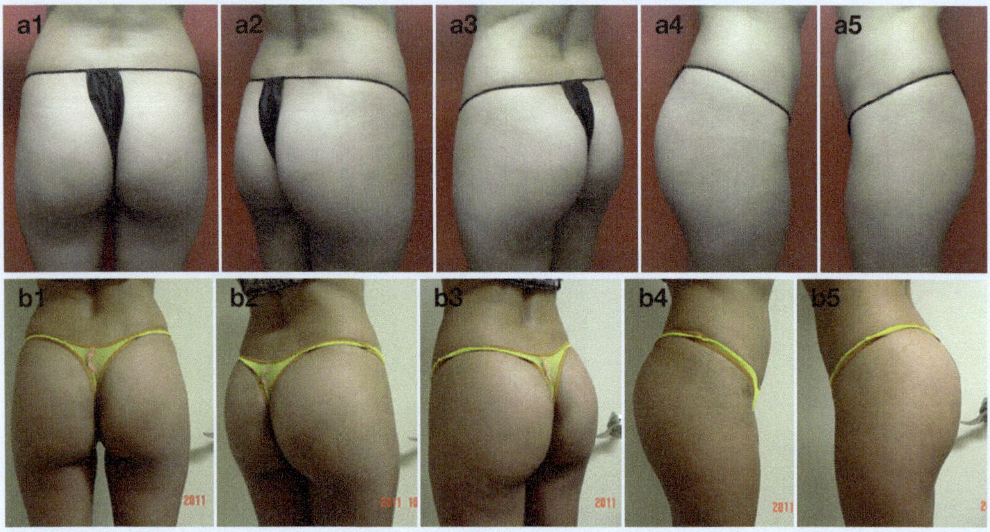

Fig. 6.49 (**a**) Preoperative. (**b**) Postoperative

Case 7 (Fig. 6.50)

A 30-year-old female underwent buttock augmentation with style 3, size 7 implants along with liposuction of the hips with aspiration of 400 mL fat. The patient is seen preoperatively and 2 months postoperatively.

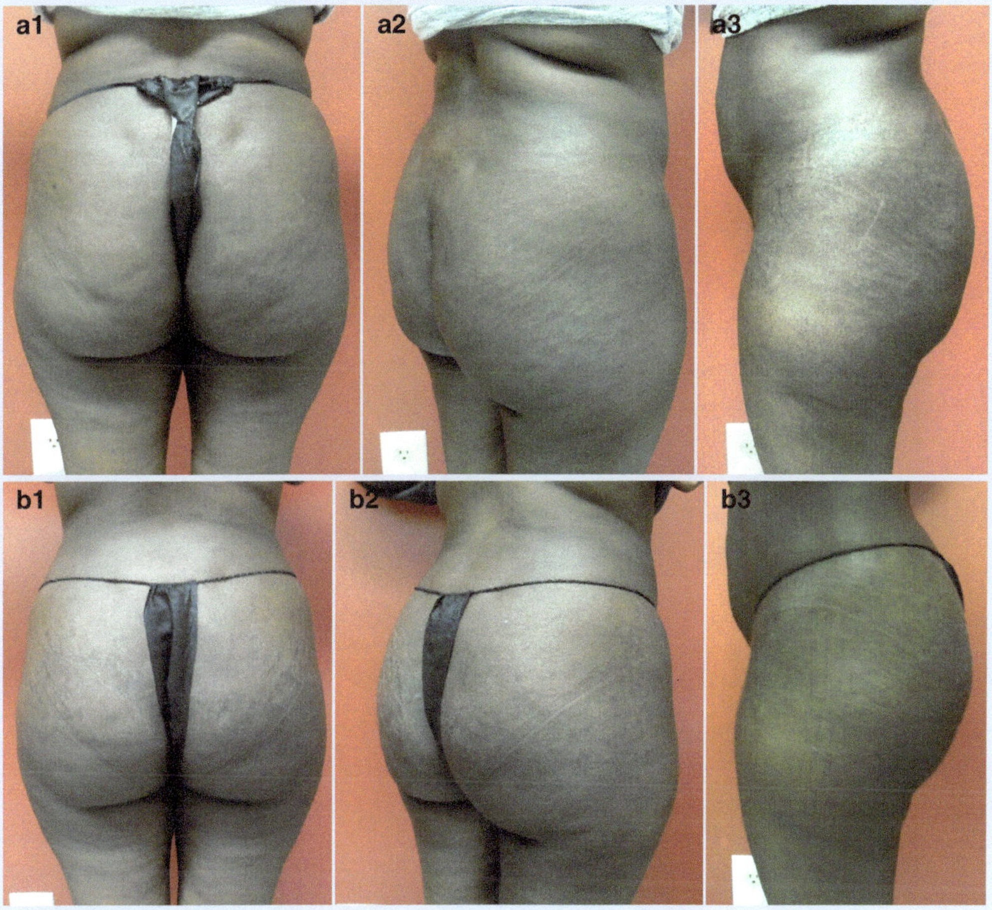

Fig. 6.50 (**a**) Preoperative. (**b**) Postoperative

Case 8 (Fig. 6.51)

A 27-year-old female underwent buttock augmentation with style 3, size 8 implants. She is seen preoperative and 2 months postoperative.

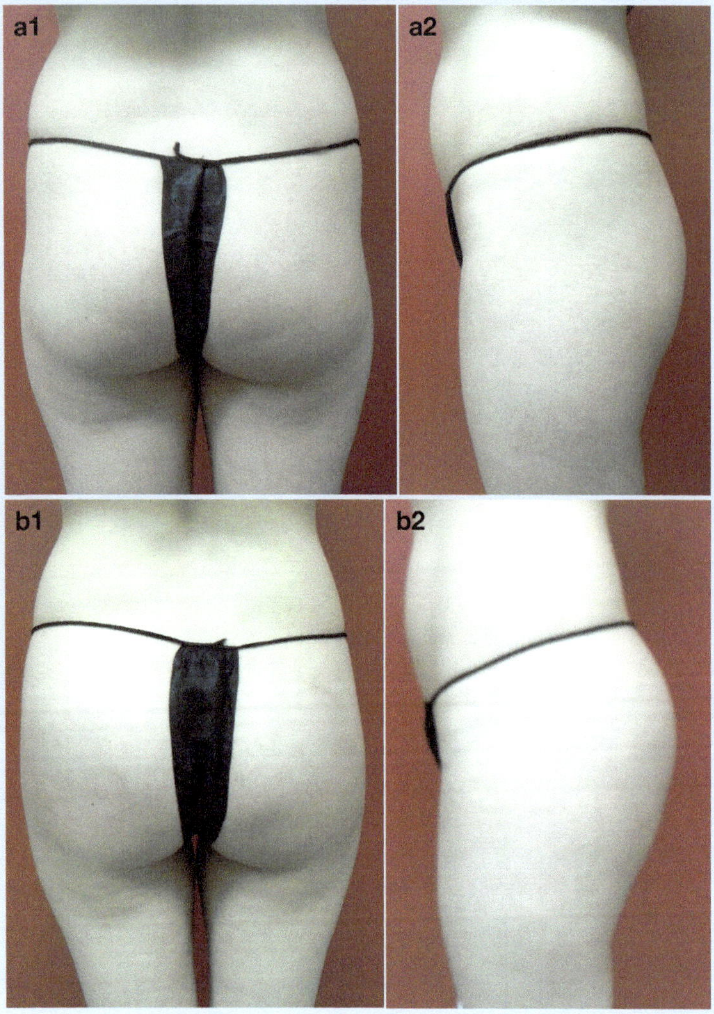

Fig. 6.51 (**a**) Preoperative. (**b**) Postoperative

Case 9 (Fig. 6.52)
A 21-year-old female underwent buttock augmentation with style 3, size 4 implants. She is seen preoperative and 1 month postoperative. The patient declined liposuction of the hips/flanks and thighs which may have improved her overall result.

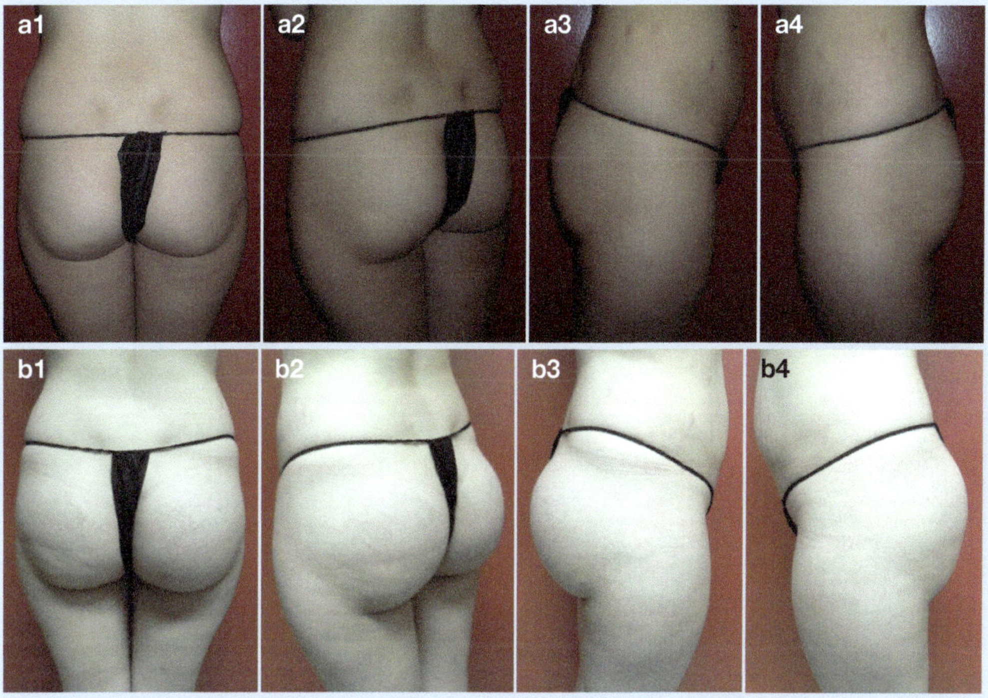

Fig. 6.52 (**a**) Preoperative. (**b**) Postoperative

Case 10 (Fig. 6.53)

A 38-year-old female underwent buttock augmentation with style 3, size 7 implants. Note excellent improvement superiorly but there is still deficiency in the lower buttock. This is typically corrected in later operations with liposuction and/or fat grafting as the implants do not extend so far caudally. The patient is seen preoperative and 2 months postoperative.

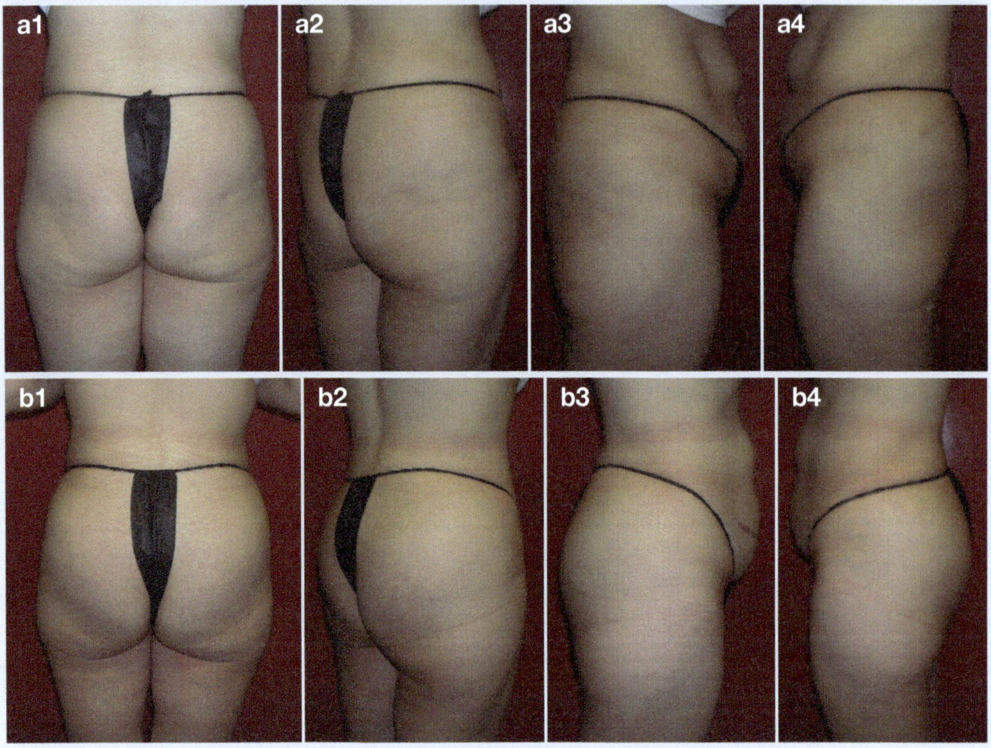

Fig. 6.53 (**a**) Preoperative. (**b**) Postoperative

Case 11 (Fig. 6.54)

A 40-year-old gay male presented with significant loss of volume in the buttocks after significant weight loss secondary to testicular cancer and his battle with HIV. He underwent augmentation with style 3, size 2 implants. The patient is seen preoperative and 2 months postoperative.

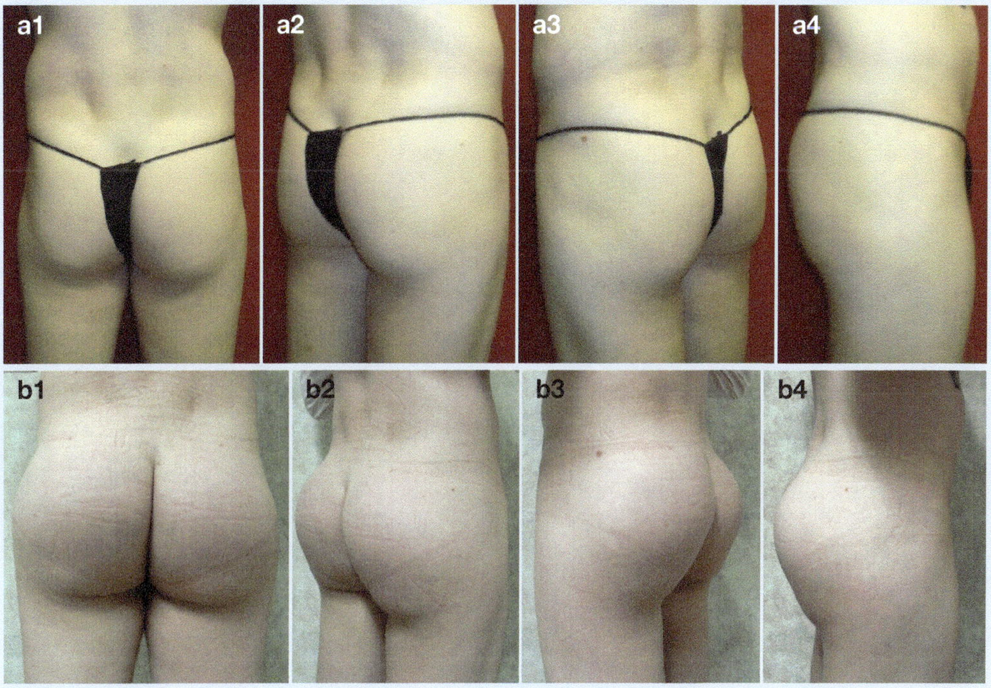

Fig. 6.54 (**a**) Preoperative. (**b**) Postoperative

Case 12 (Fig. 6.55)

A 30-year-old female underwent buttock augmentation with style 3, size 8 implants along with liposuction of the back and hips. The patient is seen preoperative and 1 month postoperative.

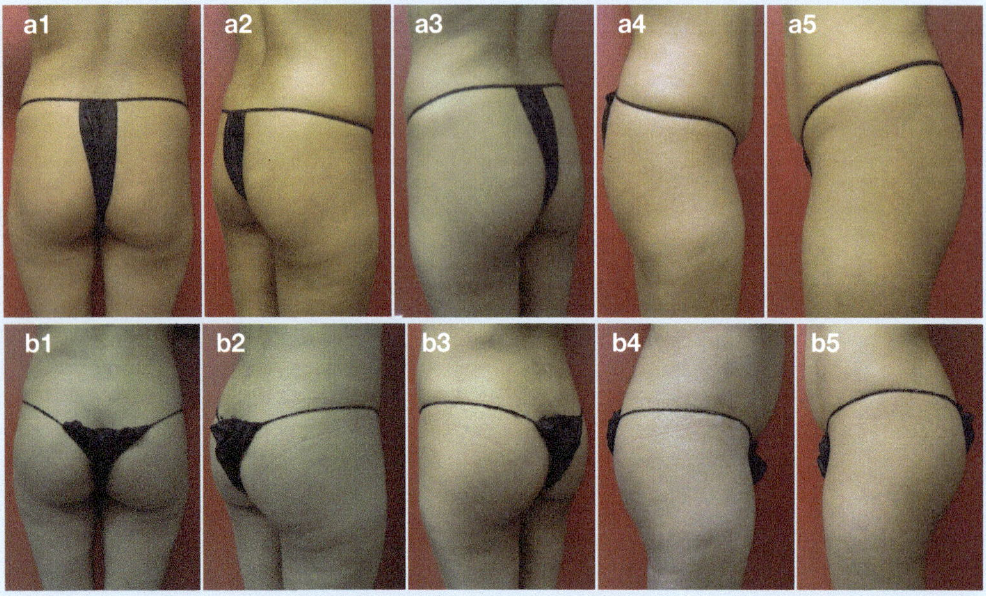

Fig. 6.55 (**a**) Preoperative. (**b**) Postoperative

Case 13 (Fig. 6.56)
A 27-year-old female underwent buttock augmentation with style 3, size 7 implants with minor liposuction of the waist (300-mL fat aspirated). The patient is seen preoperative and 1 month postoperative.

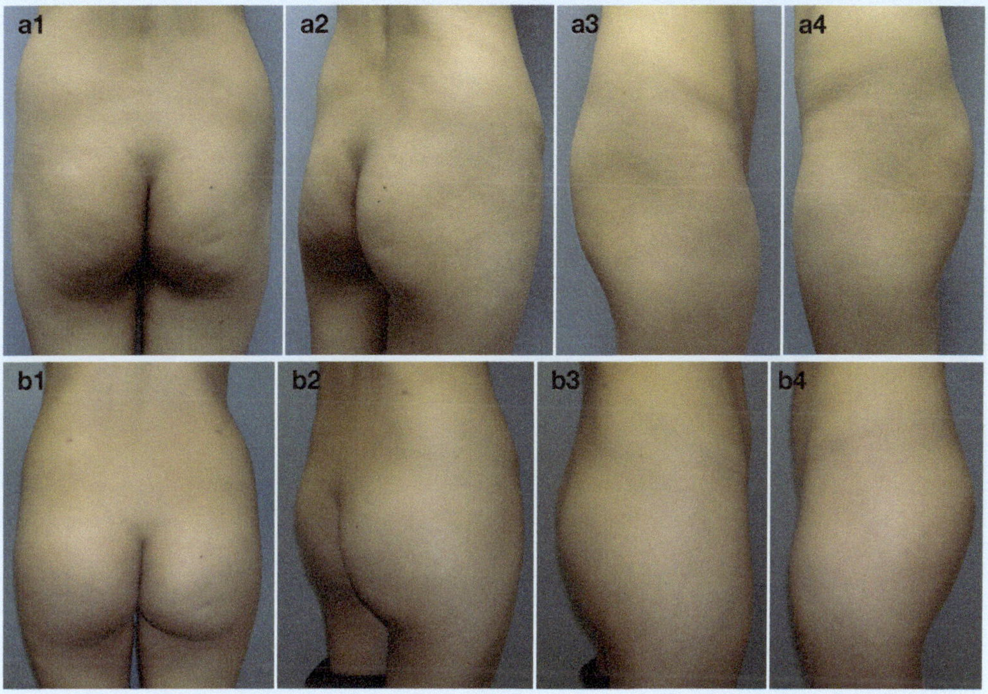

Fig. 6.56 (**a**) Preoperative. (**b**) Postoperative

Case 14 (Fig. 6.57)
A 49-year-old male underwent buttock augmentation with style 3, size 7 implants to achieve greater projection and roundness to the buttocks. The patient is seen preoperative and 1 month postoperative.

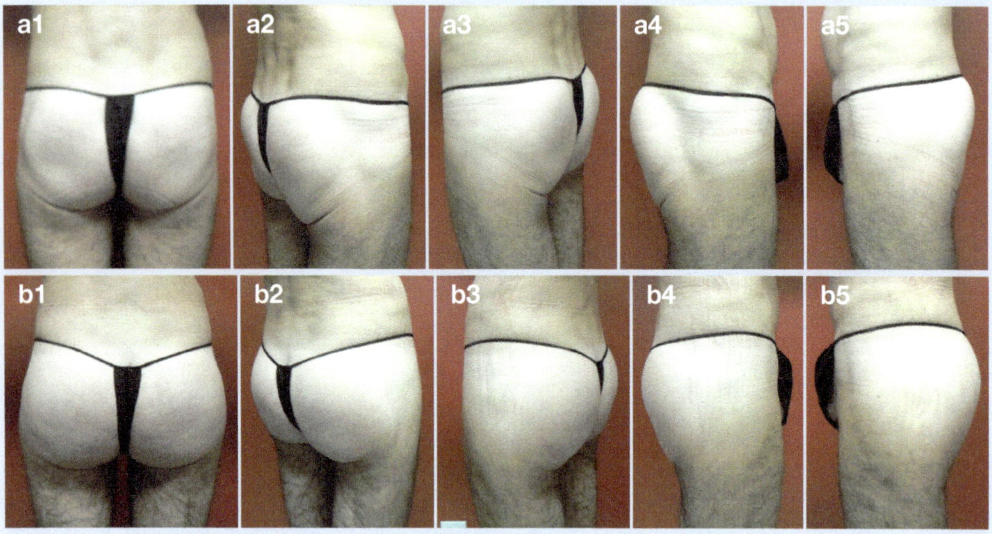

Fig. 6.57 (**a**) Preoperative. (**b**) Postoperative

Case 15 (Fig. 6.58)

A 29-year-old female underwent buttock augmentation with style 3, size 8 implant along with liposuction of the hips/flanks and fat grafting to the lateral thigh and butt (100 mL to the left side and 150 mL to the right side). The patient is seen preoperative and 6 months postoperative.

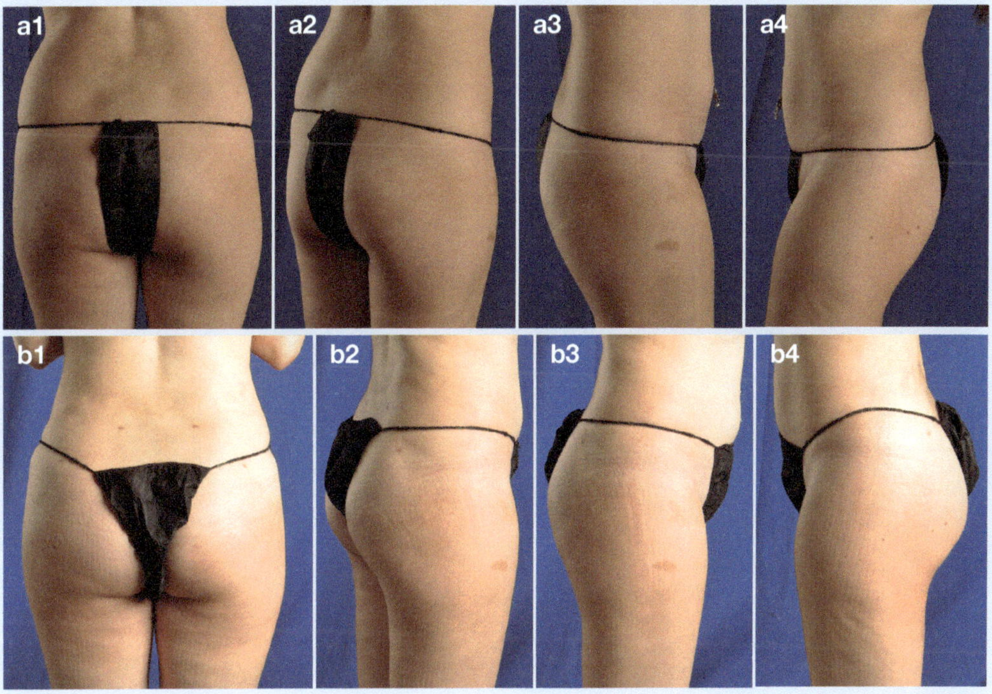

Fig. 6.58 (**a**) Preoperative. (**b**) Postoperative

Case 16 (Fig. 6.59)

A 24-year-old female underwent buttock augmentation with style 3, size 7 implants. The patient is seen preoperative and 5 months postoperative.

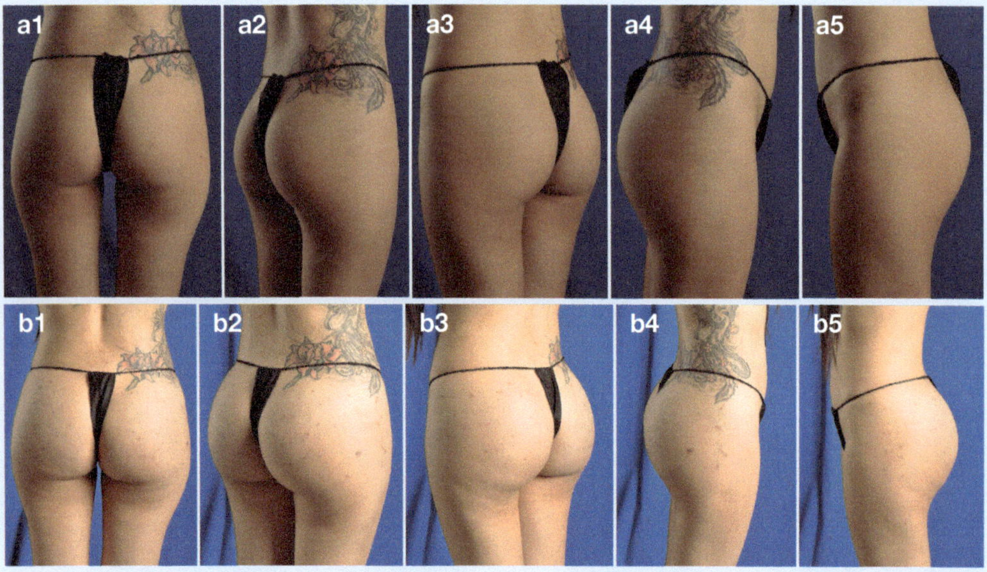

Fig. 6.59 (**a**) Preoperative. (**b**) Postoperative

Case 17 (Fig. 6.60)

A 69-year-old female underwent buttock augmentation to help correct sagging skin and significant cellulite. She had style 3, size 3 implants placed and is noted to have less dimpling of the skin and a much smoother contour. Although not a perfect solution, patients with sagging skin may benefit from augmentation to fill out the region. The patient is seen preoperative and 4 months postoperative.

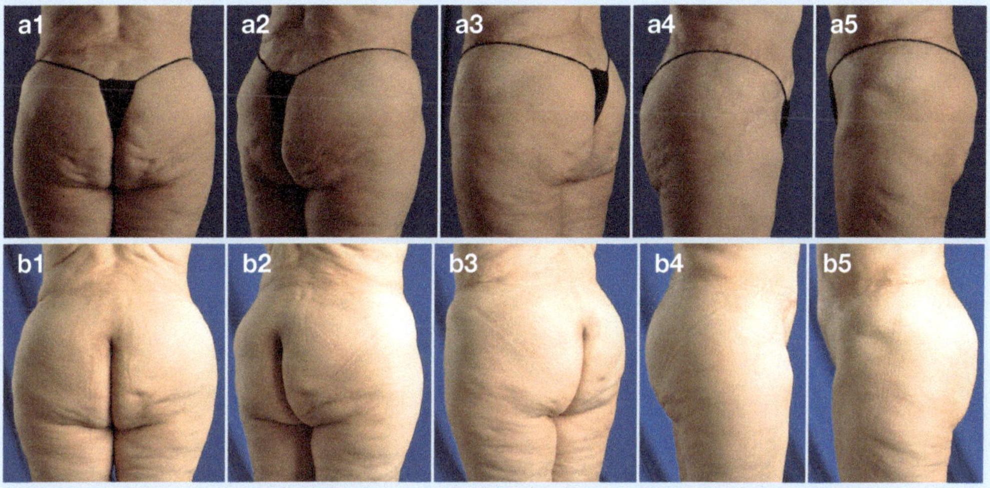

Fig. 6.60 (**a**) Preoperative. (**b**) Postoperative

Case 18 (Fig. 6.61)

A 22-year-old female underwent liposuction of the hips (300 mL of fat) along with buttock augmentation with style 3, size 2 implants. The patient is seen preoperative and 1.5 months postoperative.

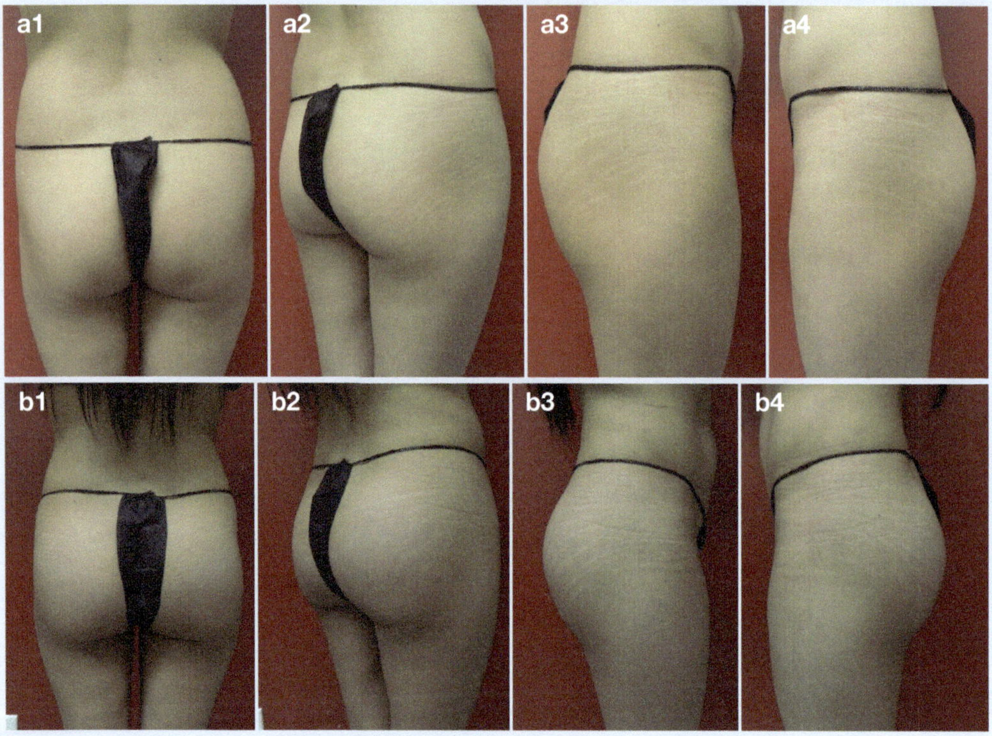

Fig. 6.61 (**a**) Preoperative. (**b**) Postoperative

Case 19 (Fig. 6.62)

A 28-year-old female presented for consultation after having lost 100 lb with bariatric surgery. She had significant skin laxity, sagging of the buttocks, and severely depressed trochanteric depressions. She wanted to improve the contour of her buttocks and did not want to undergo a buttock lift with significant scarring. She elected to proceed with buttock augmentation with style 3, size 3 implants. She is seen preoperative and 5 months postoperative.

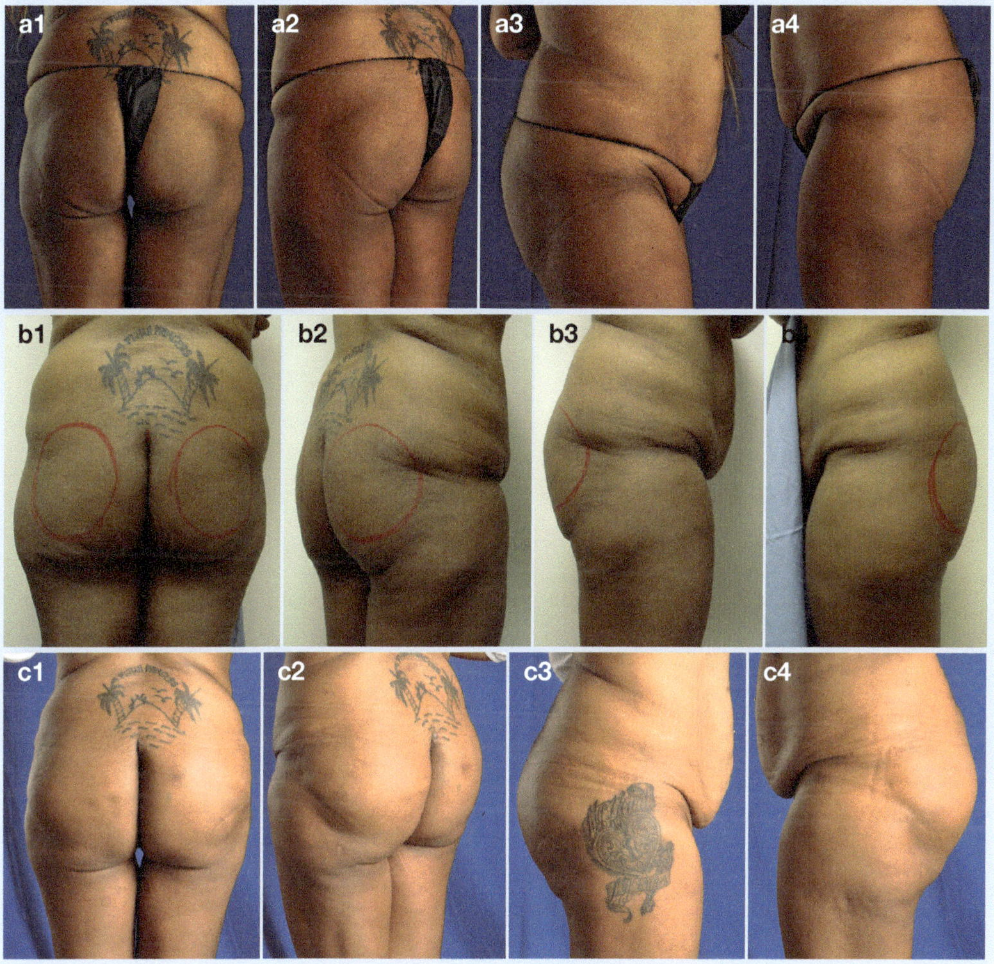

Fig. 6.62 (**a**) Preoperative. (**b**) Marking. (**c**) Postoperative

Case 20 (Fig. 6.63)
A 28-year-old gay male underwent buttock augmentation to have a rounder bottom. He had style 3, size 7 implants placed. The patient is seen preoperative and 3 months postoperative.

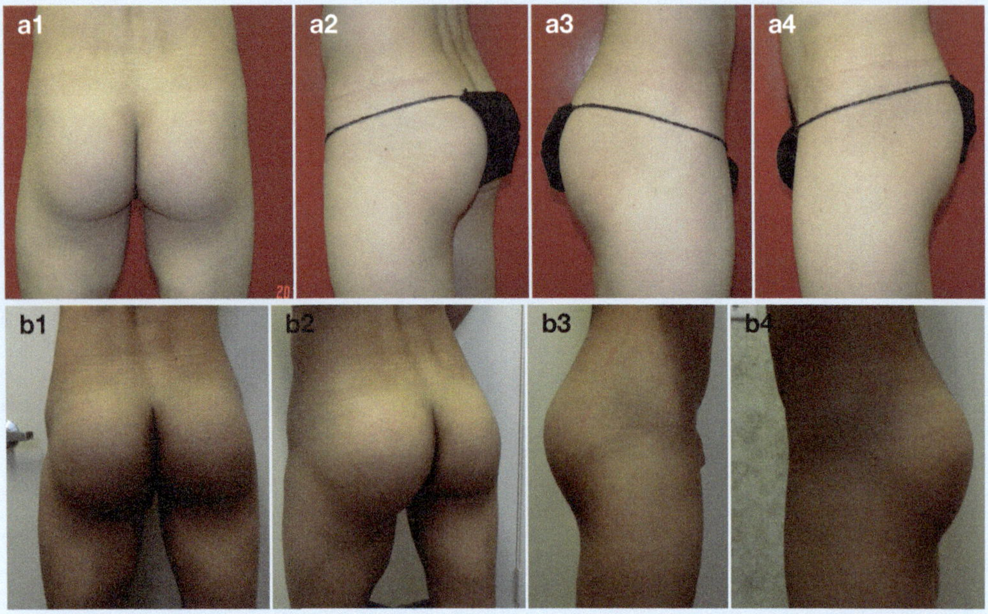

Fig. 6.63 (**a**) Preoperative. (**b**) Postoperative

Case 21 (Fig. 6.64)
A 23-year-old female underwent buttock augmentation with style 3, size 3 implants. The patient is seen preoperative and 1 month postoperative.

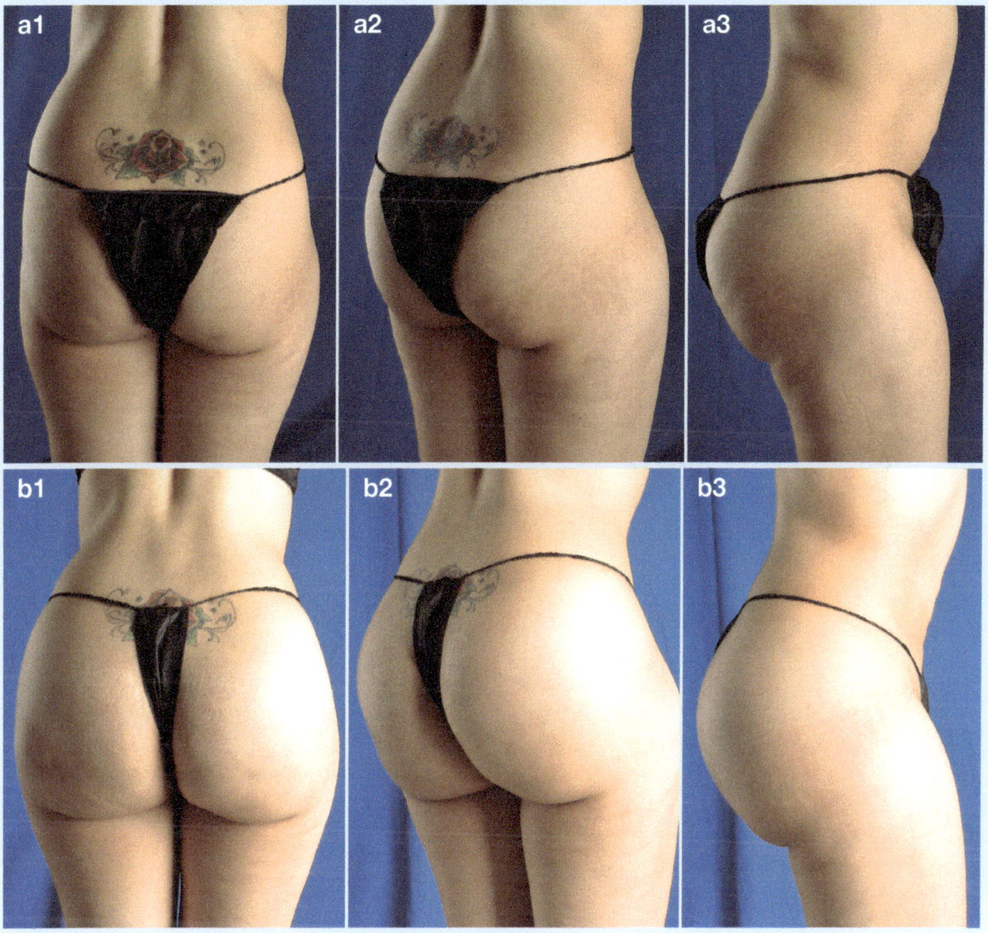

Fig. 6.64 (**a**) Preoperative. (**b**) Postoperative

Case 22 (Fig. 6.65)

A 52-year-old male underwent buttock augmentation with style 3, size 7 implants. He is seen preoperative and 3 months postoperative.

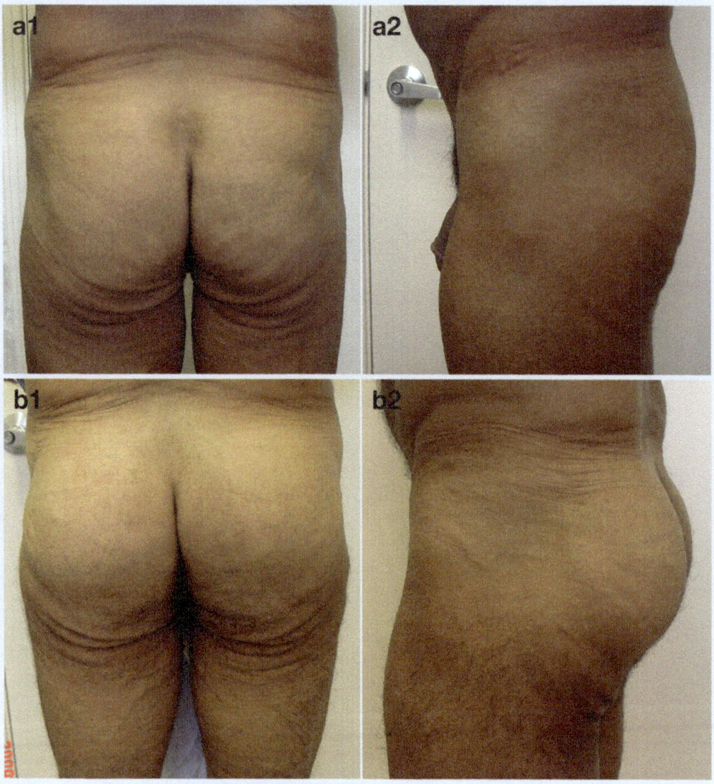

Fig. 6.65 (**a**) Preoperative. (**b**) Postoperative

Case 23 (Fig. 6.66)

A 31-year-old female underwent buttock augmentation with style 3, size 3 (379 mL) implant. One year later she was unhappy with the size of her butt and elected to exchange the implants for larger implants, moving to a style 3, size 9 implant (485 mL), giving her a slightly wider and more projected look. With any case of patients wishing to achieve a greater augmentation, we always have a discussion about staged procedures. It is unlikely that the patient would have tolerated a size 9 implant at the initial augmentation. Staged operations can be performed at an interval of 3–6 months at minimum, allowing sufficient stretch of the pocket to accommodate a larger implant.

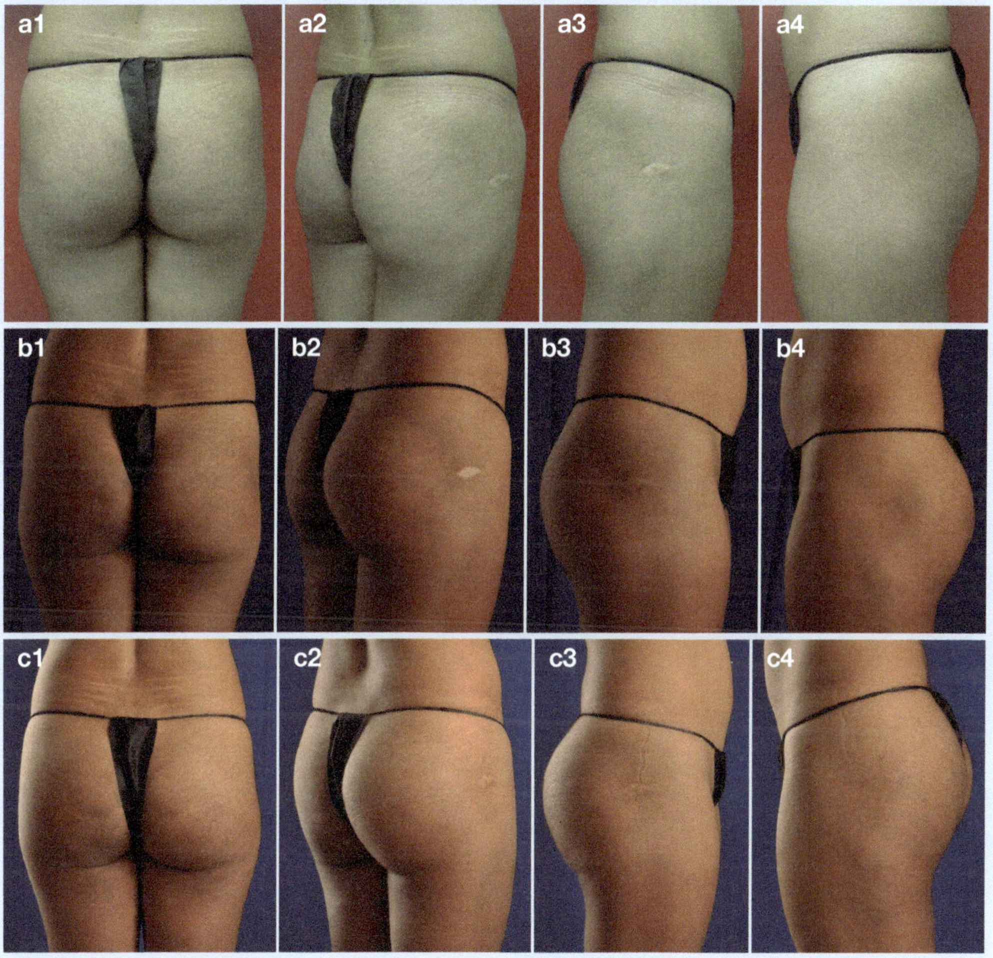

Fig. 6.66 (**a**) Preoperative. (**b**) One year postoperative following first buttock augmentation. (**c**) Postoperative following exchange of implants to larger size

Case 24 (Fig. 6.67)

A 59-year-old male underwent buttock augmentation with style 3, size 3 (379 mL) implants as he felt there was excessive laxity in his buttock region and he had "lost his butt." The patient is seen preoperative and 2 months postoperative.

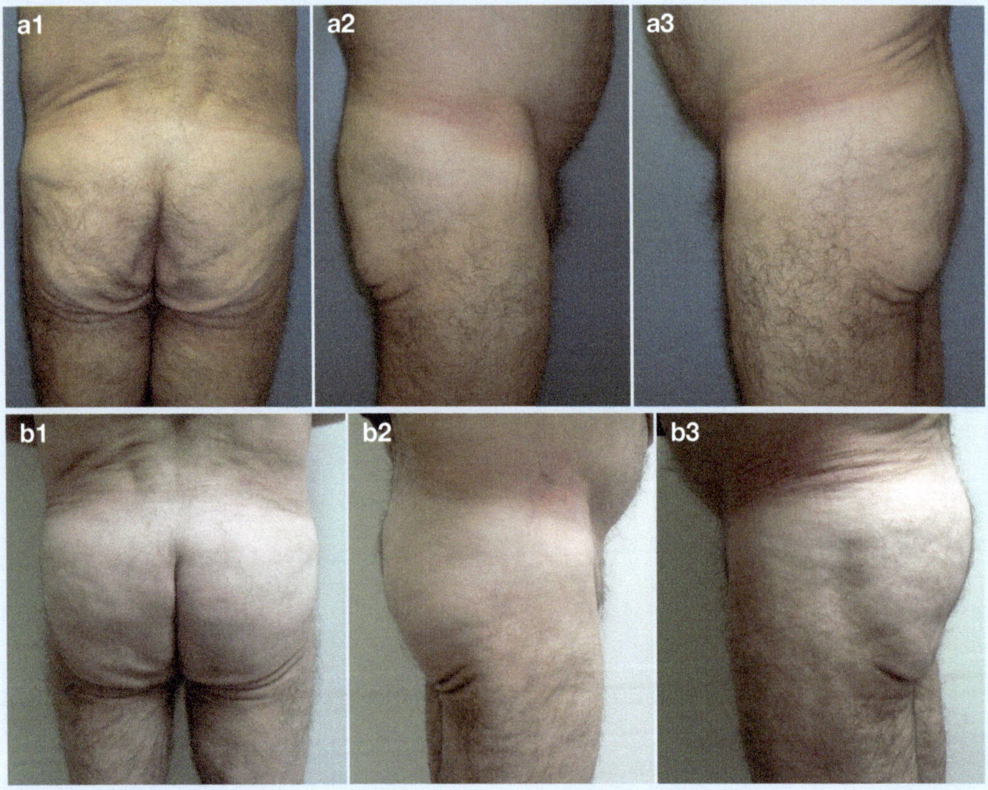

Fig. 6.67 (**a**) Preoperative. (**b**) Postoperative

Case 25 (Fig. 6.68)

A 30-year-old male underwent buttock augmentation with style 3, size 7 implants as he felt that he had no buttock projection. He is seen preoperative and 1 year postoperative.

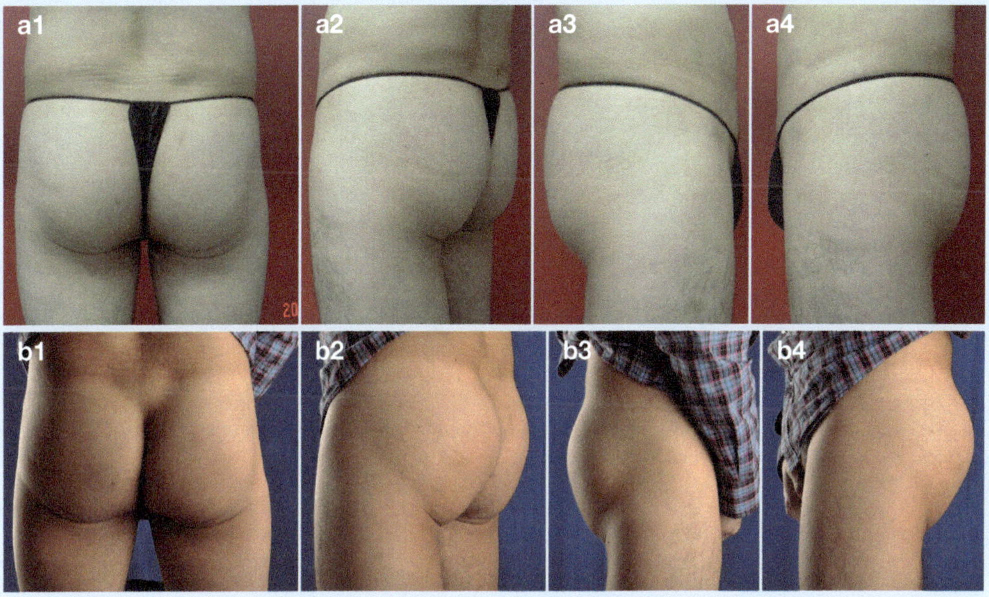

Fig. 6.68 (**a**) Preoperative. (**b**) Postoperative

Conclusions

Buttock augmentation has evolved dramatically from its infancy in the 1970s. Currently the surgeon has several positions to choose from for implant placement: subcutaneous (not recommended), submuscular, intramuscular, intermuscular, and subfascial. The intermuscular position is our preferred technique due to the ample space possible for augmentation, significant implant coverage afforded, and the decreased risk of sciatic injury. While there are various possibilities for incision placement, the intergluteal fold incision affords the best hidden and aesthetically pleasing scar. When considering buttock augmentation, the patient has the option of implant augmentation or augmentation with fat grafting, and the patient should be counseled on the risks and benefits of one procedure over another. Lastly, surgeons should always keep in mind adjunctive procedures to help accentuate the augmentation procedure performed for the patient.

References

1. ASAPS. 2006 Cosmetic Surgery National Data Bank Statistics. New York: ASAPS; 2007.
2. 2012 Plastic surgery statistics report. http://www.plasticsurgery.org/Documents/news-resources/statistics/2012-Plastic-Surgery-Statistics/full-plastic-surgery-statistics-report.pdf. Accessed 14 Sept 2013.
3. 2008 American Academy of Cosmetic Surgery Procedural Census. http://multivu.prnewswire.com/mnr/aacs/36867/docs/36867AACS2008ProceduralSurveyResults.pdf. Accessed 14 Sept 2013.
4. Singh D. Universal allure of the hourglass figure: an evolutionary theory of female physical attractiveness. Clin Plast Surg. 2006;33(3):359–70.
5. Lee EI, Roberts TL, Bruner TW. Ethnic considerations in buttock aesthetics. Semin Plast Surg. 2009;23(3):232–42.
6. Cardenas-Camarena L, Paillet JC. Combined gluteoplasty: liposuction and gluteal implants. Plast Reconstr Surg. 2007;119(3):1067–74.
7. Centeno RF. Gluteal aesthetic unit classification: a tool to improve outcomes in body contouring. Aesthetic Surg J. 2006;26(2):200–8.

8. Mendieta CG. Classification system for gluteal evaluation. Clin Plast Surg. 2006;33(3):333–46.
9. Bartels RJ, O'Malley JE, Douglas WM, Wilson RG. An unusual use of the Cronin breast prosthesis. Plast Reconstr Surg. 1969;44(5):500.
10. Cocke WM, Ricketson G. Gluteal augmentation. Plast Reconstr Surg. 1973;52(1):93.
11. Douglas WM, Bartels RJ, Baker JL. An experience in aesthetic buttocks augmentation. Clin Plast Surg. 1975;2(3):471.
12. Buchuk L. Gluteoplastia de aumento. Cir Plast Iberolatinoamericana. 1980;6(1):29.
13. Robles JM, Tagliaprietra JC, Grandi MA. Gluteoplastia de aumento: implantes submusculares. Cir Plast Iberolatinoamericana. 1984;10:4.
14. Gonzalez Ulloa M. Gluteoplasty: a ten year report. Aesthetic Plast Surg. 1991;15(1):85–91.
15. Vergara R, Amezcua H. Intramuscular gluteal implants: 15 years' experience. Aesthet Surg J. 2003;23(2):86–91.
16. Gonzalez Ulloa M. A review of the present status of the correction for sagging buttocks. In: Annals of the IV Congress of the International Society of Aesthetic Plastic Surgery, Mexico City, Apr 1977.
17. Chugay N. Modification of buttock augmentation. Am J Cosmet Surg. 1997;14(4):405–11.
18. Vergara R, Marcos M. Intramuscular gluteal implants. Aesthetic Plast Surg. 1996;20(3):259–62.
19. Bortoluzzi Daniel MJ, Maluf I. What is the durability of gluteal prostheses? Rev Bras Cir Plast. 2012;27(1):93–6.
20. Peren PA, Gomez JB, Guerrerosantos J, Salazar CA. Gluteus augmentation with fat grafting. Aesthetic Plast Surg. 2000;24(6):412–7.
21. de la Pena JA. Subfascial technique for gluteal augmentation. Aesthet Surg J. 2004;24(32):265–73.
22. Gonzalez R. Augmentation gluteoplasty: the XYZ method. Aesthetic Plast Surg. 2004;28(6):417–25.
23. Mendieta C. Intramuscular buttock implant augmentation. In: Presented at the annual meeting of the American Society of Plastic Surgery, Chicago, 27 Sept 2005.
24. Badin A, Vieira J. Endoscopically assisted buttocks augmentation. Aesthetic Plast Surg. 2007;31(6):651–6.
25. De la Pena JA, Rubio OV, Cano JP, Cedillo MC, Garces MT. History of gluteal augmentation. Clin Plast Surg. 2006;33(3):307–19.
26. Rocha R. Surgical anatomy of the gluteal region's subcutaneous screen and its use in plastic surgery. Aesthetic Plast Surg. 2001;25(2):140–4.
27. Gray H. Anatomy of the human body. Philadelphia: Lea & Febiger; 1918.
28. Pan WR, Taylor GI. The angiosomes of the thigh and buttock. Plast Reconstr Surg. 2009;123(1):79–86.
29. Clawson DK, Seddon HJ. The late consequences of sciatic nerve injury. J Bone Joint Surg. 1960;42(2):213–26.
30. Senderoff DM. Buttock augmentation using solid silicone implants. Aesthet Surg J. 2011;31(3):3200–327.
31. Mendietta CG. Gluteoplasty. Aesthetic Surg J. 2003;23(6):441–55.
32. Ford RD, Simpson WD. Massive extrication of traumatically ruptured buttock silicone prosthesis. Ann Plast Surg. 1992;29(1):86–8.
33. Alperovich M, Schreiber J, Singh NK. Infection after augmentation gluteoplasty in a pregnant patient. Aesthet Surg J. 2007;27(6):622–5.
34. Buchuk L. Complication with gluteal prosthesis. Plast Reconstr Surg. 1986;77(6):1012.
35. Chugay PN, Chugay NV. Buttock augmentation with implants and fat grafting: a comparative study. Am J Cosmet Surg. 2012;29(3):180–6.
36. Bruner TW, Roberts 3rd TL, Nguyen K. Complications of buttocks augmentation: diagnosis, management and prevention. Clin Plast Surg. 2006; 33(3):449–66.
37. Cardenas-Camarena L, Lacouture AM, Tobar-Losada A. Combined gluteoplasty: liposuction and lipoinjection. Plast Reconstr Surg. 1999;104(5): 1524–31.
38. Wang HD, Zheng JH, Deng CL, Liu QY, Yang SL. Fat embolism syndromes following liposuction. Aesthetic Plast Surg. 2008;32(5):731–6.
39. Mellor A, Soni N. Fat embolism. Anesthesia. 2001; 56(2):145–54.
40. Henson JT, Roberts CS, Giannoudis PV. Gluteal compartment syndrome. Acta Orthop Belg. 2009;75(2): 147–52.
41. Coleman SR. Long-term survival of fat transplants: controlled demonstration. Aesthetic Plast Surg. 1995;19(5):421–5.
42. Aiache AE. Gluteal re-contouring with combination treatments: implants, liposuction, and fat transfer. Clin Plast Surg. 2006;33(3):395–403.
43. Coleman SR. Structural fat grafting: more than a permanent filler. Plast Reconstr Surg. 2006;118(3 Suppl): 108S–20.
44. Coleman SR. Facial augmentation with structural fat grafting. Clin Plast Surg. 2006;33(4):567–77.
45. Niechajev I, Sevcuk O. Long term results of fat transplantation: clinical and histological studies. Plast Reconstr Surg. 1994;94(3):496–506.
46. Cardenas-Camarena L, Silva Gavarrete JF, Arenas-Quintana R. Gluteal contour improvement: different surgical alternatives. Aesthetic Plast Surg. 2011;35(6): 1117–25.
47. Pereira LH, Radwanski HN. Fat grafting of the buttocks and lower limbs. Aesthetic Plast Surg. 1996;20(5):409–16.
48. Harrison D, Selvaggi GJ. Gluteal augmentation surgery: indications and surgical management. Plast Reconstr Aesthet Surg. 2007;60(8):922–8.
49. Pedroza LV. Fat transplantation to the buttocks and legs for aesthetic enhancement or correction of deformities: long term results of large volumes of fat transplant. Dermatol Surg. 2000;26(12):1145–9.
50. Restrepo JC, Ahmed JA. Large volume lipoinjection for gluteal augmentation. Aesthetic Surg J. 2002; 22(1):33–8.
51. Murillo WL. Buttock augmentation: case studies of fat injection monitored by magnetic resonance imaging. Plast Reconstr Surg. 2004;114(6): 1606–14.
52. Har-Shai Y, Lindenbaum ES, Gamliel-Lazarovich A, Beach D, Hirshowitz B. An integrated approach for increasing the survival of autologous fat grafts in the treatment of contour defects. Plast Reconstr Surg. 1999;104(4):945–54.
53. Guerrerosantos J. Autologous fat grafting for body contouring. Clin Plast Surg. 1996;23(4):619–31.

Hip/Thigh Augmentation

7

Introduction

Over the course of time, what makes a woman beautiful and sexually attractive has changed. In the days of antiquity, a woman's worth or beauty was largely attached to her ability to produce offspring. Since ovulation is not something that can be visualized by the naked eye, men have long used external cues to determine fecundity and health in females. Women with wider, "childbearing" hips were noted to be more attractive. This fascination with the curvaceous female is well demonstrated in the art of the Baroque era. Peter Paul Rubens (1577–1640) was a German-born Flemish Baroque painter and a proponent of an extravagant Baroque style that emphasized movement, color, and sensuality. He was made famous for his love of portraying full-figured women that were curvaceous in their form, giving rise to the term "Rubenesque" when referring to plus-sized women. Over time, the concept of beauty changed from the more full-figured, curvaceous woman depicted by Rubens to an appreciation of the smaller figured, slender female [1]. Western cultures particularly began to idealize slimness and associated this with elegance, attractiveness, self-control, and youth. These women have been immortalized in the fashion magazines of the 1970s, 1980s, and 1990s. However, it seems of late that there has been a renewed interest in women with a more natural and curvaceous figure. Popular music and television icons such as Shakira, Jennifer Lopez, and Kim Kardashian have produced resurgence in the idea that the attractive woman has a more curvy appearance. A woman with a round bottom and curvy hips and thighs has again become sexy and a sign of true femininity. Although the amount of total fat that determines a maximally attractive female can vary from society to society and between time periods, it is clear that a curvy rather than straight female figure is still very important in identifying an attractive female form. For that reason, liposculpture has remained one of the top 5 most sought after cosmetic procedures among women, according to the American Society of Plastic Surgeons and the American Academy of Cosmetic Surgery [2, 3]. Liposculpture allows a surgeon to carve out a more pleasing figure even if the body mass index is not significantly changed. However, some women do not have the underlying boney and muscular structure to give them the desired curvy look or perhaps do not have sufficient fat to allow for lipo-contouring. To that end, hip implants have been introduced to help give women curves in the hip and lateral thigh area which could not have otherwise been created due to existing patient anatomy.

Waist-to-Hip Ratio

When discussing the curves that are deemed attractive in a female, one must have a discussion of the waist-to-hip ratio. The waist-to-hip ratio (WHR) is the ratio of the circumference of the waist to that of the hips. The World Health Organization (WHO) recommends that the waist

N.V. Chugay et al., *Body Sculpting with Silicone Implants*,
DOI 10.1007/978-3-319-04957-1_7,

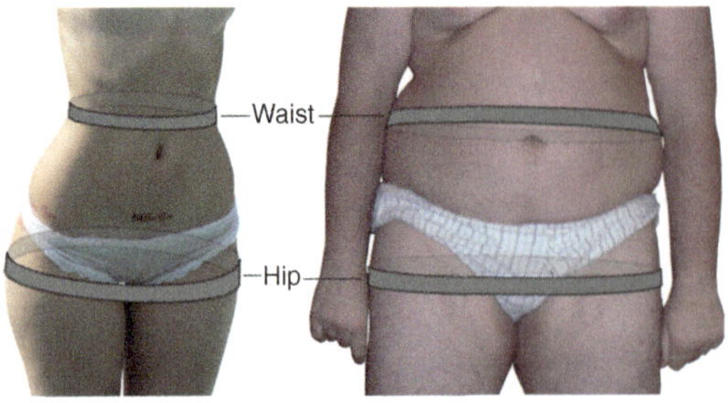

Fig. 7.1 Measurement of waist-to-hip ratio: in a lean person (*left*), the waist can be measured at its narrowest point, while for a person with a convex waist (*right*), it may be measured at about one inch above the navel. The hip is measured at its widest portion of the buttocks at *left* and at the greater trochanters at *right*

circumference be measured at the midpoint between the lower margin of the last palpable rib and the top of the iliac crest. Hip circumference should be measured around the widest portion of the buttocks or at the level of the greater trochanter (Fig. 7.1) [4, 5].

The WHR is frequently used as a measure of health risk as noted by the WHO and National Institute of Diabetes and Digestive and Kidney Diseases (NIDDK) [9]. A healthy WHR is between 0.67 and 0.80 in a healthy premenopausal woman and between 0.85 and 0.95 for a healthy adult male. The WHO and NIDDK have determined that a WHR above 0.95 in males and above 0.85 in females is associated with obesity and an increased risk of major diseases such as diabetes mellitus and coronary artery disease. Studies have found that women with a WHR of approximately 0.7 had optimal levels of estrogen and are less susceptible to diabetes, cardiovascular disorders, and ovarian cancers [6]. There has even been research that has found that the WHR was a more efficient predictor of mortality in older patients than waist circumference or body mass index [7]. Yusuf et al. [8], based on his evaluation of 27,000 participants, noted that if obesity were redefined using WHR instead of BMI that the proportion of people categorized as at risk of heart attack worldwide increases by threefold.

Along with being a method of assessing general health, the WHR has long been used as a measure of attractiveness. Due to hormonal changes during puberty, women preferentially deposit fat in the gluteofemoral region, while men tend to have an inhibition of fat deposition in the gluteofemoral region and deposit preferentially in the abdomen. This then gives women a low WHR closer to 0.7, while men typically have WHR closer to 0.9. As women age and fertility declines, skin laxity increases and the shape of the gluteal region usually changes as the content and distribution of fat and muscle change. The female hourglass shape fades and the waist-to-hip ratio approaches 1.0, similar to men, which in studies has been shown to give the female a less attractive score when evaluated by study participants [9]. Singh, an evolutionary psychologist, has argued in multiple articles since 1993 that the WHR is a significant measure of female attractiveness. Looking back at the women of ancient civilizations globally, female representations were most often in the range of a WHR of 0.6–0.7, suggesting a preference toward lower WHR in females. In the modern era, women who have a ratio near 0.7 are usually rated more attractive by men from European cultures [10]. Icons of the silver screen such as Marilyn Monroe and Sophia Loren, long touted as pinnacles of beauty, had a WHR close to 0.7 [10–12]. Singh [11] proposed a hypothesis to explain how WHR influences female attractiveness and its role in mate selection, citing evidence from studies of the WHR of Playboy playmates and Miss America winners over the past 30 years to support her work. Her hypothesis was plain and simple: regardless of time period or culture, a female with an hourglass figure as defined by the WHR near 0.7 was sexually attractive in practically all human societies. In a 2010 article, Platek and Singh [13] used functional magnetic resonance imaging (MRI) to demonstrate that male participants looking at naked female bodies with an ideal WHR (approx 0.7) showed excitation in the anterior cingulate cortex, an area associated with reward processing and decision making. To further evaluate the WHR as a signal of attractiveness, Dixson et al. [14] conducted a study using eye-tracking techniques to evaluate men's fixation on digitally altered photographs of the same women. When asked to evaluate attractiveness, the men reliably chose women that had a larger breast size. However, regardless of breast size, women who had a WHR of 0.7 were rated as the most attractive. These studies all point to the premise that men appreciate curvy women and help us understand the change in modern culture toward the desire for a more shapely and voluptuous woman.

Women have gone to great lengths in the past to alter their WHR. The corset during the Victorian era (despite internal injuries caused to women) was popular as a tool to reduce a woman's waist size to make her more physically attractive. Some women have resorted to hip and buttock padding to increase the apparent size of the hips and buttocks. Female cosmetic patients routinely employ liposculpture to help redefine their waist area. Of late, buttock augmentation with both fat and implants has been another means by which a woman can increase the curves in the lower pole of the body to help achieve a more aesthetically pleasing figure. Now, there is a way of providing a permanent solution for women who wish to increase their hip size to better suit the remainder of their figure and thereby alter their existing waist-to-hip ratio, potentially making them more attractive.

History of the Procedure

Based on a review of the literature, it seems that many physicians around the globe have been working concurrently in the past 2 years to produce a more aesthetic appearance to the hip/lateral thigh region using silicone prostheses [15–18].

The idea of reconstructing the thigh with a prosthesis was first introduced in 1995 by Kon et al. [19]. At that time, he published a paper explaining his experience with placement of a new type of implant for augmentation of the lateral thigh. A paraplegic patient was noted to have significant lateral thigh deficiency and was deemed a suitable candidate for reconstruction with a silicone prosthesis, measuring 29×7 cm. This implant was placed below the fascia lata. In 2005, Anger [20] presented his work on three patients who had medial thigh augmentation with calf implants for asymmetric medial thigh regions. He placed calf implants in the medial thigh via incisions made in the gluteal fold. The implants themselves were placed in a space that was dissected between the gracilis and adductor magnus muscles. Two patients received implants measuring 180 mL and a third patient received an implant with a volume of 140 mL. There were no complications noted and the results were satisfactory.

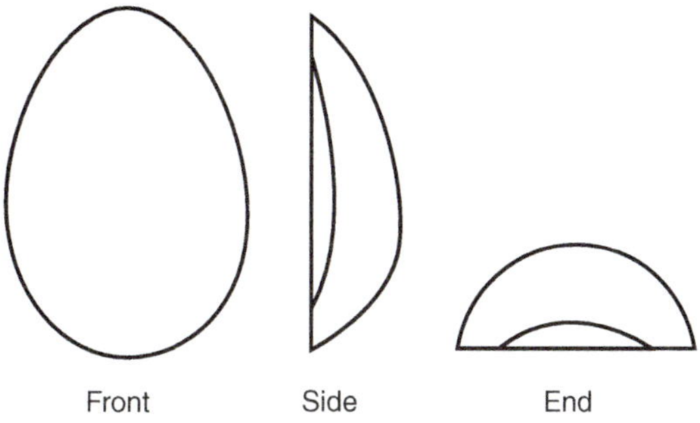

Fig. 7.2 Chugay hip prosthesis

In 2011, several surgeons presented the results of their work over the preceding years, making it clear that thigh augmentation was definitely a surgery in evolution [16–18]. The first of the three studies to be published was our own institutions initial description of the procedure published in 2011 [18]. The authors evaluated the results of 18 hip augmentations since first beginning the procedure in 2010. In that paper the results were discussed with placement of a semirigid silicone prosthesis below the fascia lata via a lateral hip incision and noted only one significant complication: a case of suspected compartment syndrome. All 18 patients, however, had excellent aesthetic results and were happy with the procedure performed once recovery was complete. The implant used in our study was an oblong-shaped implant, designed by Nikolas Chugay, specifically for addition of volume and curvature to the lateral hip/thigh region (Fig. 7.2). In 2011, Netto [16] published his work on 68 patients who had placement of a silicone prosthesis in the lateral hip/thigh region. His work is a mix of patients being treated for poliomyelitis and those seeking more shapely thighs for purely aesthetic reasons. His paper also differs in the fact that the majority of his patients (94 %) had placement of medial thigh prostheses, and only four patients (6 %) had implants placed in the lateral aspect. Implants used in his procedures were of an elliptical shape, similar to those seen for calf augmentation. His implants varied in dimensions from 23 to 29 cm in length and 4–6 cm in width. His implants ranged in volume from 140 to 290 mL. In 2011 Cardak et al. [17] reported on his lateral thigh augmentation with a suprafascial approach to implant placement. The patient described was a 42-year-old female who had suffered a thigh deformity because of childhood orthopedic surgery, secondary to muscle atrophy and significant scarring. Similar to the work of Netto, Cardak used an asymmetrical silicone gel-filled calf prosthesis with more bulk at the cephalad aspect. His technique also used two incisions for placement of a 150 mL implant.

Clearly, the field of thigh augmentation is in its infancy, and further long-term and large-volume studies are necessary to fully ascertain the long-term results, determine the best position for the implant, and assess the long-term ramifications of this surgery.

Indications

The hip implant, used in the authors' practice, is designed to improve the aesthetic contour of the hip/lateral thigh region. First introduced as a means to correct a congenital anatomic deformity, the hip implant can be used to treat deformities due to trauma, disease, or after surgical procedures. Transgender patients are excellent candidates for hip augmentation to correct a naturally male form and produce more curvature in the lateral portion of the hip/thigh region. Asian women frequently lack fullness in the hips and do not have sufficient fat to perform a fat grafting procedure are excellent candidates for hip augmentation. Although a depression over the greater trochanter is natural, many females wish to accentuate this region and fill out the area to give them a more prominent curvature and benefit from the use of a hip implant.

Contraindications

A relative contraindication to placement of a hip implant would be a patient who is very thin and has little adipose tissue. This contraindication is relative only because it may allow for a palpable implant postoperatively, which is an often undesired complication of muscle augmentation surgery. Also, another relative contraindication would be previous surgery in the lateral hip/thigh region that may have compromised blood flow, as in major oncologic procedures or surgery after trauma. It is at the surgeon's discretion to determine if a particular candidate can safely undergo surgery without major risk of compromise to tissues in the area.

Limitations

The surgeon is limited in the extent to which the lateral hip/thigh compartment can be augmented only by the implants currently available. Through work with our implant manufacturer, we have been able to create custom implants to augment larger segments of tissue. This, however, does come at an increased cost to the patient.

Relevant Anatomy

The anatomy in the lateral hip/thigh region that is encountered in the typical dissection is the area of relevant anatomy.

The tensor fascia lata (TFL) is a small muscle that lies in the middle and upper outer thigh. It arises from the anterior part of the outer lip of the iliac crest and inserts along the iliotibial tract at the middle third of the thigh. The tensor fascia lata then becomes continuous with the iliotibial band, which is a thick band of fascia that extends along the lateral thigh from the iliac crest to the knee (Fig. 7.3). The iliotibial band is inserted into the lateral condyle of the tibia (Gerdy's tubercle). The tensor fascia lata assists in flexion and abduction of the thigh. It counteracts the posterior pull from the gluteus maximus muscle on the iliotibial tract. The innervation of the TFL is via the superior gluteal nerve which exits the pelvis at the greater sciatic foramen above the piriformis muscle [21]. It is below this muscle/band that the implant is placed snuggly against the femur to attain a seamless augmentation without high risk of implant palpability.

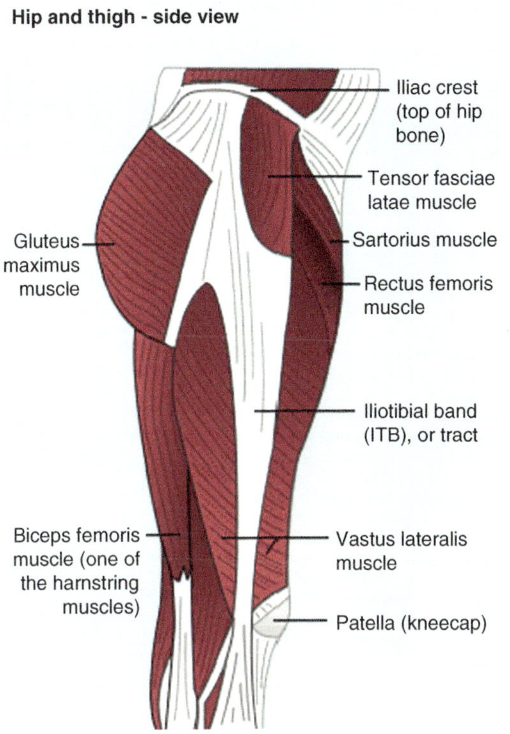

Fig. 7.3 Anatomy of the iliotibial band and tensor fascia lata

The nerve with the greatest potential for injury in this procedure is the lateral femoral cutaneous nerve of the thigh. It is a nerve of the lumbar plexus, arising from the dorsal branches of L2 and L3. The nerve exits the spine and courses anteriorly to cross under the inguinal ligament approximately 2 cm medial to the anterior superior iliac spine (ASIS). Once outside the pelvis, the nerve bifurcates into anterior and posterior branches approximately 5 cm below the ASIS on the surface of the sartorius muscle. The anterior branch becomes superficial about 10 cm below the inguinal ligament, and then it divides into branches that are distributed to the skin of the anterior and lateral parts of the knee. The posterior branch pierces the fascia lata and supplies the skin from the level of the greater trochanter to the middle of the thigh posteriorly [22]. The nerve is subject to injury at the time of dissection of the implant pocket below the fascia lata (Fig. 7.4).

Blood supply to the lateral hip/thigh region is primarily derived from branches of the femoral artery, of which the lateral circumflex femoral artery is the largest contributor (Fig. 7.5). This artery arises from the lateral side of the profunda femoris artery and passes horizontally behind the sartorius and rectus femoris, giving off three branches: ascending, transverse, and descending. The ascending branch then anastomoses with the superior gluteal and deep circumflex iliac artery to ensure a rich blood supply to the lateral hip/thigh region. These vessels are relatively remote from the area of dissection and are not at significant risk of injury if careful blunt dissection is performed and excessive medial dissection is avoided.

Consultation/Implant Selection

A thorough history and physical are paramount to preventing complications at the time of hip/thigh augmentation. During the consultation, patient's expectations are managed and assessment of the patient's mental state is undertaken. It is made clear to the patient the expected augmentation that can be seen with implant placement and limitations of the procedure are also explained.

After completion of the history portion of the consultation, an evaluation of the patient's hip/thigh is made. Any asymmetries or defects are pointed out to the patient. The patient's muscles are then evaluated. The skin and fat content are similarly assessed at this time as a patient with minimal adipose and thin skin is more at risk for implant palpability. Measurements of the patient's thighs and hips are then taken: (1) circumference of the midportion of the thigh, (2) circumference of the waist, (3) circumference around the hips (level of the greater trochanters), and (4) length of the lateral leg from the greater trochanter to the mid-thigh (suspected insertion of the tensor fascia lata). Depending on the patient's physical dimensions and desire for more volume in the lateral thigh regions, three different types of implants can be placed in the subfascial plane (small, medium, large). AART (Aesthetic and Reconstructive Technologies, Inc., Reno, NV) has been able to develop three different implants for the authors' needs measuring 207, 250, and

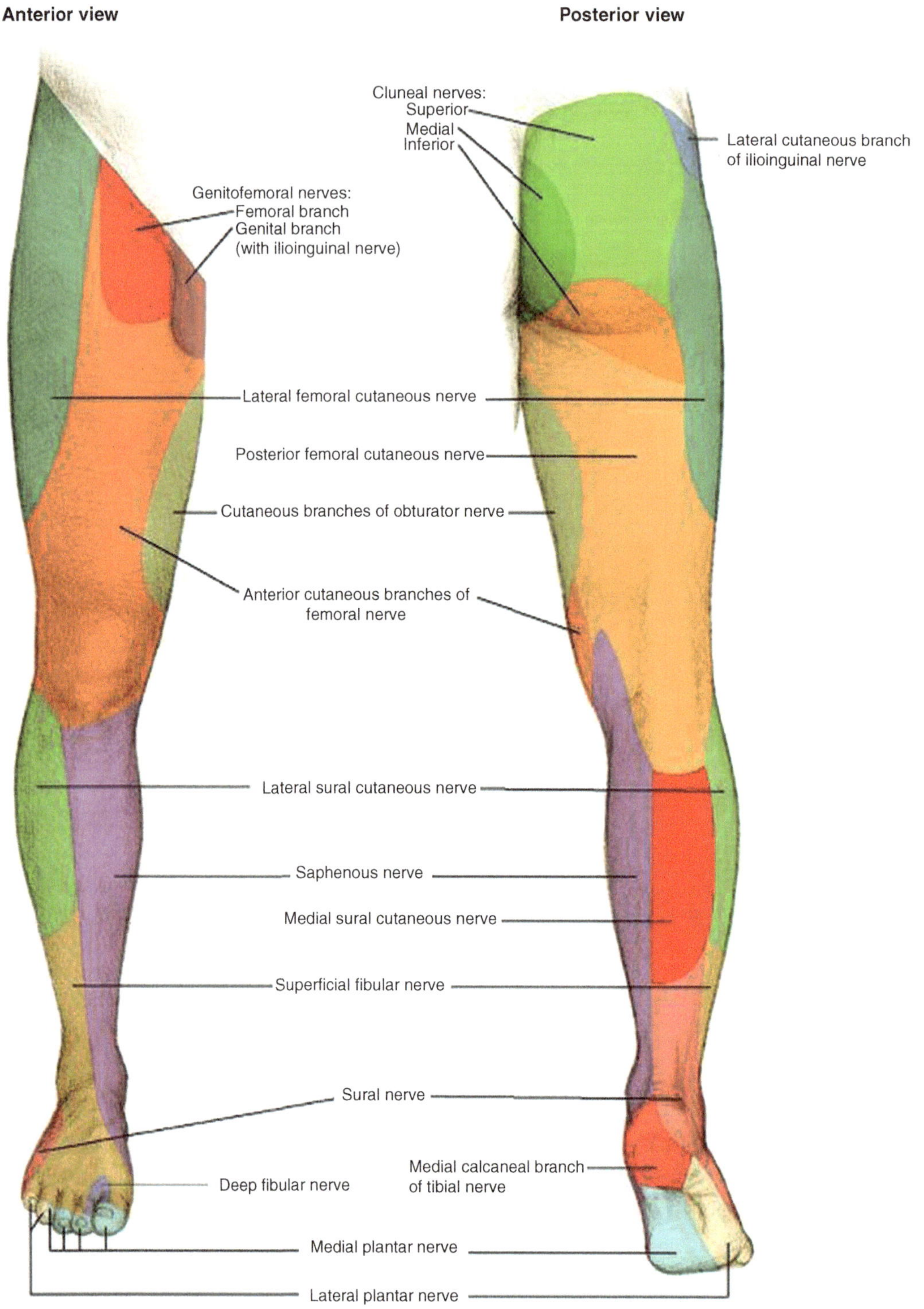

Fig. 7.4 Sensory dermatomes of the lower extremity. Take note of the dermatome relating to the lateral femoral cutaneous nerve as it is the most frequently involved in neuropathy post hip/thigh augmentation

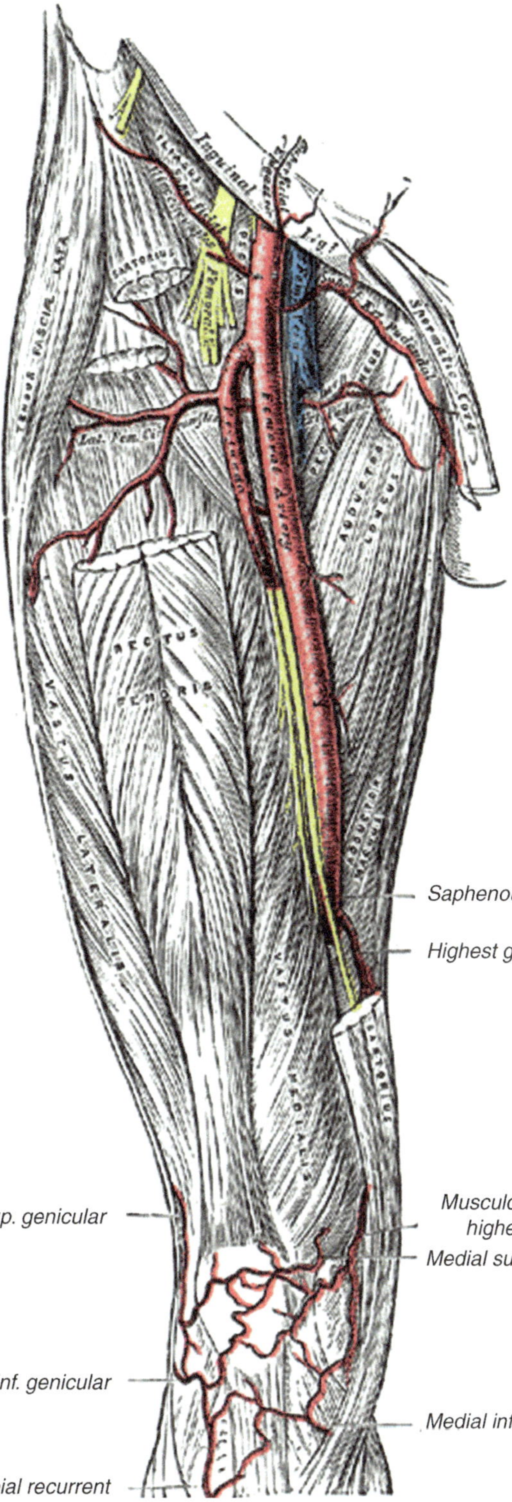

Fig. 7.5 Distribution of the femoral artery. Take note of the lateral branch of the femoral artery, the lateral femoral circumflex artery. It is this artery and its smaller branches that may be inadvertently damaged in the dissection of a pocket for the hip/thigh implant if one is not careful and dissection is carried too far medially

Table 7.1 Hip implants with sizes, dimensions, and volume

Size	Catalog #	Width	Length	Projection	Size (cc)
1	501–101	10.4	15.0	2.5	207
2	501–102	11.0	15.6	3.1	250
3	501–103	13.5	18.0	4.6	545

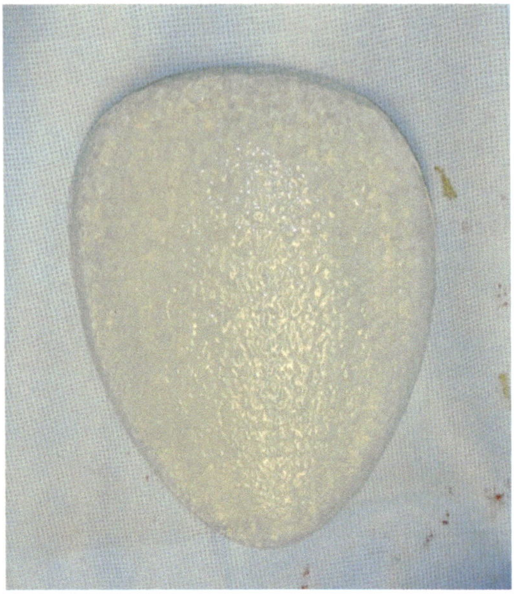

Fig. 7.6 Hip implant prior to implantation

545 mL (Table 7.1) (Fig. 7.6). The ability to place a larger implant is largely based on the length of the leg from the trochanter to the insertion of the tensor fascia lata, and implants should not be chosen that exceed this length.

Preoperative Planning and Marking

On the day of the surgery, the patient is met in the preoperative holding area. It is here that the patient's consent is verified and again risks, benefits, and alternatives are reviewed with the patient. With the patient in the erect position, the proposed site of incision is marked, measuring approximately 5–7 cm. The site of incision should be in line with the patient's bikini line/panty line so as to make the incision as well hidden postoperatively as possible (Fig. 7.7). Once the site of the incision is marked, the site of the proposed implant is marked taking into account the patient's anatomy and existing deficit along with the desires of the patient.

Operative Technique

A 3 cm incision is made in the high lateral aspect of the thigh in a transverse orientation, using a No. 15 Bard-Parker blade (Fig. 7.8). Dissection through the subcutaneous tissues is performed using both blunt and sharp dissection down to the level of the fascia (Fig. 7.9). A transverse incision is made in the fascia overlying the fascia lata muscle using a No. 15 blade (Fig. 7.10). This incision is lengthened using Metzenbaum scissors, and 2-0 Vicryl stay sutures are placed in the fascia lata on both sides (Fig. 7.11). A hemostat is used to divide the fascia lata muscle in line with its fibers. Dissection beneath the fascia lata is performed in a blunt fashion using finger dissection at first, taking care to achieve a level right on top of the femur (Fig. 7.12). A spatula dissector and a hockey-stick dissector are used to further expand the pocket to the edges of the pre-marked implant site just as in gluteal augmentation. Hemostasis is now assessed and attained as necessary with electrocautery. Once the pocket has been completed over the shaft of the femur, it is irrigated with a solution containing Betadine, normal saline, 1 g of cefazolin, and 80 mg of gentamicin. This is suctioned. 10 mL of 0.5 % Marcaine is instilled into the pocket to aid with postoperative pain control. A custom Chugay lateral thigh prosthesis is then placed (Fig. 7.13). Attention is now turned to the other side (Fig. 7.14). The second implant is placed and symmetry is assessed. Adjustments to the implants or the pockets are performed at this time to ensure as symmetric a result as possible. The fascia is then reapproximated using 2-0 Vicryl suture and the subcutaneous tissues are brought together using 3-0 Vicryl suture. The skin is then closed with 4-0 Vicryl suture in subcuticular fashion. The patient is awakened from anesthesia and taken to the recovery room.

During the course of utilizing the hip augmentation technique, the primary surgeon has worked to perfect the technique and has used alternative methods of positioning and incision placement. As an alternative to placement of the incision in

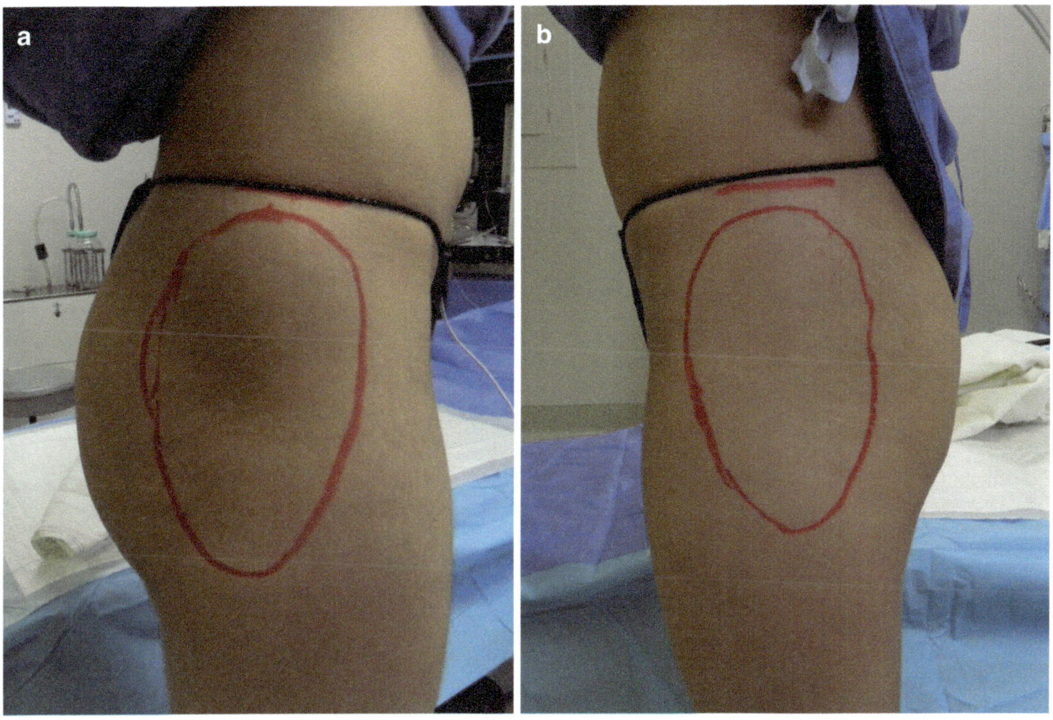

Fig. 7.7 (**a**, **b**) Preoperative markings with locations of incisions and proposed sites of implants

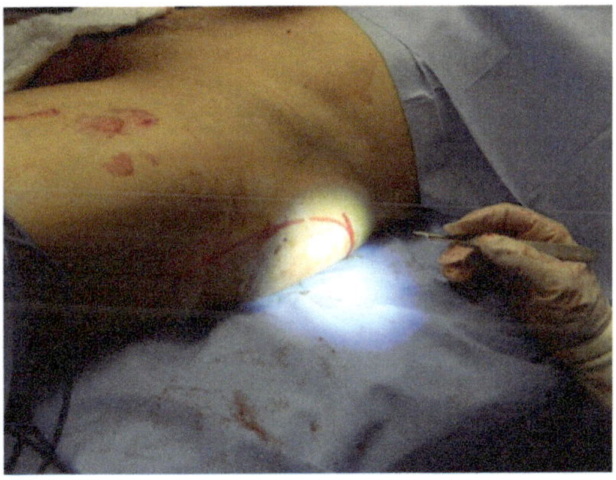

Fig. 7.8 Incision made in the lateral aspect with the site of the proposed implant similarly marked

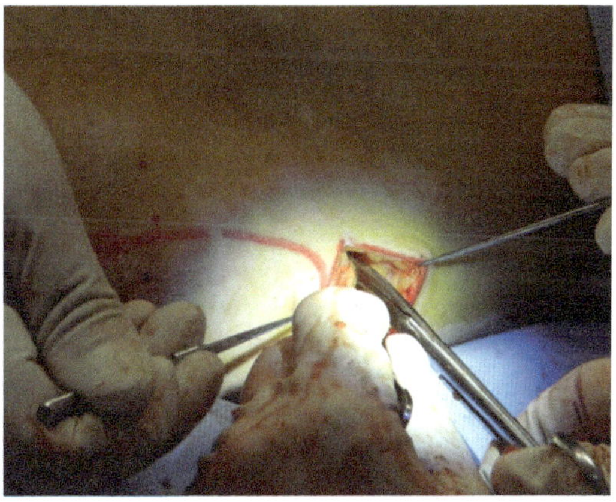

Fig. 7.9 Sharp dissection through the subcutaneous tissues using scissors and electrocautery down to the level of the fascia lata

the lateral hip region, the primary author has used a previous abdominoplasty incision as the site of incision with subsequent dissection laterally to the hip region for placement of the implant (Fig. 7.15). This technique proved to be quite challenging as the placement of the implant was not facile due to the angles created around the edge of the pelvis and greater trochanter. The patient's results were satisfactory; however, the primary author (NVC) has begun to think twice about future uses of the abdominoplasty incision unless the incision has been previously carried wide onto the hips as the dissection over the trochanter, from the anterior aspect, can prove to be quite challenging.

Another variation of the technique has been placement of the patient in the prone position (Fig. 7.16). This technique allows the surgeon

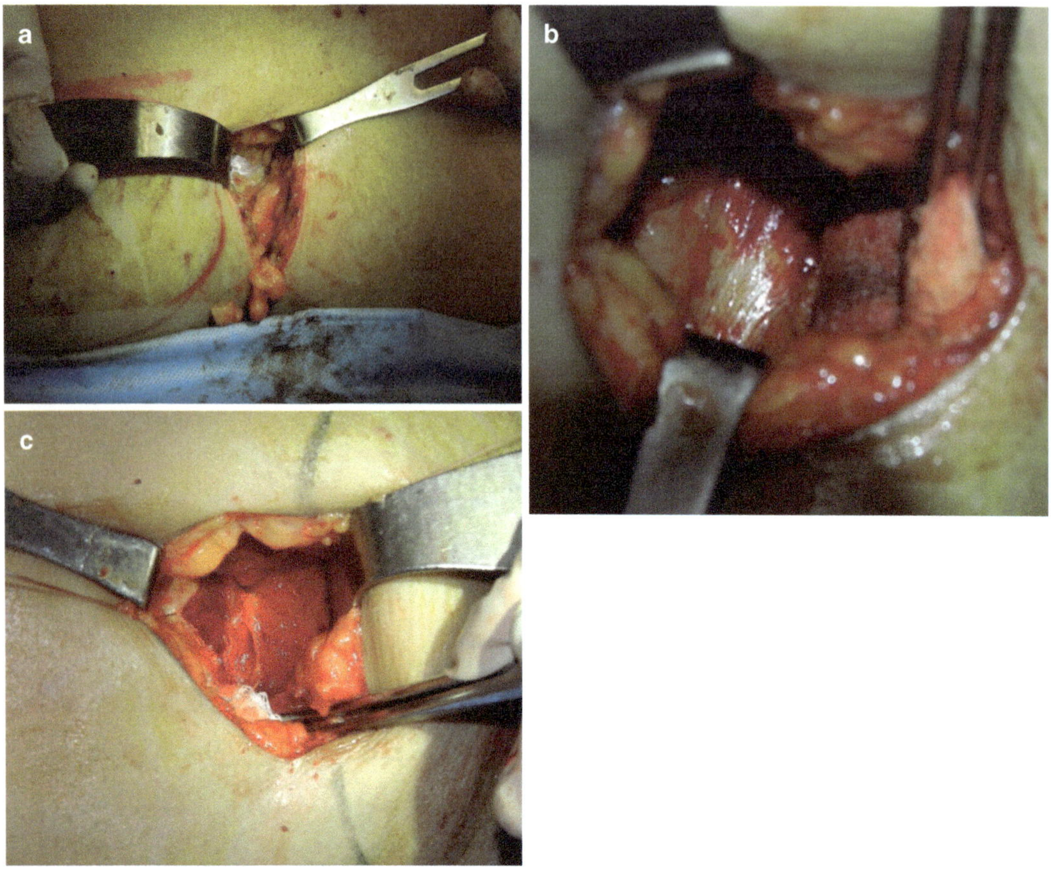

Fig. 7.10 (**a**) Fascia overlying the tensor fascia lata is exposed (glistening). (**b**) Close-up of fascia overlying the tensor fascia lata. (**c**) Incision in fascia exposing the horizontally oriented fibers of the fascia lata muscle (seen at 9 o'clock position with stitch in overlying fascia)

to better dissect in the anterior direction, potentially allowing the surgeon to seat the implant in a more anterior position. This technique was used in a patient who wished to have more prominence anteriorly rather than squarely placed in the lateral aspect of the hip. The patient's results were also noted to be satisfactory, and this remains an option for the surgeon needing to redirect an implant more anteriorly.

Postoperative Care/Instructions

Postoperatively, the patient may begin ambulating starting on the evening of the procedure. They may shower the first postoperative day, making sure to keep dressings clean and dry the Robbins tape with a hair dryer on a low heat setting. If permanent sutures were used by the surgeon, they may be removed at the 1-week-after visit (Fig. 7.17). Patients are then allowed to begin light activity at week 2 and full unrestricted activity at weeks 4–6. Patients are asked to wear an elastic compression garment for 4 weeks postoperatively to prevent dead space, thereby helping to reduce the risk of seroma formation. The legs are to be elevated as much as possible to allow for better lymphatic/venous drainage. Patients are prescribed both narcotic analgesics along with muscle relaxants (diazepam 5 mg every 8 h as needed for spasm) to assist with postoperative pain.

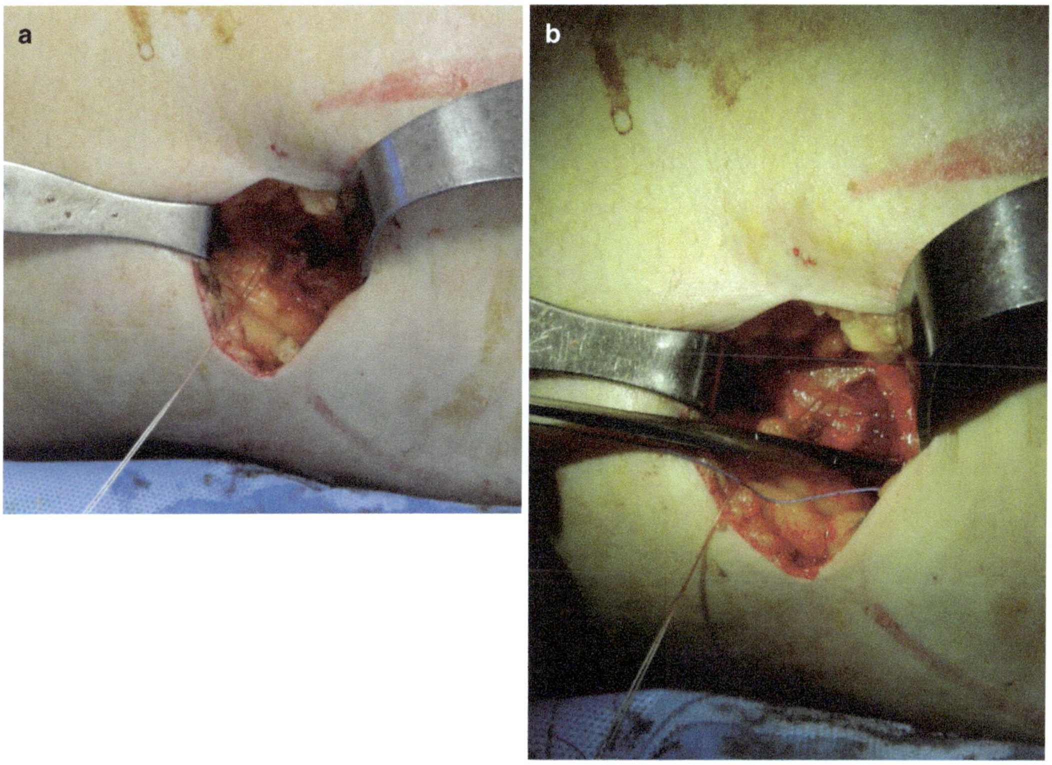

Fig. 7.11 Placement of stay sutures in the fascia overlying the tensor fascia lata. (**a**) Undyed Vicryl suture placed in the upper portion of the fascia (patient's head at 9 o'clock position and feet at 3 o'clock). (**b**) Dyed suture placed in caudal portion of fascia (down)

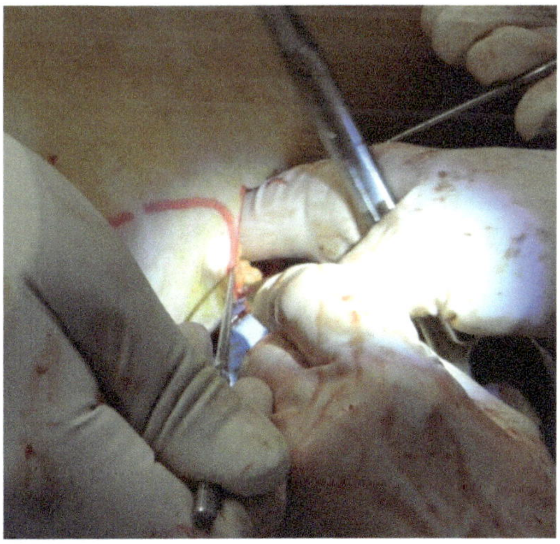

Fig. 7.12 Finger dissection of the pocket below the fascia lata taking care to identify the femur and stay along it

Complications

In performing hip augmentation, there is a host of complications that can arise (Table 7.2).

Infection

Infection, either superficial or deep, is a possibility in hip/lateral thigh augmentation surgery. The most likely culprits would be *Staphylococcus aureus* and *Staphylococcus epidermidis*, relatively common skin flora. Prior to making incision, standard practice should be the administration of 2 g of intravenous (IV) Ancef (or 300 mg IV clindamycin in a penicillin- or cephalosporin-allergic patient). During the procedure, irrigation of the pocket with a standard antibiotic solution

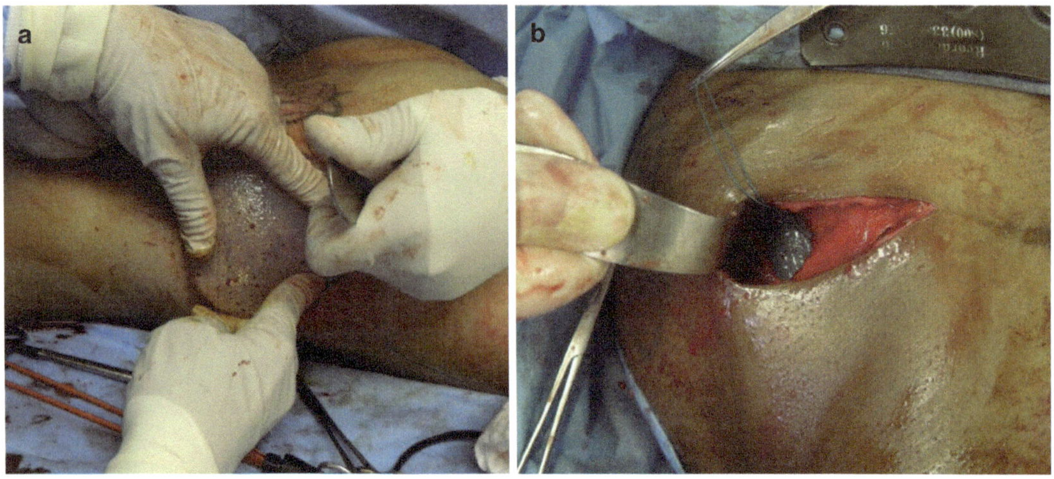

Fig. 7.13 (**a**) Implant being advanced into position. (**b**) Implant in position below the fascia lata muscle

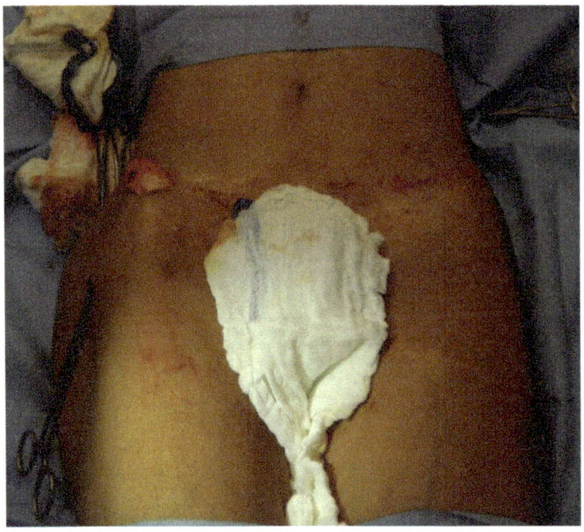

Fig. 7.14 Patient in the supine position with incisions having been made in the previous abdominoplasty incisions. The right side has been augmented and now attention is turned to the contralateral side

containing normal saline, Betadine, Ancef, and gentamicin should be performed. Postoperatively, a 5-day regimen of oral antibiotics covering normal skin flora should be administered (the authors prefer ciprofloxacin 500 mg twice daily for its broad coverage). If a deep infection occurs, the standard of practice is removal of the implant, closure, and possible reimplantation in 3–6 months. There are reports in other forms of implant surgery that conservative management and implant salvage are possible. This should be left at the discretion of the surgeon and performed with careful counseling of the patient.

Seroma

Seromas are statistically the most common complication occurring in implant surgeries. They typically present as new onset pain, swelling, or asymmetry. The treatment of choice remains percutaneous aspiration using aseptic technique. This complication is best prevented with patient compliance with compression garments and proper implant placement at the time of surgery, thereby minimizing dead space.

In the authors' practice, there was one patient with a delayed seroma/hematoma. A 28-year-old female presented 5 years after lateral buttock/hip augmentation with a large seroma development in the right lateral buttock/hip region. The patient had been playing with her niece when the little girl fell on top of her. Shortly thereafter, the patient noted significant swelling in the area that developed over several days. She was taken to the operating room (OR) for removal of hip/lateral buttock implants and was noted to have a significant seroma/hematoma of the right hip region (Fig. 7.18). The patient likely suffered a small capsular tear that produced the hematoma/seroma. No active bleeding was appreciated.

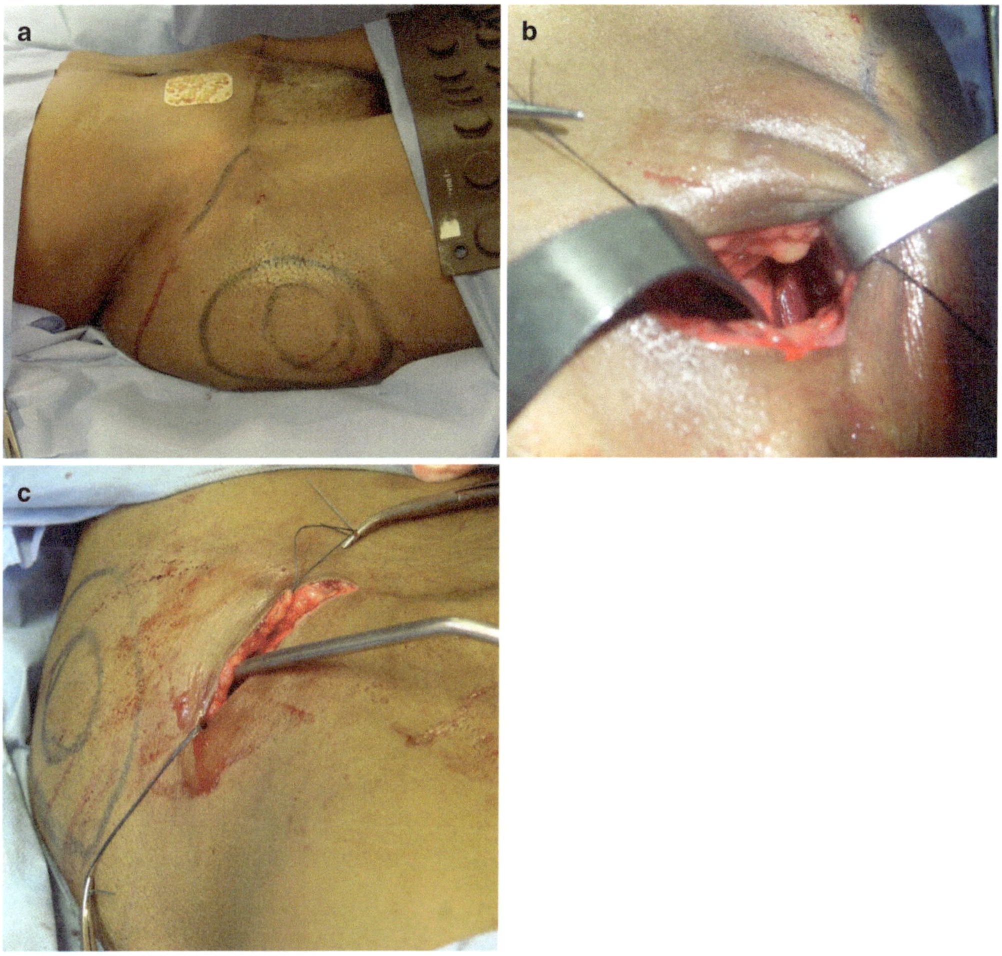

Fig. 7.15 Using abdominoplasty incision for site of entry for hip augmentation. (**a**) Markings delineating site for implant placement and the site of the incision in the skin (in line with tail end of patient's abdominoplasty incision). (**b**) Dissection through subcutaneous tissues and through the fascia of the leg demonstrates the anterior border of the tensor fascia lata muscle at 3 o'clock. (**c**) Dissection of the implant pocket with the aid of a spatula dissector

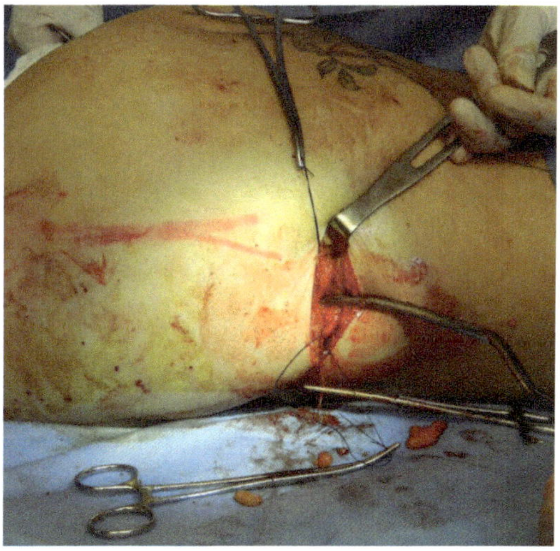

Fig. 7.16 Hip augmentation with the patient in the prone position when a more anterior position of the implant is desired by the patient

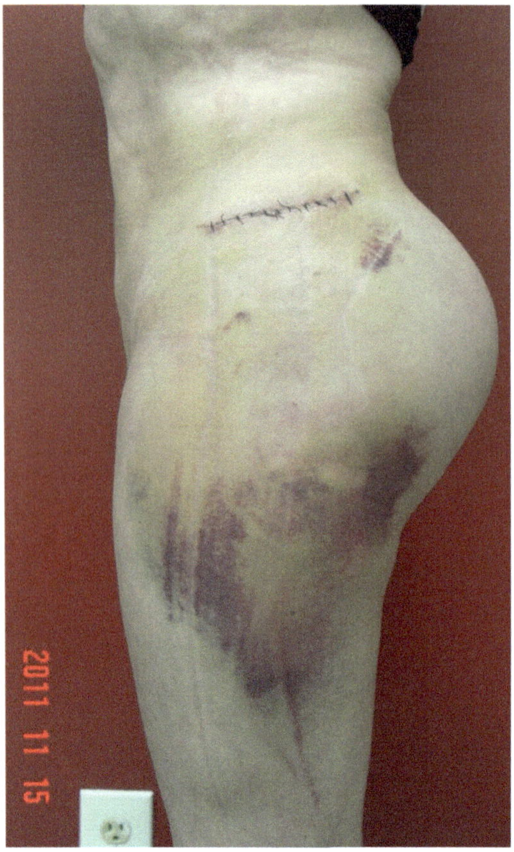

Fig. 7.17 Typical bruising at 1 week after surgery. Permanent sutures noted in position as per surgeon's preference. Since the wound appears clean, removal of the sutures at this time would be appropriate

Table 7.2 Potential complications of hip/thigh augmentation

Potential complications of hip/thigh augmentation surgery
Infection
Seroma
Hematoma
Asymmetry
Implant visibility
Implant migration
Hypertrophic scarring
Hyperpigmentation of the scar
Capsular contracture
Wound dehiscence
Nerve injury (permanent or temporary, motor or sensory)
Compartment syndrome

Hematoma

Although a rare occurrence due to the relatively avascular plane of dissection for the hip augmentation procedure, a hematoma is always a possibility in surgical procedures. Small branches of the lateral circumflex femoral artery, a branch of the profunda femoris, can be injured during the dissection for hip augmentation. In the event of a hematoma, rapid evacuation, pocket irrigation, and reimplantation are the mainstays of therapy. This complication is best prevented by meticulous hemostasis at the time of surgery and good compression of the thigh post-op to prevent potential space creation.

Asymmetry

This can occur as a product of preexisting variability in the patient's legs or variability in dissection of the pocket bilaterally. This is best minimized by good preoperative photography and noting any asymmetries preoperatively. To avoid creation of asymmetry, it is important to maintain the same pattern of dissection and pocket creation bilaterally.

Implant Visibility

Due to the submuscular placement of the implant, this is indeed a rare complication. However, those patients that have very thin and atrophic legs to begin with may suffer from implant palpability and visibility. Patients should be counseled on this fact preoperatively if there is a feeling that the patient could be at risk.

In the authors' practice, there was one patient that had noticeable implants shortly after surgery. A 62-year-old female underwent hip augmentation with style 1, size 1 implants. The implants were not placed deep below the fascia lata but beneath the superficial fascia of the thigh (Fig. 7.19). This resulted in the implant outline being visible, requiring removal as the patient did not wish to undergo deeper placement of the implants. For this reason, we routinely employ the shaft of the femur as our landmark for depth

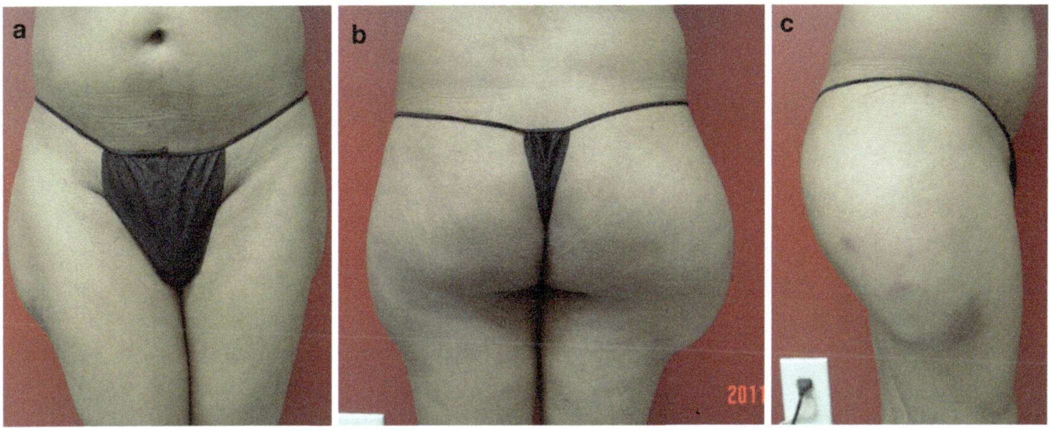

Fig. 7.18 (**a–c**) Patient presented with a delayed hematoma of the right hip likely secondary to a minor capsular tear

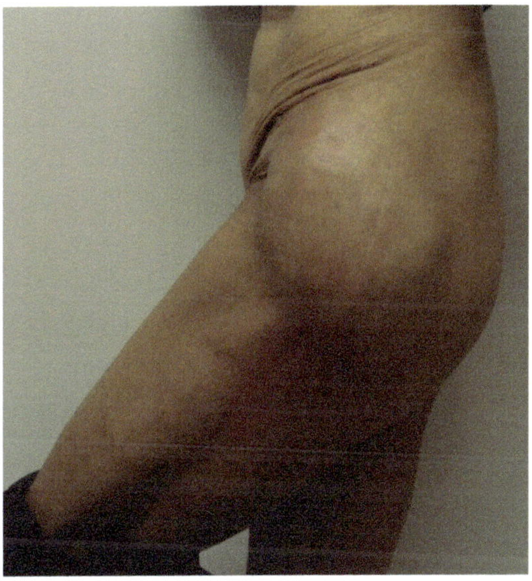

Fig. 7.19 A patient with a superficial implant that is easily palpable. At the time of surgery, the implant was placed in a more superficial plane rather than being below the fascia lata muscle. This was confirmed at the second operation (implant removal)

when placing the implant. If the femoral shaft cannot be palpated, then the implant is being placed in too superficial a plane.

Implant Migration

While it is true that any implant can shift with time, the placement of an implant very near the hip joint which is constantly moving likely places hip implants at a higher risk of implant migration. If it occurs, a return to the operating room with implant repositioning may be an option. However, due to the deep position of the implants, significant malposition may warrant implant removal. If the patient wishes to have the implants replaced, they can be replaced 3–6 months after implant removal.

In the one case of implant migration that we have noted, a 32-year-old female presented 4 months postoperatively with implants that had shifted out of position. She had undergone hip augmentation with style 1, size 1 implants and had a protracted course with postoperative seromas for 2 months. These were drained percutaneously without incident and with resolution of the seroma by 2 months. However, she presented at 4 months with a left implant that was significantly shifted out of position, with the left implant shifting inferiorly (Fig. 7.20). Due to the complications she had suffered up to that point, she elected to have the implants removed.

Scar Hyperpigmentation and Hypertrophy

The key to reduction of these problems is careful layered closure. Patients with a history of keloid or hypertrophic scar formation may require the use of steroid injected at the site of incision in the perioperative period. When placing the hip/thigh

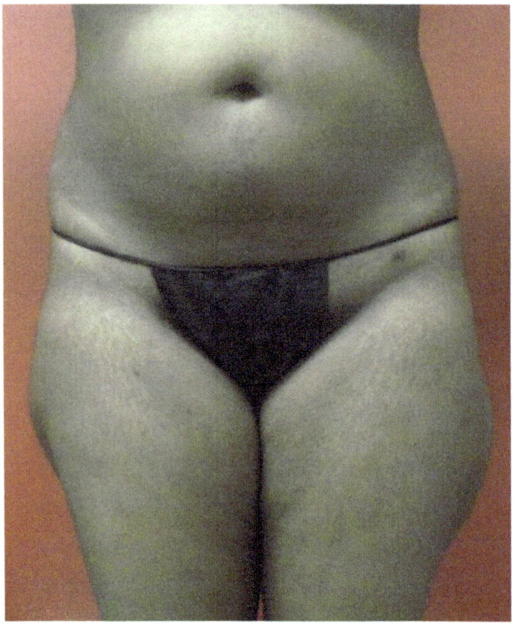

Fig. 7.20 Implant malposition. Note the inferiorly displaced left hip implant

augmentation incision, care should be taken to place the scar in the bikini line to best hide the incision. Unfortunately, this incision is one of the hardest incisions to hide in all of the muscle augmentation procedures that we perform. Using a previous abdominoplasty incision is an option when it is available; however, the dissection is a bit more complex owing to the need to dissect over the trochanter from the anterior aspect. When the incision is closed in layered fashion and good wound care is provided postoperatively, patients have the potential to achieve excellent scars and can all but avoid noticeable scars (Fig. 7.21).

Capsular Contracture

This is a possible late sequelae of any implant placement, most frequently described in the breast augmentation literature. In the event that a patient presents with signs/symptoms of capsular contracture (e.g., induration of the implant site, tightness in the leg, new onset pain, new onset swelling), ultrasound or CT evaluation of the affected extremity is warranted. If a capsule is identified, typically characterized by calcifications, then a partial or complete capsulectomy is warranted. Capsulotomies are a better option if the capsule is not easily accessible, as in most implant procedures. Capsular contracture is best prevented by meticulous hemostasis, good sterile technique, and avoidance of bleeding in the postoperative period. There may be a role for Accolate (zafirlukast) use to help soften a newly forming thick capsule. If identified early, our practice is to place patients on zafirlukast 10 mg bid for 3 months.

Wound Dehiscence

Wound dehiscence is a product of poor wound closure under too much tension typically. In order to prevent this, meticulous closure in three layers is paramount: fascia, deep dermis, and skin.

Nerve Injury

Due to the avascular and relatively structure-free dissection performed in the vast majority of cases, permanent nerve injury is rarely a problem. It is quite common for patients to complain of some numbness over the area of the posterolateral thigh postoperatively; however, this subsides within 1–3 months postoperatively. This complaint of numbness is likely a result of traction injury to the lateral femoral cutaneous nerve. The posterior branch of the lateral femoral cutaneous nerve pierces the fascia lata in the upper to mid-thigh region and supplies the skin from the level of the greater trochanter to the middle of the thigh posteriorly. Careful dissection of the fascia lata and use of blunt dissection below the fascia allow for the creation of a pocket with minimal risk of injury to the nerve.

Injury to the lateral femoral cutaneous nerve, when due to compression by the implant or significant inflammation of the thigh, results

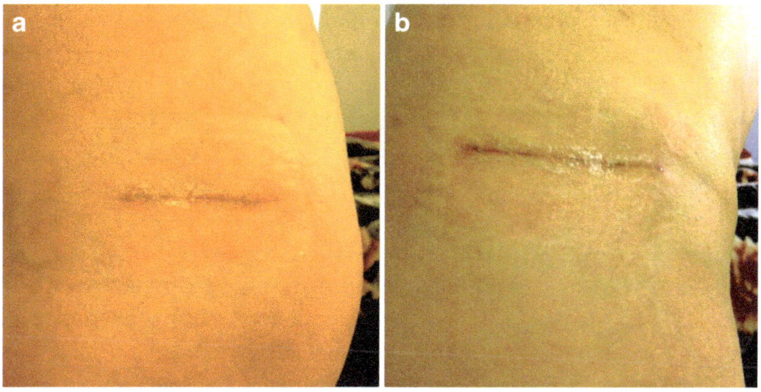

Fig. 7.21 These scars are shown 1 month postoperatively. There is a shine to them as the patient has been religious about application of silicone sheeting and liquid silicone bandages to her incision. This has resulted in a well-healed scar that will only improve with the coming months. (**a**) Depicts a picture of the patient's left hip and (**b**) depicts a picture of the patient's right hip

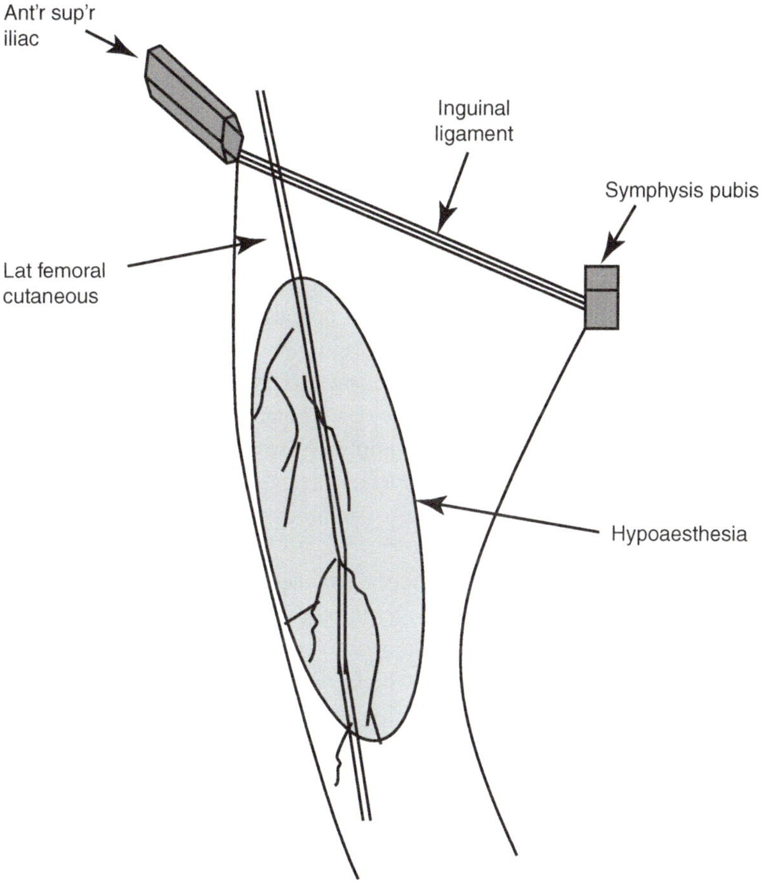

Fig. 7.22 Meralgia paresthetica and the course of the lateral femoral cutaneous nerve

in a syndrome named meralgia paresthetica (Fig. 7.22) [23–25]. First described by Bernhardt, in 1878 [25], the syndrome is primarily characterized by pain on the outer side of the thigh, occasionally extending to the lateral knee. There may also be a burning sensation, tingling, or numbness in the same area. Patients will at times complain of multiple beesting-like pains in the area of distribution of the nerve. Lastly, patients may complain of hypersensitivity to heat, with even lukewarm water feeling like it is scalding hot. The cause most frequently cited in the literature is compression and stretching injury to the nerve due to obesity, pregnancy, ascites, tight garments, seat belts, braces, direct trauma, leg length changes, scoliosis, and muscle spasm [26]. Diagnosis is largely based on patient description of the characteristics of the syndrome with a temporal relationship to recent surgical intervention. CT, MRI, or electromyography are examples of adjunctive studies but are rarely required. The mainstay of treatment is removal of the cause of compression (the hip implant) if it is felt that the nerve is intact. The use of NSAIDs and narcotic pain medications is very common in addition to rest of the lower extremity. In some cases, the physician may offer a local nerve block at the inguinal ligament, using a combination of lidocaine and corticosteroids to help ease the discomfort and decrease significant inflammation surrounding the nerve. Pain medications used in the treatment of neuralgia pain (e.g., gabapentin and pregabalin) may be employed to help with symptoms of pain. Should medical measures be unsuccessful, the surgeon should strongly consider implant removal. If the nerve has been completely severed, then treatment is largely supportive as most patients have a permanent sense of numbness, which is painless.

The probability of lateral femoral cutaneous nerve injury is best approximated by the reported incidence in the Smith-Petersen approach (anterolateral) for total hip replacement, which has a path of dissection that approximates that for lateral hip augmentation. Hussel [27] in his evaluation of various surgical approaches for periacetabular osteotomy found that the incidence of lateral femoral cutaneous nerve injury was approximately 30 % and largely attributed to blunt force trauma due to retractors and traction. Similarly, the patients that the authors have treated with hip augmentation have a reported incidence of numbness in the lateral thigh region of approximately 20 %. This has been self-limited in these cases and has lead to no permanent deficits. The femoral nerve itself is far removed from the area of dissection in this procedure as it is located in the anterior thigh, medial to the sartorius.

Compartment Pressure Problems/ Compartment Syndrome

Compartment syndromes, typically seen in trauma, involve an acute increase in pressure inside a closed space, thereby impairing blood flow to the affected space and potentially putting the limb at risk for loss. Clinical signs of compartment syndrome include the 6 Ps: pain, poikilothermia, pallor, paresthesias, paralysis, and pulselessness. In conscious patients, pain out of proportion to examination is the prominent symptom. Pain with passive range of motion is particularly troubling. In the authors' experience with hip augmentation since 2010, there has been only one patient who had a near compartment syndrome:

In that case, a 35-year-old female presented for hip augmentation secondary to a flattened lateral thigh/hip region. The patient's surgery was uneventful with placement of 250 mL implants into the hip region. One week after surgery, she presented with complaints of tightness over the lateral thigh region on the right side. The skin was dusky and several vesicles were noted. Because of the lack of obvious signs of limb compromise, observation with daily wound checks were performed to evaluate for possible evolution of compartment syndrome. Daily wound care to the vesicles consisted of Betadine to help dry the area overlying the vesicles with regular use of Neosporin to prevent bacterial colonization. Within 4 days, the duskiness improved and the vesicles had subsided. The patient's condition was likely a near compartment syndrome secondary to a tight submuscular pocket for a medium-sized implant. This patient was one of the early patients treated with a hip implant, and since that time, it has been the authors' standard practice to perform a slightly more generous pocket dissection in the anteroposterior dimension to minimize the risk of having an overly tight pocket. However, refrain from over-dissecting in the craniocaudal direction as this can produce a significant problem with sliding of the implant in the vertical dimension.

Authors' Practice Experience

To date, the authors have performed a total of 40 hip augmentations using the lateral thigh/hip prosthesis since 2010. Aesthetic results have been good in the majority of cases with a patient satisfaction rate of 82.5 % (33/40). For those that were dissatisfied with the results of the procedure, the dissatisfaction arose largely from the patient feeling that the augmentation was insufficient and should have been more dramatic (5/7). This again reinforces the need to determine if the patient's initial expectations are realistic. Because of this dissatisfaction with size, 4 pairs out of the 40 pairs of implants (10 %) were removed at a later surgery. The other two patients were dissatisfied with asymmetry that was clearly apparent requiring revision surgery. Of the implants placed, the majority of patients received size 1 (207 mL) implants (Table 7.3).

The complications actually observed are noted in Table 7.4, with the most frequent complication being seroma accumulation followed by temporary nerve injury resulting in loss of sensation over the distribution of the lateral femoral cutaneous nerve. For those patients that did see a seroma accumulate, it was noted that 50 % were noncompliant with strict garment use and activity restriction in the postoperative period. Strict adherence to postoperative instructions can minimize the risk of seroma formation, especially when coupled with conservative pocket dissection. Patients are advised to wear a compression garment 24/7 as much as possible for 1 month. In addition, vigorous activity is restricted until 4–6 weeks after surgery.

Table 7.3 Implants used between 2010 and 2013

Implant size	Number ($n=40$)	Percentage (%)
#1 (207 mL)	32	80
#2 (250 mL)	7	17.5
#3 (545 mL)	1	2.5

Table 7.4 Complications observed with hip augmentation 2010 to present

Complication	Number ($n=40$)	Percentage (%)
Infection	0	0
Seroma	10	25
Hematoma	0	0
Asymmetry (minor or major)	6	15
Implant migration	1	2.50
Hypertrophic/hyperpigmented scarring	1	2.50
Capsular contracture	0	0
Nerve injury (temporary)	8	20
Nerve injury (permanent)	0	0
Post operative pain 8–10	4	10
Wound dehiscence	0	0
Unhappy with size of implants	5	12.50

Patient Cases

Case 1 (Fig. 7.23)
A 39-year-old transgender patient underwent hip augmentation with style 1, size 1 hip implants. In addition to providing a more feminine form, there was improvement in overall symmetry of the legs as there was noted to be a minor defect in the left lateral hip/buttock region. Liposuction of the waist was also performed to further narrow the patient's waist and improve the overall projection of the hip implant.

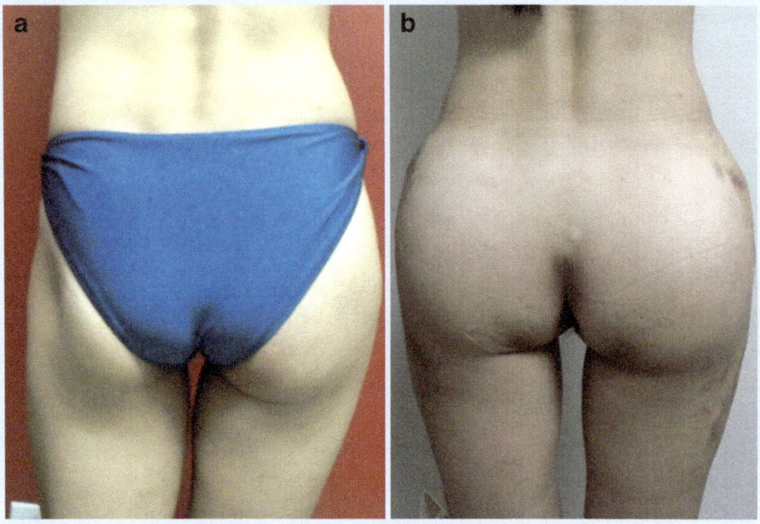

Fig. 7.23 (**a**) before, (**b**) 1 week postop hip augmentation with style 1, size 1 implant bilaterally

Case 2 (Fig. 7.24)
A 28-year-old transgender patient underwent hip augmentation initially with style 1, size 2 implants (250 mL). Six months later the patient underwent a second operation to achieve a more curvy figure. In her second operation she received the only style 1, size 3 implant that we have placed to date. The patient is shown preoperative, before her first surgery, and 6 months later after completion of the second augmentation.

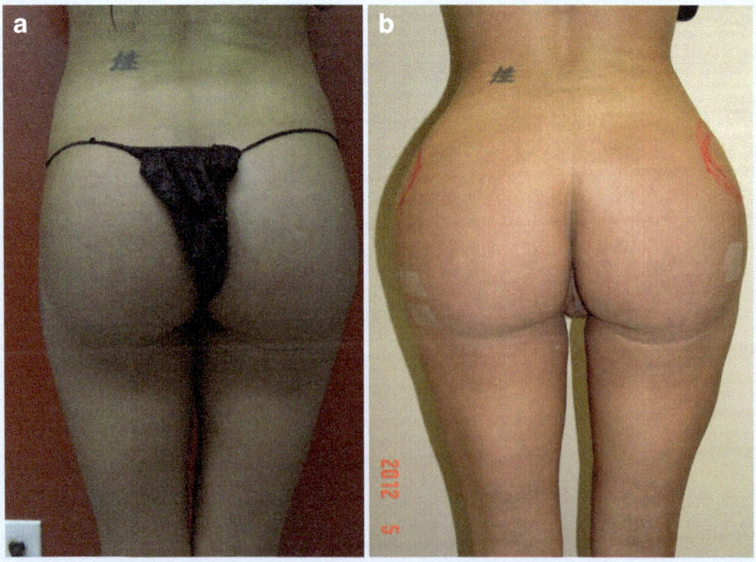

Fig. 7.24 (**a**) Preop hip augmentation and lipo to the hips. (**b**) The patient is show 6 months after completion of the second augmentation with style 1, size 3 implants and having undergone liposuction of the hips/waist

Case 3 (Fig. 7.25)

A 36-year-old female presented to have hip implants placed for increased curves and to eliminate the depression at the trochanters. She underwent augmentation with style 1, size 1 implants and is noted to have an improved contour to the lateral hip/buttock region, eliminating the notable trochanteric depressions.

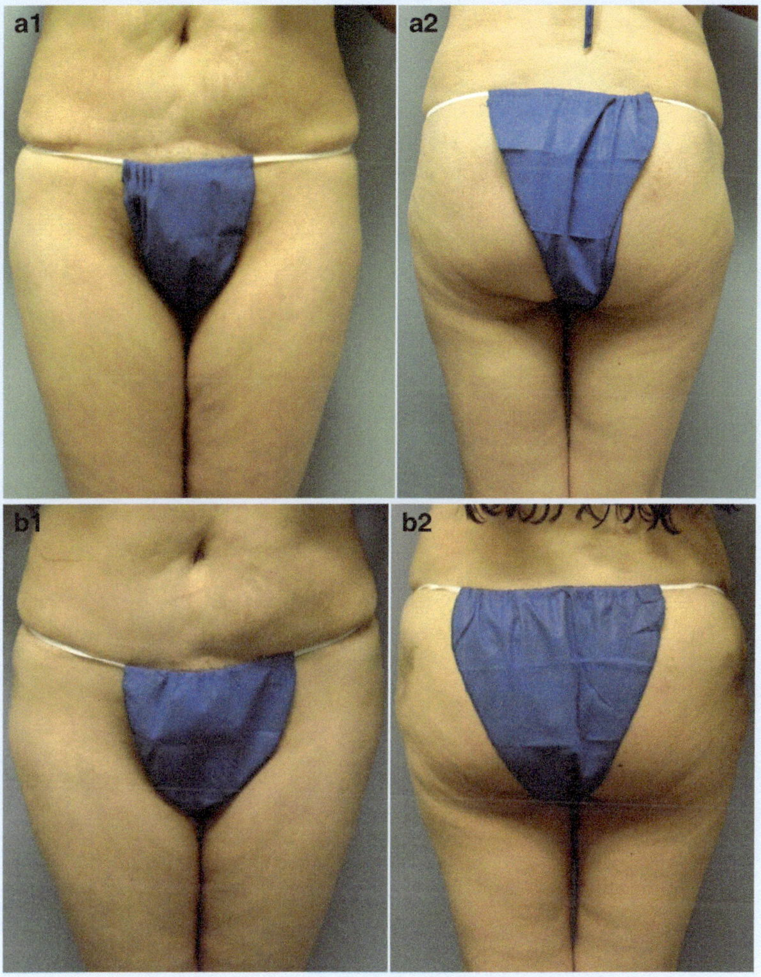

Fig. 7.25 (**a1**, **a2**) preop AP and PA views of the patient. (**b1**, **b2**) Postop AP and PA views 3 weeks after hip augmentation with style 1, size 1 hip implants bilaterally

Case 4 (Fig. 7.26)

A 33-year-old female underwent hip augmentation surgery with style 1, size 1 implants. She had previously undergone buttock augmentation 3 months prior without sufficient improvement in the lateral hip region and wanted more projection in the lateral aspect to complement her improved bottom side. The patient is shown preoperatively, having undergone her buttock augmentation successfully, and 1 week after hip augmentation.

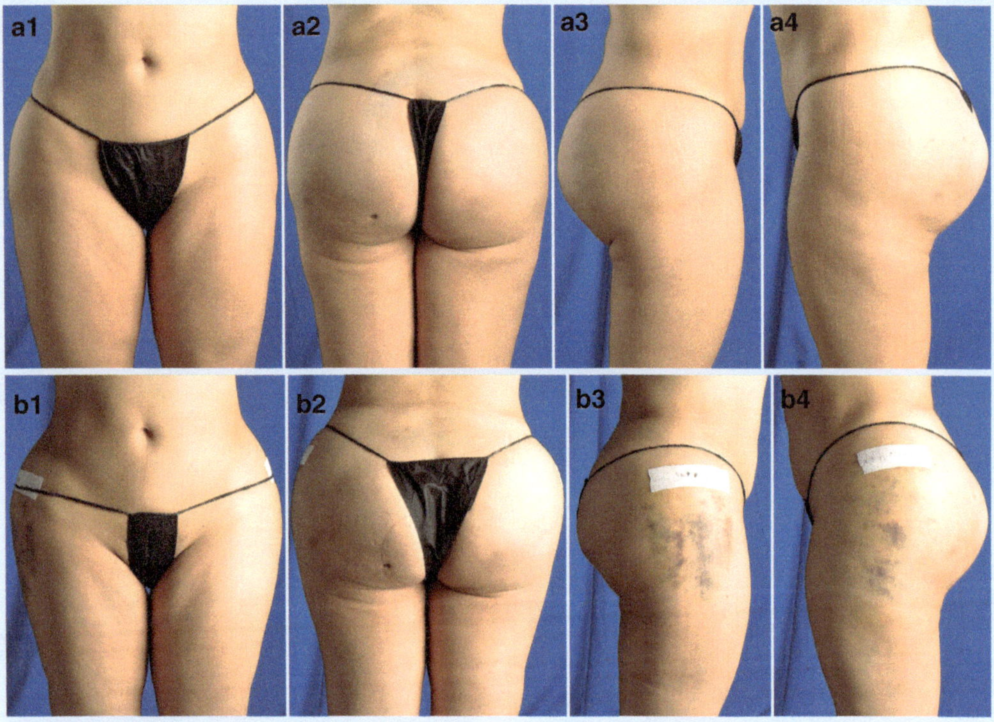

Fig. 7.26 **a1**–**a4** AP, PA, Lateral views of the patient 3 months after buttock augmentation seeking further curve in the lateral hip region. **b1**–**b4** Postop AP, PA, Lateral views of patient 1 week after hip augmentation with style 1, size 1 implant with increased projection to create a more significant lateral curvature

Case 5 (Fig. 7.27)

A 43-year-old female had previously undergone liposuction of the lateral thigh with another surgeon. This created a lateral thigh defect. She attempted fat grafting to the area without improvement. She presented for hip/lateral thigh augmentation to improve the contour of her leg. She underwent augmentation with style 1, size 1 lateral hip prosthesis and was happy with the improvement in her lateral thigh region. She is shown preoperatively and 3 months postoperatively.

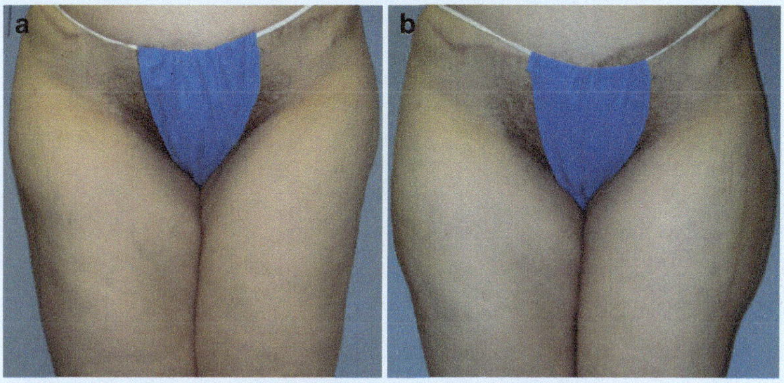

Fig. 7.27 (**a**) Preop AP view of patient prior to implant placed to augment lateral thigh to correct liposuction defect. (**b**) 3 months post lateral thigh augmentation with style 1, size 1 hip/thigh implant

Case 6 (Fig. 7.28)

A 25-year-old female underwent hip augmentation for hypoplastic hips with style 1, size 2 hip implants. The patient is shown preoperative and 2 months postoperative.

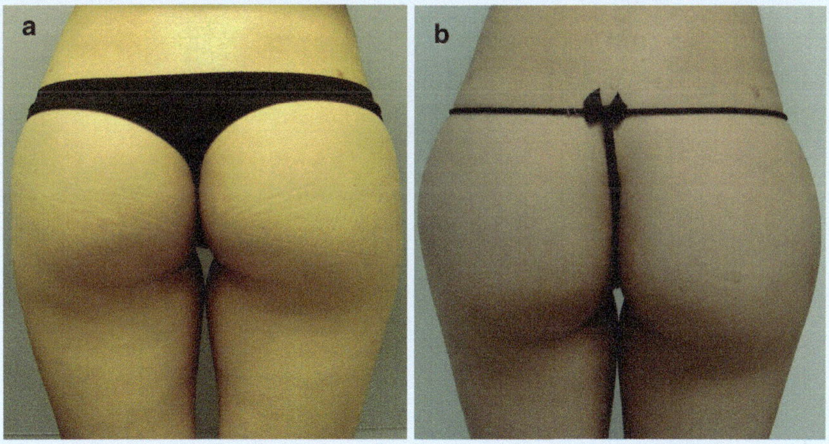

Fig. 7.28 (**a**) Preop PA view of patient prior to hip augmentation. (**b**) 2 months postop hip augmentation, producing more projection in hip area to give more curvy figure

Case 7 (Fig. 7.29)

A 28-year-old female underwent hip augmentation with style 1, size 2 hip implants for hypoplastic hips. She is shown preoperative and 1 month postoperative.

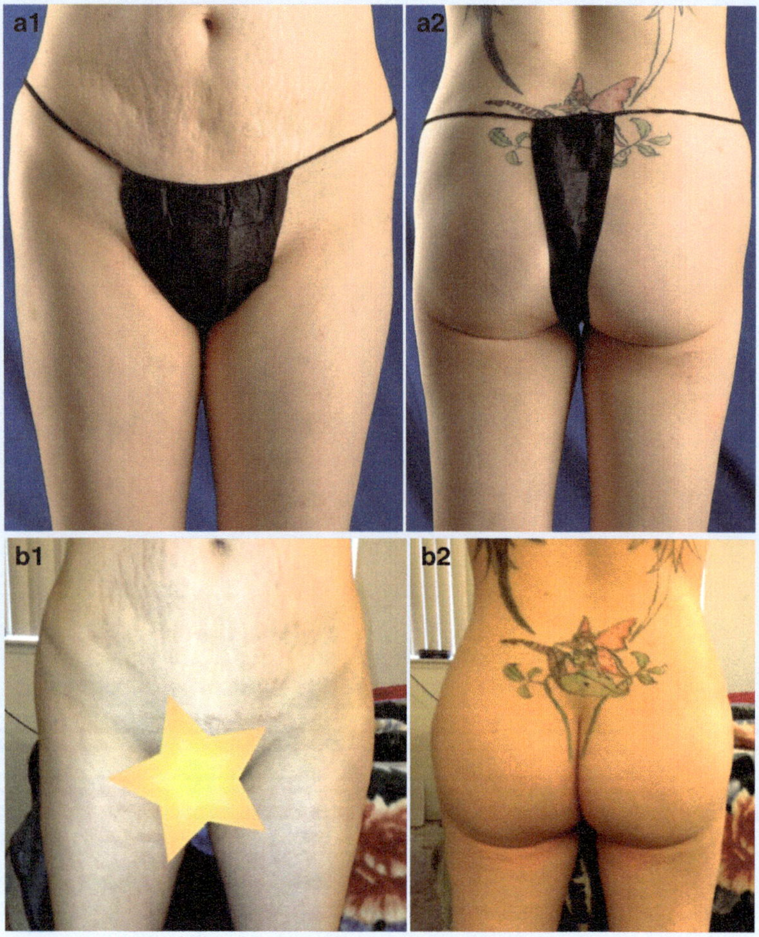

Fig. 7.29 (**a1**, **a2**) Preop AP and PA views prior to hip augmentation and liposuction to the hips/waist. (**b1**, **b2**) 1 month postop from hip augmentation with style 1, size 2 implants and liposuction

Case 8 (Fig. 7.30)

A 30-year-old transgender underwent hip augmentation with style 1, size 2 hip implants to achieve a more feminine and curvy figure. The patient is shown preoperative and 4 months postoperative.

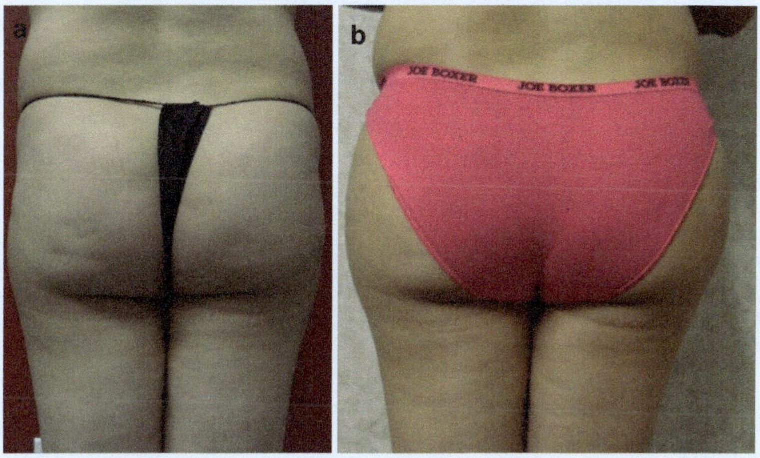

Fig. 7.30 (**a**) PA view preop. (**b**) PA view postop after hip augmentation with style 1, size 2 implants demonstrating more curvy figure

Conclusions

Augmentation of the lateral hip/thigh region with a silicone prosthesis is a great way to aesthetically enhance a woman's body. It is a procedure that does have a steep learning curve and requires repetition to achieve aesthetically pleasing and reproducible results. However, once a surgeon becomes adept at the procedure, it is useful in enhancing the lateral aspect of the leg and giving the female patient curves "in all the right places."

References

1. Garner D, Garfinkel P, Schwartz D, Thompson M. Cultural expectations of thinness in women. Psychol Rep. 1980;47(2):483–91.
2. Plastic Surgery Statistics Report. 2012. http://www.plasticsurgery.org/Documents/news-resources/statistics/2012-Plastic-Surgery-Statistics/full-plastic-surgery-statistics-report.pdf. Accessed 14 Sept 2013.
3. American Academy of Cosmetic Surgery Procedural Census. 2008. http://multivu.prnewswire.com/mnr/aacs/36867/docs/36867AACS2008ProceduralSurveyResults.pdf. Accessed 14 Sept 2013.
4. Waist Circumference and Waist-Hip Ratio, Report of a WHO expert consultation. WHO. 2008. http://whqlibdoc.who.int/publications/2011/978. Accessed 14 Sept 2013.
5. Brown JE, Potter JD, Jacobs Jr DR, Kopher RA, Rourke MJ, Barosso GM, Hannan PJ, Schmid LA. Maternal waist-to-hip ratio as a predictor of newborn size: results of the Diana project. Epidemiology. 1996;7(1):62–6.
6. Marlowe FW, Apicella CL, Reed D. Men's preferences for women's profile waist-hip-ratio in two societies. Evol Hum Behav. 2005;26:458–68.
7. Price GM, Uauy R, Breeze E, Bulpitt CJ, Fletcher AE. Weight, shape, and mortality risk in older persons: elevated waist-hip ratio, not high body mass index, is associated with a greater risk of death. Am J Clin Nutr. 2006;84(2):449–60.
8. Yusuf S, et al. Obesity and the risk of myocardial infarction in 27,000 participants from 52 countries: a case control study. Lancet. 2005;366(9497):1640–9.
9. Cuenca-Guerra R, Quezada J. What makes buttocks beautiful? A review and classification of the determinants of gluteal beauty and the surgical techniques to achieve them. Aesthetic Plast Surg. 2004;28(5):340–7.
10. Singh D, Young RK. Body weight, waist-to-hip ratio, breasts, and hips: role in judgments of female attractiveness and desirability for relationships. Ethol Sociobiol. 2001;16:483–507.
11. Singh D. Adaptive significance of female physical attractiveness: role of waist-to-hip ratio. J Pers Soc Psychol. 1993;65(2):293–307.
12. Singh D. Body shape and women's attractiveness: the critical role of waist-to-hip ratio. Hum Nat. 1993;4:297–321.

13. Platek S, Singh D. Optimal waist-to-hip ratios in women activate neural reward centers in men. PLoS One. 2010;5(2):e9042.
14. Dixson B, Grimshaw G, Liklater W, Dixson A. Eye tracking of men's preferences for waist–to-hip ratio and breast size of women. Arch Sex Behav. 2011;40(1):43–50.
15. Anger J. Letters to the editor. Rev Bras Cir Plast. 2011;26(4):718–9.
16. Netto NM. Aumento das coxas com implantes de silicone. Rev Bras Cir Plast. 2011;26(2):306–13.
17. Cardak N, Filinte G, Gonullu M, Akoz T. Thigh augmentation with calf prosthesis: a case report. Eur J Plast Surg. 2012;35(7):561–3.
18. Chugay NV, Chugay PN. Thigh augmentation: giving the average woman curves in the right places. Am J Cosmet Surg. 2011;28(4):255–60.
19. Kon M, Baert CM, de Lange MY. Thigh augmentation. Ann Plast Surg. 1995;35(5):519–21.
20. Anger J. Thigh augmentation: submuscular placement of a silicone gel-filled prosthesis. Aesthet Surg J. 2005;25(1):44–8.
21. Gottschalk F, Kourosh S, Leveau B. The functional anatomy of tensor fascia latae and gluteus medius and minimus. J Anat. 1989;166:179–89.
22. Grothaus MC, Hold M, Mekhail AO, Ebraheim NA, Yeasting RA. Lateral femoral cutaneous nerve: an anatomic study. Clin Orthop Relat Res. 2005;437:164–8.
23. Ivins GK. Meralgia paresthetica, the elusive diagnosis. Ann Surg. 2000;232(2):281–6.
24. Pearce JMS. Meralgia paraesthetica (Bernhardt-Roth syndrome). J Neurol Neurosurg Psychiatry. 2006;77(1):84.
25. Bernhardt M. Neuropathologische beobachtungen. Deutsch Arch fur Linische Medicin. 1878;22:362–93.
26. Williams PH, Trzil KP. Management of meralgia paresthetica. J Neurosurg. 1991;74(1):76–80.
27. Hussell JG, Mast JW, Mayo KA, Howie DW, Ganz R. A comparison of different surgical approaches for the periacetabular osteotomy. Clin Orthop. 1999;363:64–72.

8 Calf Augmentation

Introduction

Men and women alike wish to have a more muscular and toned physique, and the calf region is not exempt from this. Despite vigorous exercise and body building, some people are unable to attain the definition that they desire in the calf. Many patients who present for consultation want to look good in shorts and skirts but due to a hypoplastic calf say that they are unable to do so. To that end, calf implants of various shapes and sizes have been created to increase volume in the calf. In addition to calf implants, there has been increasing interest in the use of fat to augment the calf in order to avoid foreign body placement [1].

Calf Aesthetics

While the perception of an aesthetic calf may vary from culture to culture and time period to time period, the anatomy is consistent and ultimately gives the basis for calf aesthetics. The shape of the calf is defined primarily by the volume of the gastrocnemius and soleus muscles. In addition, the crural bones and the subcutaneous fat work in tandem with the muscles to further define the calf. While the bones cannot be altered easily to adjust the aesthetics of the calf, there is liposuction available to treat the subcutaneous fat and implants to address the muscle volume.

Over the years multiple physicians and mathematicians have tried to define beauty and what constitutes a beautiful human form. It was Howard [2] who first described the ideal length proportions of the calves, basing his paper's findings on the drawings of Leonardo da Vinci. Howard defined the golden ratio of calf aesthetics to exist when the distance between the ankle and the lower border of the gastrocnemius muscle was equal to the distance between the knee and the most prominent point on the medial curvature of the gastrocnemius muscle; and the entire length of the gastrocnemius should be 1.6 times the former value. This golden ratio correlated to the golden section of 1:1.618 as defined by the Italian mathematician Bonacci or what German astronomer and physicist Johannes Kepler called the "divine proportion" (Fig. 8.1) [3].

Szalay [4], based on his 12 years of experience with calf augmentation, also helped to define the aesthetics of the calf by determining that the attractive range for female calf circumference is between 33 and 36 cm. Values outside this range were considered aesthetically unattractive [4, 5].

History of the Procedure

Over the course of the last 40 years since the introduction of calf augmentation for reconstructive purposes, there have been various surgeons that have proposed novel implant shapes and sizes along with varying locations for the placement of the implants [3–13]. The implant most commonly used today is largely based on the silicone gel implants of Glitzenstein [2]. However, Carlsen [14] was the first to use calf implants

N.V. Chugay et al., *Body Sculpting with Silicone Implants*,
DOI 10.1007/978-3-319-04957-1_8,

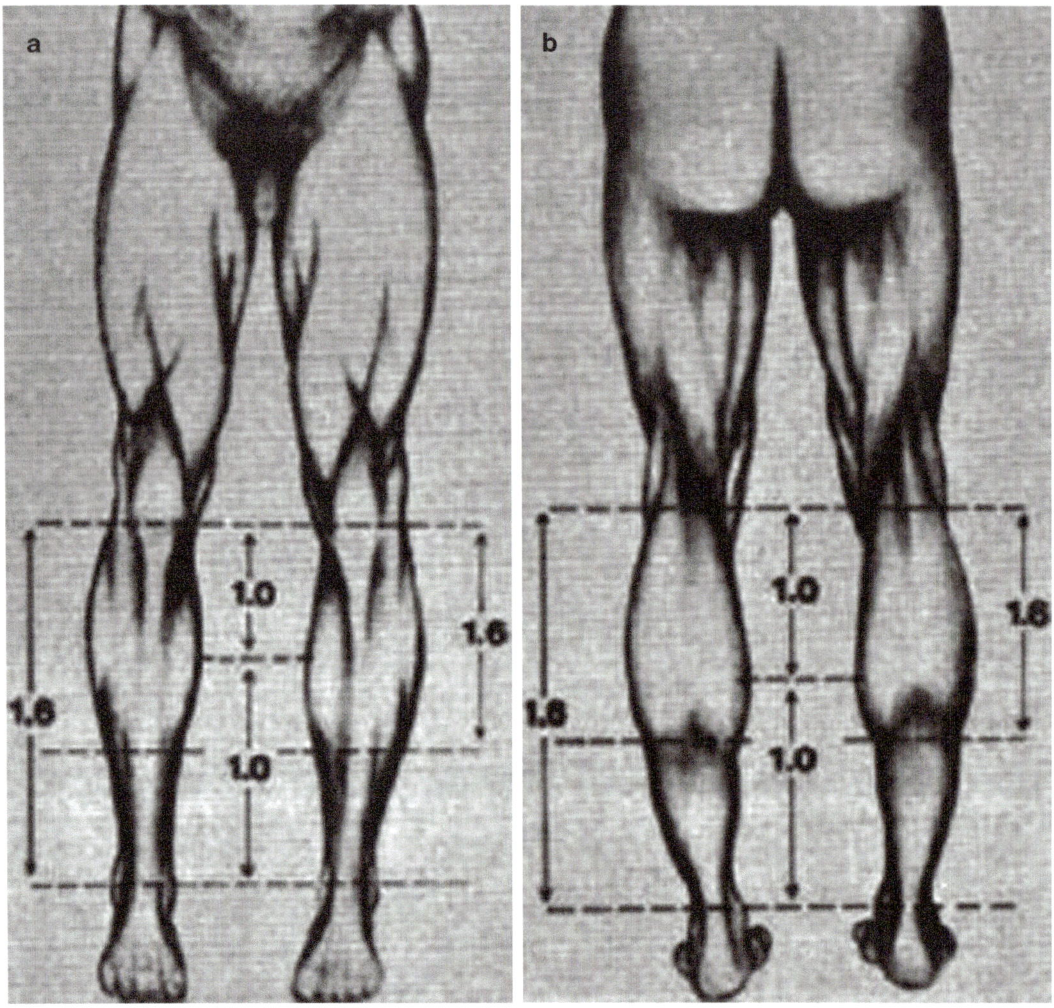

Fig. 8.1 Golden ratio of calf aesthetics [6]

back in 1972. His initial implant was made out of Silastic foam. Glitzenstein, in 1979 [2], used calf implants for patients with atrophy of the leg and muscular aplasia. Unlike Carlsen, his implants were designed from silicone gel. In 1984, Szalay [4] introduced torpedo-shaped implants that were placed beneath the fascia. In his technique, however, he did recommend the use of relaxing incisions in the fascia. Aiache in 1991 [13] introduced lenticular-shaped implants. In 2006, Gutstein [9] described a new silicone prosthesis that enhances the curved medial lower leg which he termed a "combined calf-tibial implant."

The early pioneers of the procedure, Carlsen and Glitzenstein, introduced the implant into a subfascial plane. However, in 2003 Kalixto and Vergara [8] described a calf augmentation with placement of the implant in a submuscular pocket, between the gastrocnemius and soleus muscles. The dissection that they proposed was done far away from the union of the gastrocnemius muscles where there were no vessels or nerves that could be damaged. It was noted however that these patients had a more tedious dissection and prolonged recovery than the patients who had undergone subfascial implant placement as described in previous reports. The use of muscle relaxants was paramount in these patients. The rationale for submuscular placement, according to the authors, was that they were able to gain better camouflaging of the implant. In 2004, Nunes described a method for calf augmentation that placed the implant in a supraperiosteal plane associated with fasciotomies. Ultimately, it is at the surgeon's discretion where to place the implant; however, based on anatomic studies it seems that the subfascial plane is a safe plane that allows for reproducible results with minimal risk of postoperative complications and significantly less pain from the patient's perspective [12]. It is for this reason that the authors favor a subfascial plane in the medial aspect of the calf.

Indications

Calf augmentation was originally designed to fill defects left following oncologic surgery, after trauma or infection, or due to genetic abnormalities. There are many causes for unilateral or bilateral calf deformities, and they include but are not limited to the following: (1) congenital hypoplasia due to agenesis of a calf muscle or adipose tissue reduction; (2) as a sequelae of clubfoot (talipes equinovarus), cerebral palsy, polio, and spina bifida; (3) due to poliomyelitis or osteomyelitis; and (4) following fractures of the femur and as a result of burn contractures [2, 6, 7, 14]. While calf implants do not improve function of the affected extremity, patients are pleased with the improved aesthetic appearance of the leg after implantation.

Since its initial introduction, calf augmentation surgery has become a widely popular aesthetic procedure to help patients gain more shapely legs. Whether it is a body builder that is looking to "bulk up" the leg despite a vigorous exercise regimen or the average patient who wants a more shapely calf region, there are implants of various shapes and sizes to help add volume to a hypoplastic calf.

Contraindications

Contraindications to the calf augmentation procedure are few. The first is unrealistic expectations on the part of the patient. The patient must be fully aware of the amount of augmentation that can be safely achieved. Patients that desire a more substantial augmentation may be candidates for serial operations but must be prepared for this fact up front. Secondly, patients with severe medical conditions that place the patient in a high ASA classification and at significant surgical risk are not good candidates for elective calf augmentation surgery. The surgeon must always be cognizant of the patient's circulation to the lower extremity. Compromised circulation in the postoperative period can be disastrous and cause limb loss. A patient who already has preexisting arterial or venous insufficiency may be at an increased risk of limb loss and may be a poor candidate for surgery.

Limitations

Some authors have noted that calf prostheses have the disadvantages of being unable to adequately correct ankle deformities, having a risk of displacement, having a risk of capsular contracture, and potentially having problems with extrusion. While the authors do agree that calf augmentation does not correct ankle deformities, they feel that this can be addressed with judicious fat grafting to the ankle region via small stab incisions at the medial and lateral malleoli.

Relevant Anatomy

As a result of anatomic studies [12] and operative dissections, the anatomy of the calf region is well understood. The calf is made up of two muscle groups: the gastrocnemius and the soleus (Fig. 8.2). The gastrocnemius has two heads and lies superficial to the deeper soleus muscle. The two heads of the gastrocnemius are connected to the condyles of the femur by strong tendons. The medial and larger head originates from a depression at the upper and back part of the medial condyle and from the adjacent part of the femur. The lateral head arises from an impression on the side of the lateral condyle and from the posterior surface of the femur immediately above the lateral part of the condyle. The fibers of the two heads unite at an angle in the midline of the muscle in a tendinous raphe, which expands into a broad aponeurosis. The aponeurosis, gradually contracting, unites with the tendon of the soleus and forms the calcaneal tendon (Achilles tendon). In performing

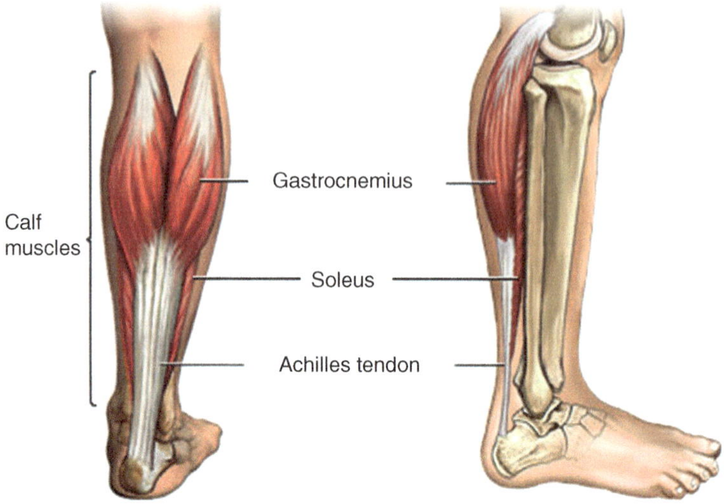

Fig. 8.2 Major muscles of the calf region: gastrocnemius and soleus

the dissection to attain a subfascial plane, the lateral and medial cutaneous nerves, branches of the peroneal nerve and tibial nerve, respectively, are potentially encountered. These nerves provide sensory innervation to the skin (Fig. 8.3). The medial sural cutaneous nerve originates from the tibial nerve of the sciatic and descends between the two heads of the gastrocnemius. It can be identified prior to diving between the heads of the gastrocnemius in the upper midline calf region. The lateral sural cutaneous nerve supplies the skin on the posterior and lateral surfaces of the leg and travels in a subcutaneous plane alongside the small (short) saphenous vein, joining with the medial sural cutaneous nerve to form the sural nerve. Major arterial, venous, and nerve structures are deep within the calf and remain undisturbed during a routine calf augmentation procedure (Fig. 8.4). The subfascial plane in the medial calf region is relatively avascular, allowing for creation of a relatively bloodless plane. Care must be taken to avoid injury to the short saphenous vein which lies deep to the investing fascia of the leg and superficial to the gastrocnemius in the midline posteriorly. This vein drains into the popliteal vein in the popliteal fossa.

Consultation/Implant Selection

The consultation begins with a thorough medical history on the patient. Special attention is taken to ask specifically about trauma to the extremity, history of surgery to the foot or ankle, history of vascular insufficiency which may put blood flow at risk, history of venous insufficiency or leg swelling which may prolong postoperative edema in the lower extremity, and any history of nerve damage or sensory deficits as may be seen in patients with diabetes mellitus. At the time of consultation, the patient is asked what specifically about their calf bothers them. Preoperative goals are assessed at this point. A patient who has unrealistic expectations and is unable to comply with the strict postoperative instructions is deemed a poor candidate for augmentation. Patients who have congenital anomalies, a significant size disparity between the two calves, or bilateral hypoplasia are informed that several surgeries may be required to attain symmetry and achieve the augmentation they desire. In the typical consultation, patients are asked if their deficiency lies primarily in the medial aspect of the calf, the lateral aspect of the calf, or whether they would like a larger calf size overall. The reason for this distinction is to help the surgeon plan the right implant style for surgery.

After completion of the history, the patient's calves are evaluated. The symmetry of the two sides is assessed and any disparity is brought to the attention of the patient. Although the majority of patients present with a preexisting asymmetry of the calves, not many patients note the difference and this can be a source of medicolegal matters in the future. If the patient suffers from

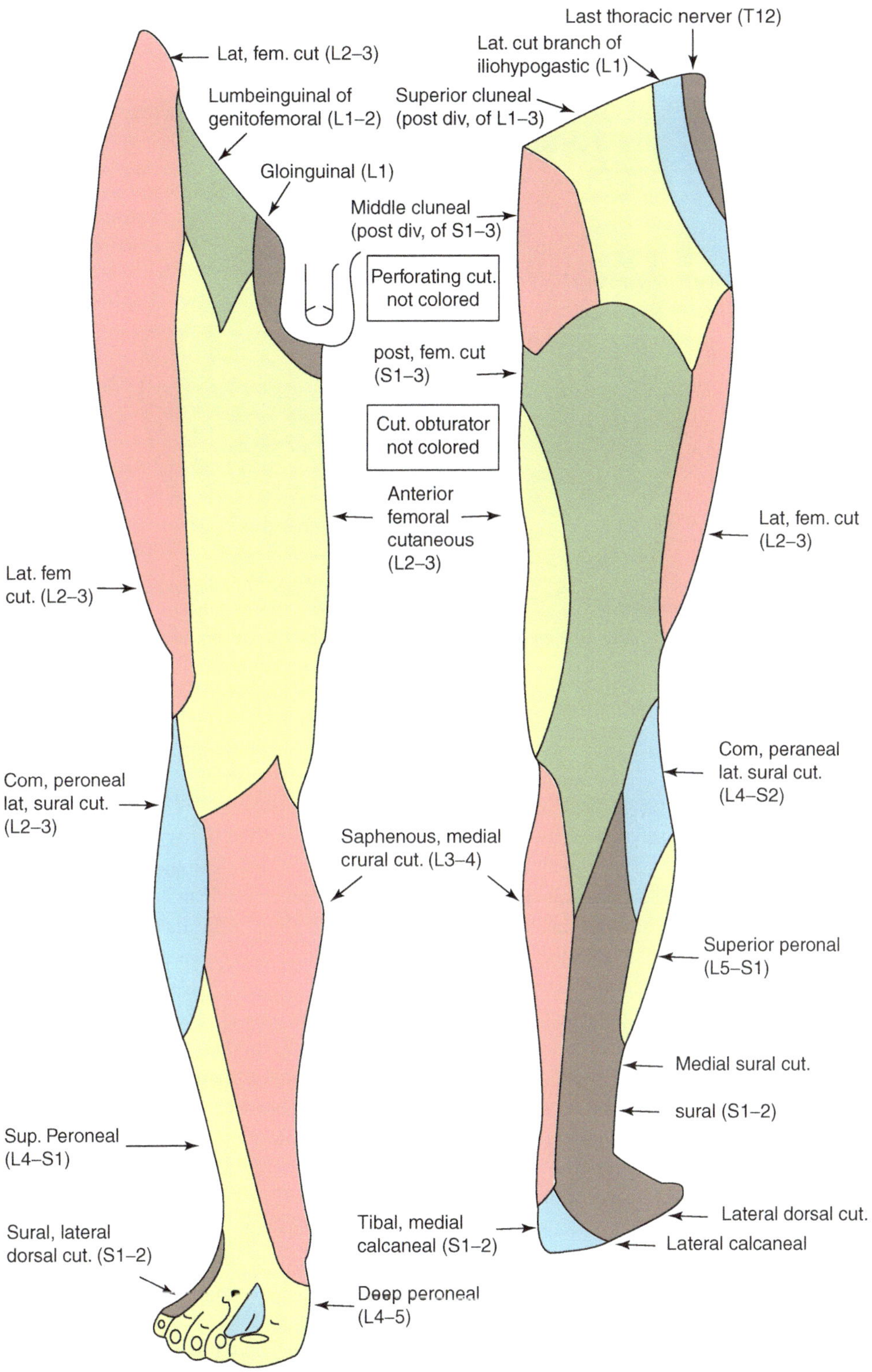

Fig. 8.3 The lateral and medial cutaneous nerve dermatomes are seen here. These are branches of the peroneal nerve and tibial nerve, respectively, and are potentially encountered in dissection for calf augmentation. These nerves provide sensory innervation to the skin in the area

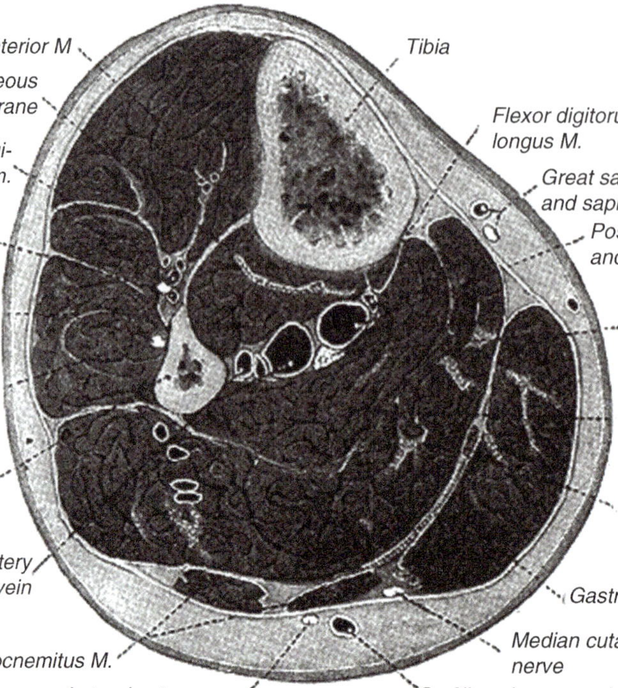

Fig. 8.4 Major neurovascular structures are seen in this cross section of the midportion of the calf. When performing a subfascial augmentation, these structures are relatively safe from injury

clubfoot deformity or a previous bout of polio, leg asymmetry is noted. The physician then evaluates the quality of the skin, subcutaneous tissue, and muscle. A person who has very thin tissues or significant hypoplasia of the calf may not be able to adequately accommodate a large implant. The patient's calves are measured in circumference at the midportion of the calf. A second measurement, from the popliteal fossa (proposed incision line) to the insertion of the Achilles tendon, is also taken. Having this second measurement allows one to assess the maximum length of implant that can be accommodated in the calf.

When determining the type of implant to use, the determination is based on the desires of the patient. However, the authors also take into account the length from the popliteal fossa to the insertion of the Achilles tendon to better define the length that will be accommodated. If the patient merely wishes to have more definition in the calf, then the style 2 implants will be used in most cases. With the style 2 calf implant, there is a greater enhancement of the medial calf muscle (Fig. 8.5). If, however, the patient wishes to have more overall volume to the calf region and is looking for more of a blocklike appearance to the calf, then the style 1 implant is favored (Fig. 8.5). With the style 1 implant, there is a greater enhancement of the entire calf region, which in our practice is best suited for patients who already have a great deal of muscle volume (e.g., body builders) and just want an overall increase in volume. Style 3 is used for lateral head augmentation and is rarely used. Each of the different style implants has a range of sizes to fit each patient need. Regardless of the implant chosen, the position of the implant is still in the subfascial plane and minimizes dissection around key neurovascular structures. With experience, the surgeon will be better able to determine the best implant for each patient.

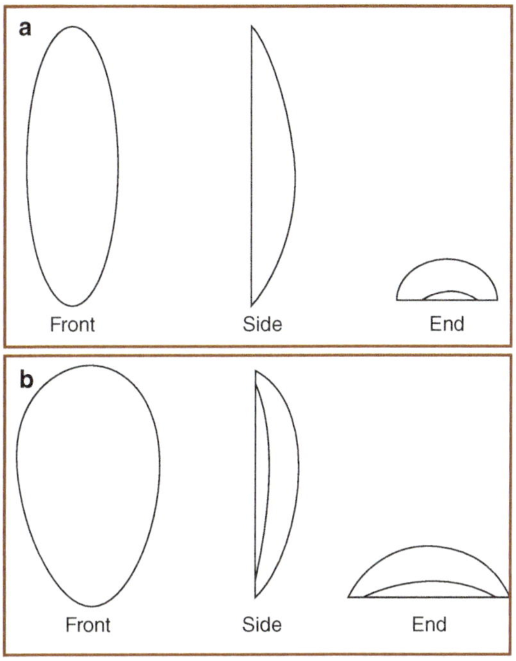

Fig. 8.5 (**a**) Calf implant style 2 (Courtesy of AART (Aesthetic and Reconstructive Technologies, Inc., Reno, NV)). (**b**) Calf implant style 1 (Courtesy of AART (Aesthetic and Reconstructive Technologies, Inc., Reno, NV))

Available Implants

Style 1 is the authors' preference for bulky calf augmentation (Table 8.1). Style 2 is the authors' preference for medial calf augmentation (Table 8.2). Style 3 is the authors' preference for lateral calf augmentation (Table 8.3).

Preoperative Planning and Marking

On the day of the surgery, the patient is met in the preoperative holding area. It is here that the patient's consent is verified and again risks, benefits, and alternatives are reviewed with the patient. With the patient in the erect position, the proposed site of incision is marked, measuring approximately 5 cm. The site of incision should be in line with the patient's natural crease in the popliteal fossa. To help accentuate this crease and make marking easier, the patient may be asked to hold on to a stationary object and flex at the knee. Once the site of the incision is marked, the site of the proposed implant is marked taking into account the patient's anatomy and existing deficit along with the desires of the patient (Fig. 8.6).

Operative Technique

Medial Calf Augmentation

The surgery can be performed under general anesthesia or under simple local anesthesia; however, our preference is to use monitored anesthesia care with propofol and ketamine. Two grams of Ancef are administered prior to the incision for prophylaxis (if allergic to penicillin or cephalosporin, then intravenous (IV) clindamycin 300 mg is administered). The patient is repositioned in the prone position after administration of anesthesia. The calves are then prepped with Betadine, and each calf is injected with a total of 50 mL of 1 % lidocaine with epinephrine in the area of proposed implant placement. The patient is then reprepped and draped in sterile fashion. A 5 cm incision is made in the popliteal fossa in line with preoperative markings (Fig. 8.7). Dissection is performed through the subcutaneous tissues using a combination of blunt dissection with gauze and a hemostat. Further dissection and hemostasis can be achieved with electrocautery (Fig. 8.8). Dissection is carried to the level of the popliteal fascia (Fig. 8.9). On reaching the fascia, a #15 blade scalpel is used to make a transverse incision. This is extended with Metzenbaum scissors medially and laterally. At this point 2-0 Vicryl stay sutures are placed in each section of the fascia (Fig. 8.9). A subfascial plane, beginning beneath the popliteal fascia and extending into the deep investing fascia of the leg, is then dissected using blunt finger dissection and a spatula dissector, ensuring an adequate plane for the implant in the medial aspect of the calf (in line with preoperative markings/patient wishes) (Fig. 8.10). While performing this dissection, care is taken to avoid injury to the short saphenous vein which runs in the midline posteriorly and lies deep to the investing fascia of the leg along the surface of the gastrocnemius. Once a sufficient pocket

Table 8.1 Style 1 (Aesthetic and Reconstructive Technologies, Inc., Reno, NV)

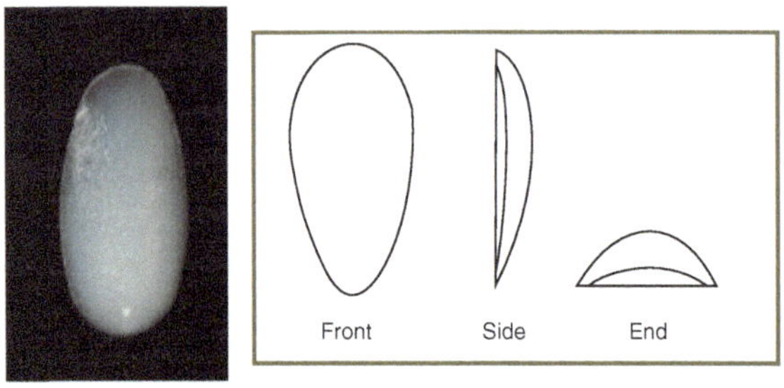

Size	Catalog #	Width	Length	Projection	Volume (cc)
1	502–101	6.2	12.7	1.6	53
2	502–102	6.9	13.9	1.7	68
3	502–103	7.8	14.2	1.9	91
4	502–104	9.5	16.3	2.0	131
5	502–105	11.3	17.3	2.7	275
6	502–106	9.5	16.3	2.5	147
7	502–107	9.7	17.2	2.3	192

Table 8.2 Style 2 (Aesthetic and Reconstructive Technologies, Inc., Reno, NV)

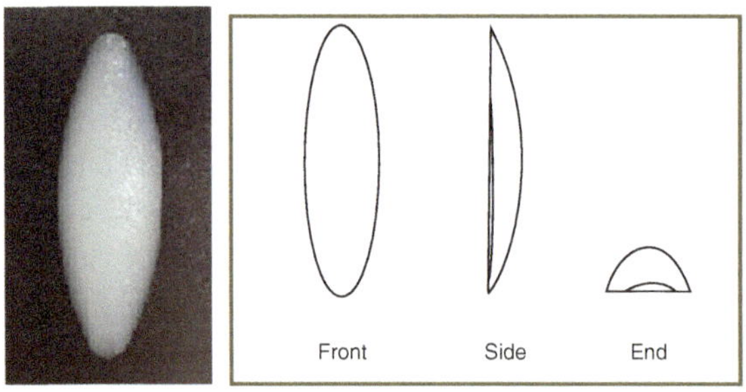

Size	Catalog #	Width	Length	Projection	Volume (cc)
1	502–201	6.1	17.4	2.1	94
2	502–202	6.5	20.7	2.3	126

is dissected, the pocket is irrigated with a solution containing normal saline, Betadine, Ancef, and gentamicin. Fifteen milliliters of 0.5 % Marcaine is injected into the pocket for postoperative analgesia. A lozenge-shaped implant is then placed into the pocket, making sure to attain symmetry (Fig. 8.11). Once the implant has been placed, symmetry is assessed. At this point closure is begun. The fascia is re-approximated with 2-0 Monocryl suture in interrupted fashion (Fig. 8.12). The deep dermis is re-approximated with 3-0 Monocryl suture in buried fashion. The skin is closed in subcuticular fashion with 4-0 Vicryl suture or with interrupted 4-0 silk sutures (based on surgeon preference). The same procedure is mirrored on the contralateral side. The legs are wrapped with Coban and the patient is then taken to the postanesthesia care unit (PACU).

Lateral Calf Augmentation

If the patient is in need of lateral calf augmentation, the same incision in the popliteal fossa may be used to augment the lateral calf. In this case, dissection is carried out below the popliteal/deep investing fascia of the leg over the lateral head of the gastrocnemius muscle. Incision is made in the same manner as described above and can be carried further lateral in the popliteal fossa to facilitate implant placement in the lateral calf. Subcutaneous dissection is carried out down to

Table 8.3 Style 3 (Aesthetic and Reconstructive Technologies, Inc., Reno, NV)

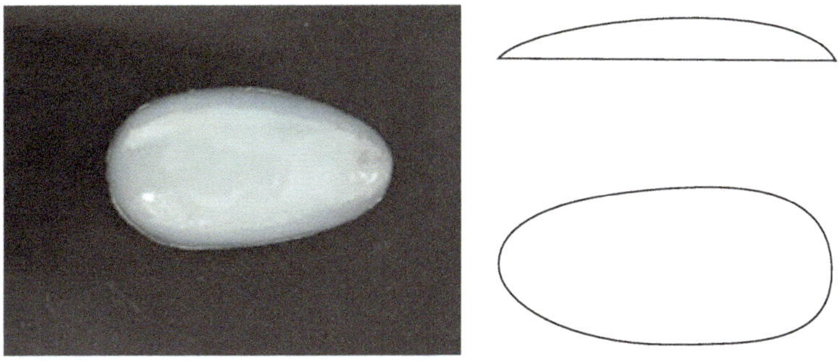

Size	Catalog #	Width	Length	Projection	Volume (cc)
0	502–300	5.2	12.5	1.5	49
1	502–301	6.5	14.0	1.7	72
2	502–302	6.7	14.3	1.8	80
3	502–303	8.0	14.6	2.0	133
4	502–304	9.5	16.5	2.2	163
5	502–305	6.2	13.5	1.6	68
6	502–306	6.5	14.5	1.8	81
7	502–307	7.9	14.7	2.0	110
8	502–308	9.1	17.1	2.0	144
9	502–309	5.7	12.4	1.5	47

the level of the deep fascia of the leg. An incision is made in the fascia and extended with Metzenbaum scissors. Stay sutures are placed in this fascia (Fig. 8.13). Dissection is performed in the subfascial plane with a combination of blunt finger dissection and a spatula-type dissector as described for medial calf augmentation (Fig. 8.14). The fibula is used as the medial extent of dissection, and as in the medial calf augmentation, dissection is carried caudally until resistance is met at the insertions of the deep investing fascia near the level of the ankle (Fig. 8.14). Just as with medial augmentation, the implant is positioned and closure is performed in layers (Fig. 8.15).

Postoperative Care Instructions

Postoperatively the patient may begin ambulating starting on the evening of the procedure. They may shower on the second postoperative day, making sure to keep dressings clean and dry the Robbins tape with a hair dryer on a low-heat setting. Patients are allowed to begin light activity at week 2 and full unrestricted activity at weeks 4–6. Patients are asked to wear compression stockings with a grading of 20–30 mmHg for 4 weeks postoperatively to prevent dead space, thereby helping to reduce the risk of seroma formation. The legs are to be elevated as much as possible to allow for better lymphatic/venous drainage. Patients are prescribed both narcotic analgesics and muscle relaxants (diazepam 5 mg every 8 h as needed for spasm) to assist with postoperative pain.

Complications

In performing calf augmentation, there is a host of complications that can arise (Table 8.4).

Infection

Infection, either superficial or deep, is a possibility in calf augmentation surgery. The literature

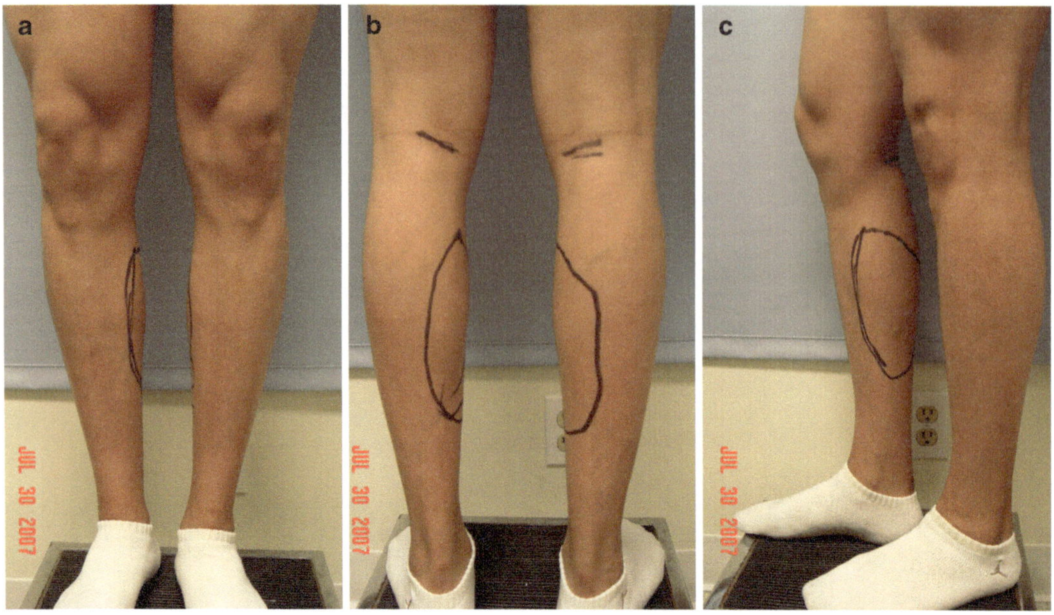

Fig. 8.6 (**a**–**c**) Preoperative markings for calf augmentation surgery. Note the site of the incision in the popliteal fossa and the outline of the site for calf augmentation. The markings for implant position are done in concert with the patient to maximize patient satisfaction postoperatively

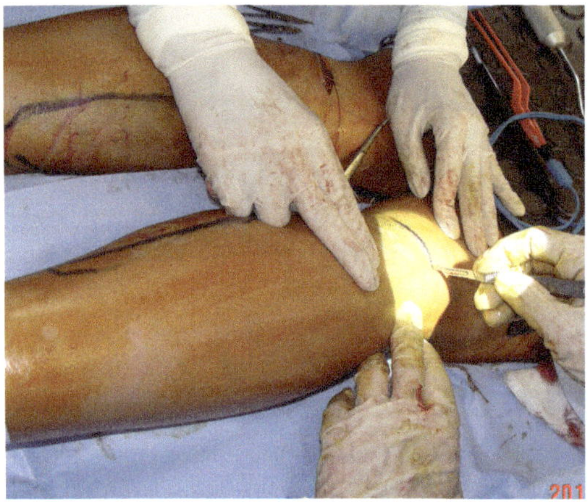

Fig. 8.7 Incision at the popliteal fossa

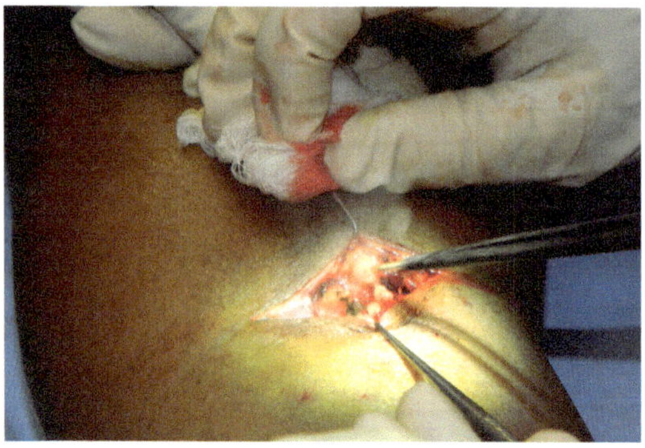

Fig. 8.8 Dissection through the subcutaneous tissues using electrocautery. Single-tooth hooks are used for retraction of the skin

reports infection rates between 0 [8] and 3.3 % [6]. Species identified in the authors' experiences were isolated to *Staphylococcus aureus* and *Staphylococcus epidermidis*, relatively common skin flora. Prior to making an incision, standard practice should be the administration of 2 g of intravenous (IV) Ancef (or 300 mg IV clindamycin in a penicillin- or cephalosporin-allergic patient). During the procedure, irrigation of the pocket with a standard antibiotic solution containing normal saline, Betadine, Ancef, and gentamicin should be performed. Postoperatively, a 7–10-day regimen of oral antibiotics covering normal skin flora should be administered. If a deep infection occurs, the standard practice is removal of the implant, closure, and possible reimplantation in 3–6 months. There are reports in other forms of implant surgery that conservative management and implant salvage are

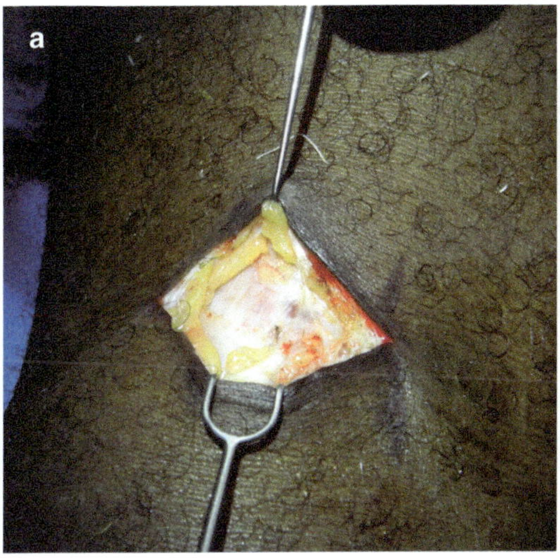

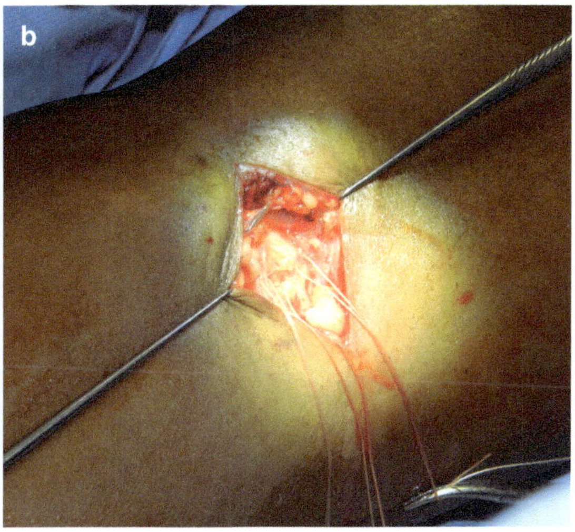

Fig. 8.9 (**a**) Deep investing fascia of the leg (glistening). (**b**) Incision has been made through the investing fascia with stay sutures being placed in the superior and inferior aspect of the cut fascia. The authors' standard is to put one up and two down as the inferior portion of the fascia tends to retract, and secure fascial sutures are key to helping re-approximation at the end of the case

possible. This should be left at the discretion of the surgeon and performed with careful counseling of the patient.

Seroma

Seromas are statistically the most common complication occurring in calf augmentation surgery, occurring in approximately 6 % of cases in most large volume studies [4, 12, 15, 16]. They typically present as new-onset pain, swelling, or asymmetry. The treatment of choice remains percutaneous aspiration. This complication is best prevented with patient compliance with compression stockings and proper implant placement at the time of surgery, thereby minimizing dead space.

Hematoma

Although this is a rare occurrence due to the relatively avascular plane of dissection for the calf augmentation procedure, a hematoma is always possible if damage is done to the vessels that perforate the investing fascia of the leg [12]. In the event of a hematoma, rapid evacuation, pocket irrigation, and reimplantation are the mainstays of therapy. This complication is best prevented by meticulous hemostasis at the time of surgery and good compression of the calf post-op to prevent potential space creation.

Old blood that has not been well absorbed by the body can be found at later dissection as a course granular material resembling fine gravel. A patient returned to the authors' practice 16 years after initial augmentation complaining of nodularity in the calves. He wished to have the calf implants out as they were too bulky for their present age. On return to the OR, the implants were removed and fine calcific material was found which explained the previously described nodularity (Fig. 8.16). Final pathology demonstrated significant calcifications and no evidence of malignancy.

Asymmetry

This can occur as a product of preexisting variability in the patient's legs or variability in dissection of the pocket bilaterally. This is best minimized by good preoperative photography

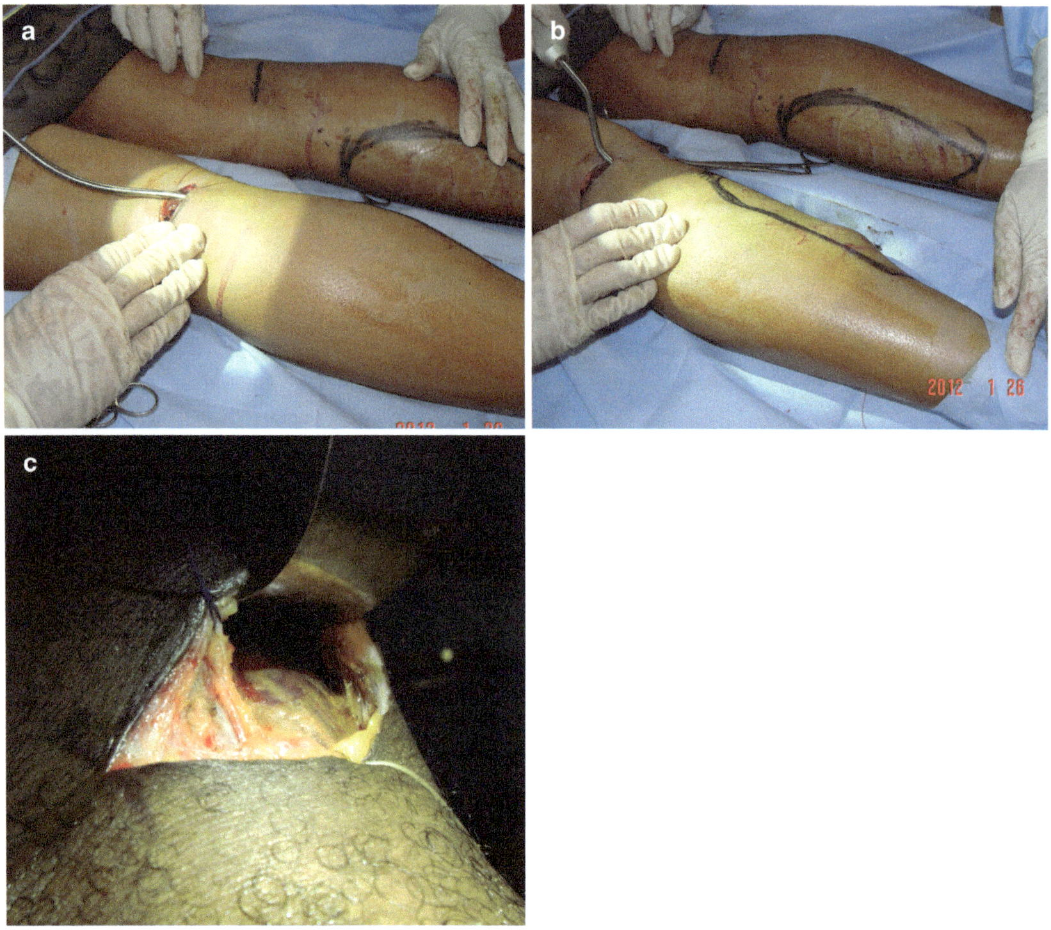

Fig. 8.10 Dissection of the subfascial pocket. (**a**) After initial dissection of the pocket using blunt finger dissection, a spatula dissector is used to further dissect the pocket. (**b**) The dissector tip is noted in the midportion of the calf tenting up the skin overlying the subfascial pocket. (**c**) At completion of dissection, there is an ample pocket that has been created with the gastrocnemius muscle seen below

and noting any asymmetries preoperatively. To avoid creation of asymmetry, it is important to maintain the same pattern of dissection and pocket creation bilaterally. Patients, like those suffering from clubfoot, must be made aware of the fact that despite multiple surgeries, they may never achieve absolute symmetry in their legs (Fig. 8.17).

Implant Visibility

Due to the subfascial placement of the implant, this is indeed a rare complication. However, those patients that have very thin and atrophic legs to begin with may suffer from implant palpability and visibility. Patients should be counseled on this fact preoperatively if there is a feeling that the patient could be at risk.

Scar Hyperpigmentation and Hypertrophy

In reviewing the primary author's (NVC) two-decade history with the procedure, the most frequent complication observed was hypertrophic or hyperpigmented scarring. This may be a function of the author's patient population which is primarily Hispanic and has a higher tendency to

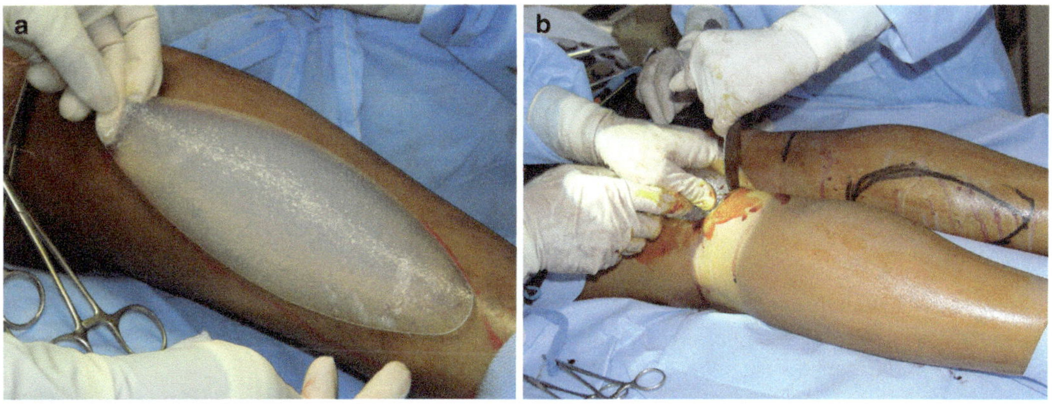

Fig. 8.11 (**a**) The implant (style 2, size 2) being demonstrated in its position in the right medial calf. (**b**) Insertion of the prosthesis into the subfascial pocket taking care to fold the implant along its long axis to facilitate positioning

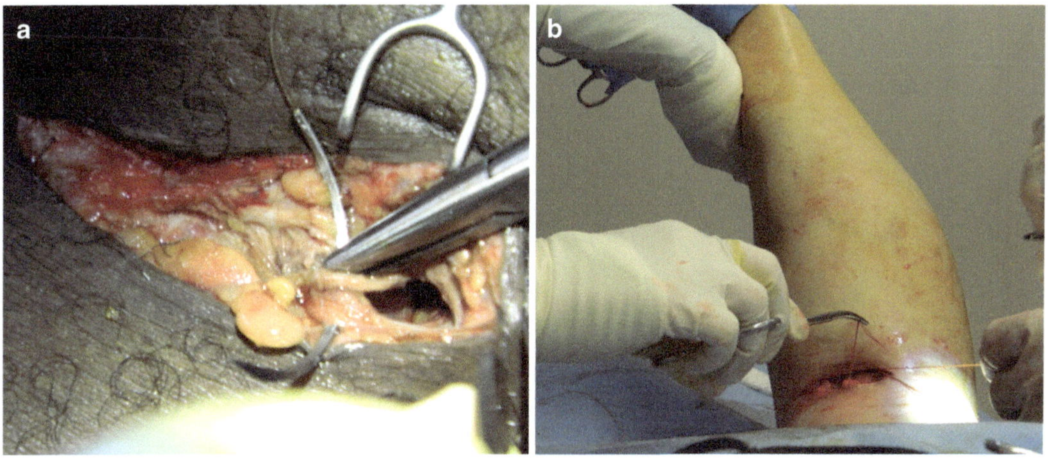

Fig. 8.12 (**a**) Closure of the deep investing fascia of the leg using 2-0 Vicryl suture. (**b**) To facilitate closure and take tension off of the ends of the fascia, the knee is flexed by the assistant

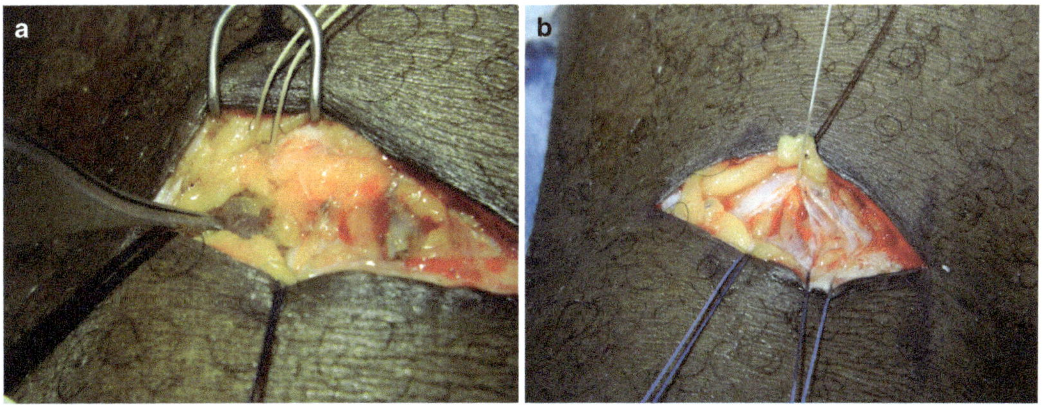

Fig. 8.13 (**a**) Incision has been made in the deep investing fascia showing the lateral head of the gastrocnemius muscle (9 o'clock). (**b**) Stay suture being placed in the fascia

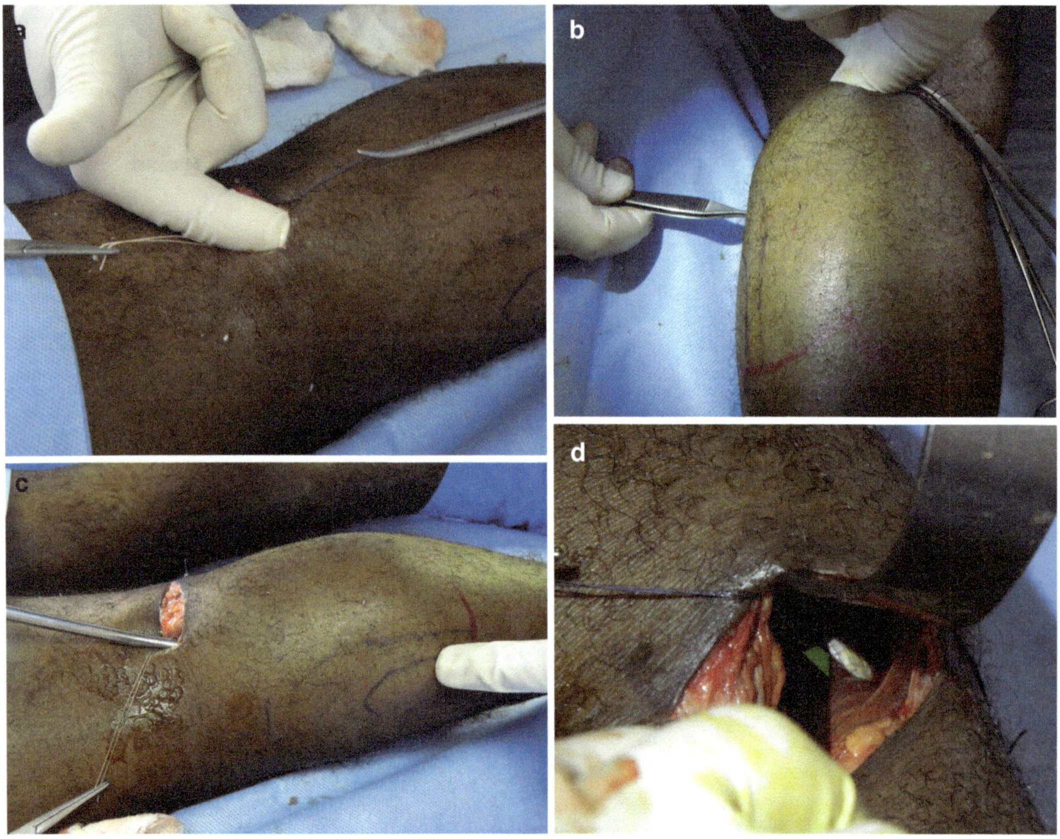

Fig. 8.14 Dissection of the subfascial pocket. (a) Dissection begins with blunt finger dissection. (b) Dissection is taken lateral to the shaft of the fibula (marked with tip of forceps). (c) Further dissection of the implant pocket is carried out with spatula dissector. (d) Demonstration of the completed subfascial pocket with the glistening lateral head of the gastrocnemius visualized

form hypertrophic and/or hyperpigmented scars. The key to reduction of these problems is careful layered closure.

Capsular Contracture

This is a possible late sequelae of any implant placement, most frequently described in the breast augmentation literature. The literature in calf augmentation has described a rate between 0 [3–5, 11] and 5 % [6]. In the event that a patient presents with signs/symptoms of capsular contracture (e.g., induration of the implant site, tightness in the leg, new-onset pain, new-onset swelling), ultrasound or CT evaluation of the affected extremity is warranted. If a capsule is identified, typically characterized by calcifications, then a partial or complete capsulectomy is warranted. An alternative might be to perform capsulotomies as the removal of the capsule may be quite difficult in the confined space of the calf.

Wound Dehiscence

Wound dehiscence is a product of poor wound closure under too much tension typically. In addition patients who do not comply with limited activity restrictions can be at increased risk of wound dehiscence. In order to prevent dehiscence, meticulous closure in three layers

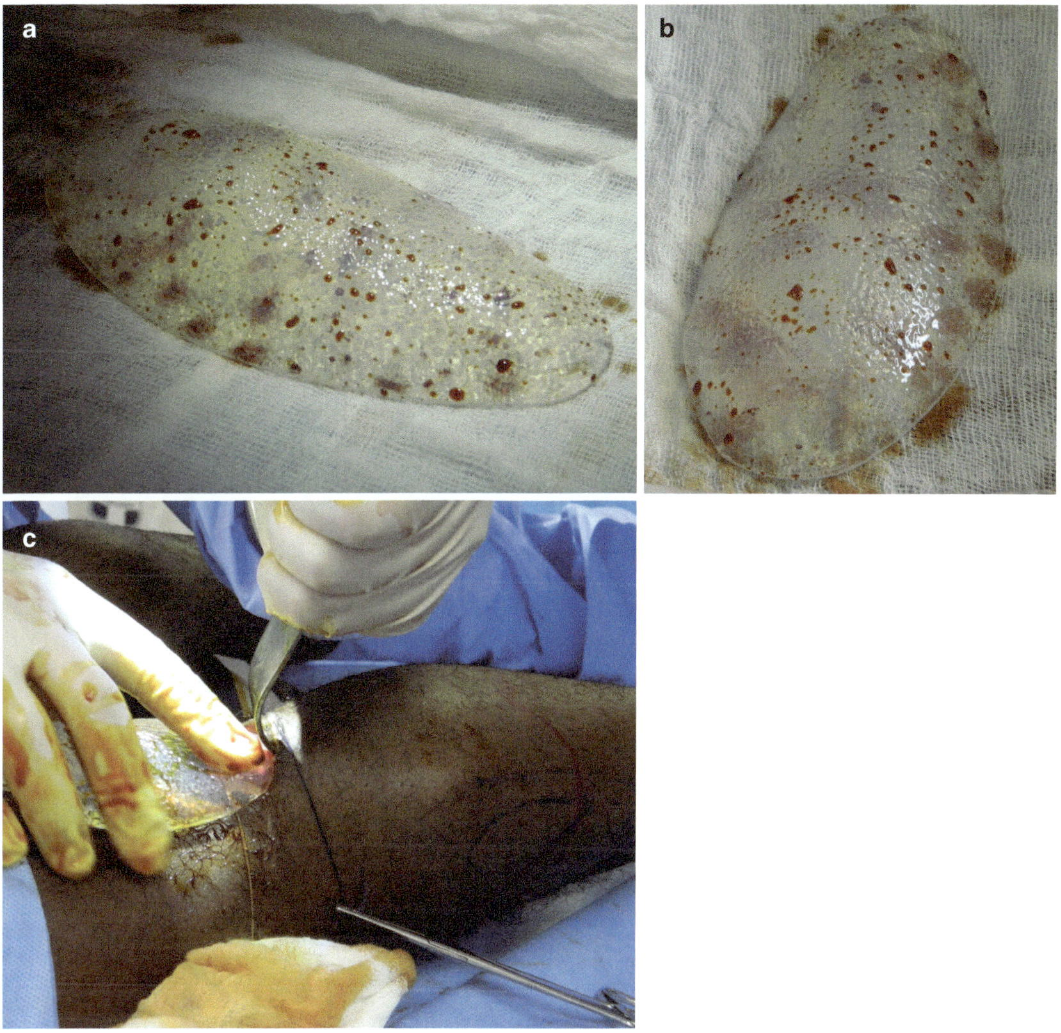

Fig. 8.15 The implant for lateral calf augmentation can be inverted if needed to give greater volume in the lower pole of the calf as in this patient who suffered from clubfoot deformity. (**a**) Natural position of the implant with bulk at the top tapering to a smaller point inferiorly. (**b**) Inverted position of the lateral calf implant (common for clubfoot patients who wish to achieve greater volume inferiorly in the leg region). (**c**) Insertion of the lateral calf implant

is paramount: fascia, deep dermis, and skin. While closing the fascia, the knee is flexed so as to bring about a good approximation of the fascia. Patient compliance with minimal activity in the first 2 weeks and light activity until the end of the first month is key. Even in the best-planned cases, dehiscence can occur and is typically found in the medial-most aspect of the incision due to the significant tension at this position (Fig. 8.18).

Nerve Injury

Due to the avascular and relatively structure-free dissection performed in the vast majority of cases, permanent nerve injury is rarely a problem. It is quite common for patients to complain of some numbness over the area of the popliteal fossa postoperatively; however, this returns within 1–3 months postoperatively. Major motor and sensory deficits can accompany

Table 8.4 Potential complications of calf augmentation

Potential complications of calf augmentation surgery
Infection
Seroma
Hematoma
Asymmetry
Implant visibility
Hypertrophic scarring
Hyperpigmentation of the scar
Capsular contracture
Wound dehiscence
Nerve injury (permanent or temporary, motor or sensory)
Compartment syndrome

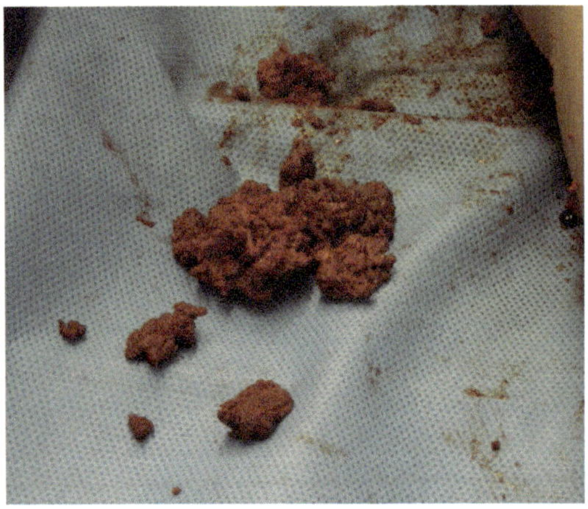

Fig. 8.16 Coarse granular material in a patient's calf region at time of implant removal 16 years after initial augmentation. The final pathology demonstrated significant calcifications but no malignancy

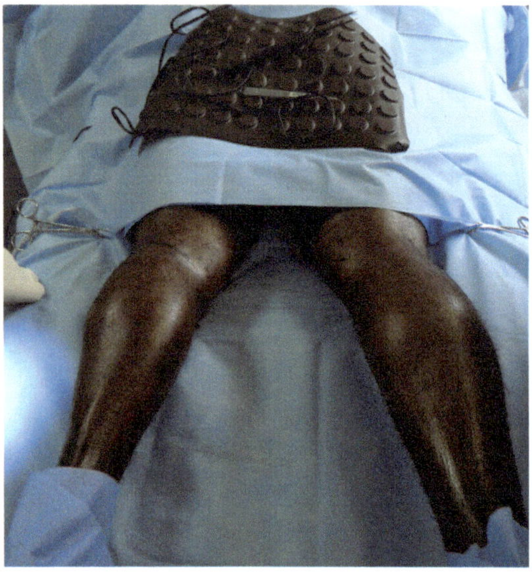

Fig. 8.17 This is a patient who suffers from left clubfoot deformity. He is athletic and wishes to have a more symmetric body. Despite a previous calf augmentation to the medial aspect of his left leg, he wishes to have further volume adjustment and is shown just prior to left lateral calf augmentation to achieve better symmetry. Even with the left lateral augmentation, there can never be a guarantee of achieving absolute symmetry

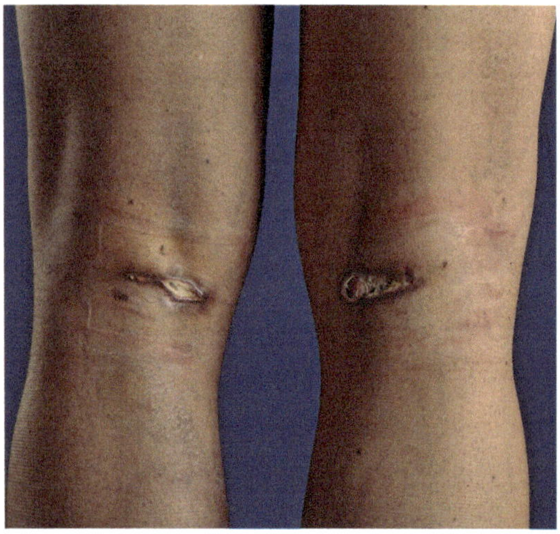

Fig. 8.18 Patient shown 2 weeks postoperatively with dehiscence of bilateral medial aspects of the popliteal incision and near complete dehiscence of the right calf incision. The patient later admitted to being more active in the first 2 weeks post-op than previously instructed, possibly resulting in his dehiscence

compartment syndrome, and this must be ruled out immediately if any significant deficits are appreciated.

Compartment Pressure Problems/ Compartment Syndrome

Compartment syndromes, typically seen in trauma, involve an acute increase in pressure inside a closed space, thereby impairing blood flow to the affected space and potentially putting the limb at risk for loss. Clinical signs of compartment syndrome include the 6 Ps: pain, poikilothermia, pallor, paresthesias, paralysis, and pulselessness. In conscious patients, pain out of proportion to examination is the prominent symptom. Pain with passive range of motion is particularly troubling. Paresthesias may also be described. In the lower extremity, numbness between the first and second toes due to compression of the deep peroneal nerve in the anterior compartment is the hallmark of early compartment syndrome. Progression to paralysis can occur, and loss of pulses is a late sign. By the time pulselessness has occurred, it may be too late for limb salvage. In patients with a compatible history and a tense extremity, clinical diagnosis may be sufficient. If the diagnosis is in doubt, compartment pressures may be measured with a handheld Stryker device. An absolute pressure greater than 30 mmHg in any compartment, a pressure within 30 mmHg of the diastolic blood pressure in hypotensive patients, and a patient with a concerning history who demonstrates the constellation of signs and symptoms of compartment syndrome are all possible indications for surgical compartment release *via* fasciotomy [17].

In the case of calf augmentation, the cause of compartment syndrome is typically due to placing too large an implant in too small a space, thereby increasing the compartment pressure and causing arterial insufficiency or venous outflow compromise. However, due to the fact that the patient is post-op, there is an implant in place and postoperative edema is present. Therefore, diagnosis may be problematic. In an affected compartment, accurate pressure readings may be difficult to obtain and may be inaccurate due to the patient's postoperative state. Clinical assessment and clinical diagnosis is the mainstay in compartment syndrome in the postoperative calf patient. Patients who are suspected of having compartment syndrome should have serial neurovascular checks, and any worsening of the patient's examination warrants surgical intervention. A patient who is clinically stable, has evidence of decreased pain or clinical improvement, and is cooperative may be a candidate for further close observation and neurovascular monitoring rather than immediate surgical intervention [18].

Both of the following cases occurred in patients who had augmentation for leg asymmetry due to clubfoot deformity. These cases point to the fact that it is the job of the physician to take special care in these types of complex cases and be ever aware of the potential for compartment syndrome.

Case 1

Near-Compartment Syndrome with Dehiscence and Resolution

This 36-year-old male patient underwent an uneventful calf augmentation of the left leg for clubfoot deformity. A style 2, size 2 AART implant measuring 126 mL was placed in a subfascial plane without difficulty. Four days postoperatively, the patient presented with pain in his calf that had been quite severe for the past days until he noted minor serosanguineous drainage. On physical examination, he demonstrated a dusky appearance to the skin over the medial calf and dorsal aspect of the foot. He had an intact dorsalis pedis pulse, sensation was intact, and motor function was grossly intact. Serosanguineous drainage from his calf incision with compression of the leg and a slight dehiscence of the wound were noted. There was indeed pain on palpation over the entirety of the calf. He was promptly admitted to the hospital for admission and urgent ultrasound to evaluate for any collections or DVT. No collections or DVT were noted. The patient had regular neurovascular checks to follow progression of the suspected compartment syndrome. Likely due to the decrease in pressure resulting from wound dehiscence at the level of the fascia (as evidenced by the rush of serosanguineous fluid), the patient was able to avoid a full-blown compartment syndrome. Three days later the patient was discharged with resolution of his pain, a strongly palpable dorsalis pedis pulse, and good motor function in the lower extremity. He had no further sequelae and is now 2 years postoperative.

Case 2 (Fig. 8.19)

Near-Compartment Syndrome

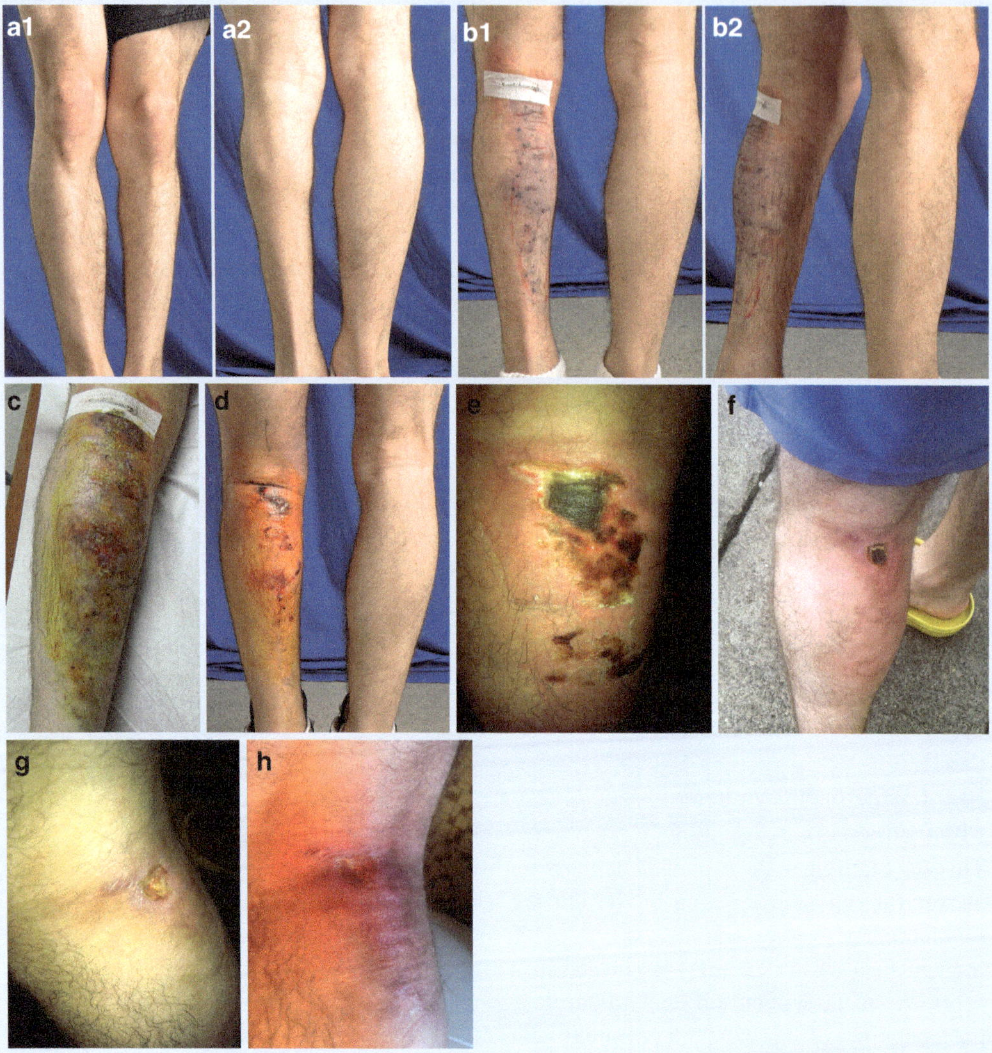

Fig. 8.19 (**a**) A preoperative 25-year-old male. (**b**) One day postoperatively, the patient is noted to have minimal bruising with a duskiness to the skin over the medial calf. The remainder of the leg is unaffected. (**c**) Two days postoperatively, the patient is shown to have more notable swelling with bruising and blistering over the medial aspect of his left leg. The leg has been painted with Betadine to help in the management of the blisters (drying them out). (**d**) Ten days postoperatively, the patient is shown with improved appearance to the leg with decreased swelling and blistering. (**e**) Two weeks after his surgery with necrosis over the site of the incision and scabbing over of the blisters. (**f**) 2.5 months after his initial surgery with significant contracture of his popliteal wound and healing of the skin in the areas that had previously blistered. (**g**) 3.5 months after his initial surgery with the scab in the popliteal fossa fallen off and continued contracture of the wound occurring. He still has no hair over the medial calf but coloration is continuing to improve. (**h**) The patient's medial calf 4 months after his initial surgery with granulation of the necrotic popliteal fossa and minor residual erythema of the leg in areas that have healed after blistering

This 25-year-old male presented with clubfoot deformity of his left leg which he had battled with since childhood. After consultation and implant selection, he had an uneventful left calf augmentation for clubfoot deformity. A style 2, size 2 AART implant, measuring 126 mL, was placed in a subfascial plane without complication. One day postoperatively, the patient presented with a foot that appeared dusky in color. His compression wrap was undone with return of color to the foot. His pain was not out of proportion to examination and the patient was ambulating on his operated leg. He had a strongly palpable pulse. His motor and sensory functions were intact except for a small area of numbness just below the site of the incision in the popliteal fossa. His foot was noted to be warm to touch. He was sent home with plans for follow-up on the next day, attributing his pale foot to a tight compression wrap postoperatively. He returned the following morning to the office with blisters over his leg and erythema of the calf region. Due to the fact that the patient desperately wanted to keep the implant if at all possible and did not have medical insurance, it was agreed in discussion with the patient and his mother that we would continue with close follow-up of the leg on a day-to-day basis. Any worsening of the condition would require prompt removal of the implant secondary to possible compartment syndrome. The patient was seen on a daily basis for wound assessment, pulse checks, evaluation of range of motion, and evaluation of sensation. The blistered areas were left intact and the calf was dressed with antibiotic ointment, as if treating any other pressure or burn wound. To minimize the risk of any additional pressure on the calf, the patient's compression garment was left off during the healing process. By postoperative day 10, the patient was much improved in the overall appearance of his leg and was ambulating and pain was minimal. He was cleared at this point to return home with plans for communication through email/phone. The patient did experience minor necrosis below the level of the popliteal fossa but had a full healing of the remainder of the skin overlying the calf. At no point in time did he ever have a complete loss of motor or distal sensory function. The foot was consistently warm and pulses were never lost. The patient was ambulating and even able to jog for short distances at 1 month post-op and continues to improve. The area of necrosis did granulate and heal by secondary intention without requirement of any further intervention by the fourth month postoperative. Once the scar has contracted, discussions will be had regarding scar revision to the affected area.

This case of near-compartment syndrome and its management may be criticized by some since there was not an immediate return to the operating room (OR) for implant removal. An open discussion was had with the patient and his mother regarding a return to the OR; however, since the patient had long wanted a corrective surgery for improvement of the aesthetics of his calf, he was willing to forego a trip to the operating room in the hope that his leg would slowly accommodate the increased volume. It was made clear that should any worsening of the patient's condition occur, we would be forced to immediately return to the OR for implant removal and limb salvage. This case clearly demonstrates the importance of a strong physician/patient relationship. To the patient's credit and to his mother's credit, they were consistently communicating with the physicians involved and took excellent care of the wounds in the postoperative period, allowing for good healing of the blisters and the popliteal fossa wound. While watchful waiting and close observation may be frustrating at times for both patient and surgeon, it is an option for those who wish to keep their implants in the face of a near-compartment syndrome. If there is deterioration of the patient or extremity at any point in time, a prompt return to the OR for implant removal is critical.

Special Cases

Reconstruction of the Hypoplastic Leg

In patients who have been afflicted with clubfoot, polio, or trauma, there is at times a noticeable discrepancy in the size of the lower extremities. For those patients wishing to achieve symmetry, a calf implant may be an ideal way to do so. However, that being said, a single augmentation may be insufficient to achieve symmetry.

Carlsen [15, 16], knowing this full well, designed a custom expander to slowly expand the calf region without having to subject the patient to multiple operations and risk possible issues of skin slough and excessively elevated compartment pressures. The expander designed had the following dimensions: 22 cm in length and 8 cm in width at the upper pole and 6 cm in the lower pole. This expander, which was filled with saline, was placed identically to the typical silicone calf implant and had a loop at the distal aspect which held a needle. Once the implant was well seated at the lower pole, near the malleolus, the needle was pushed through the skin and the implant was positioned as needed. The stitch was then cut at the skin level with the implant in position and an expander port was placed subcutaneously behind the knee. With this in place, Carlsen performed expansion every 7–10 days. At times, the expansion process could take 3–4 months, particularly in those patients with significant size discrepancies. Once the lower leg was overexpanded by 1 cm, Carlsen would remove the expander and place a solid silicone prosthesis.

While the idea of an expander makes sense, many patients are unwilling to go through a prolonged expansion period. In contrast, it has been the author's standard practice to place a smaller silicone prosthesis into position as per the technique described previously. Then 6 months later, after having stretched out the proposed implant pocket, a second procedure can be performed with either a larger standard implant or a custom-made implant. Regardless of the second operation performed, the patient is able to enjoy a fairly normal lifestyle free of return doctor visits for expansion and the possible discomfort associated with a port near the popliteal fossa. Although this method does require close attention in the postoperative period on the part of the patient and physician, it has been the author's experience that patients are much more content with the idea of this approach than the concept of slow expansion over time (Fig. 8.24). The following cases are examples of patients treated for hypoplastic legs. Staged operations are always discussed as a possibility but are not always required/desired.

Case 3 (Fig. 8.20)

A 17-year-old male was diagnosed with spina bifida occulta at birth. There was significant nerve damage due to lipomyelomeningocele which was removed at age 2 months. The patient and his mother wished to achieve greater symmetry between the left (hypoplastic) side and right side. He underwent augmentation of the left buttock (style 3, size 7) and left calf (style 2, size 1).

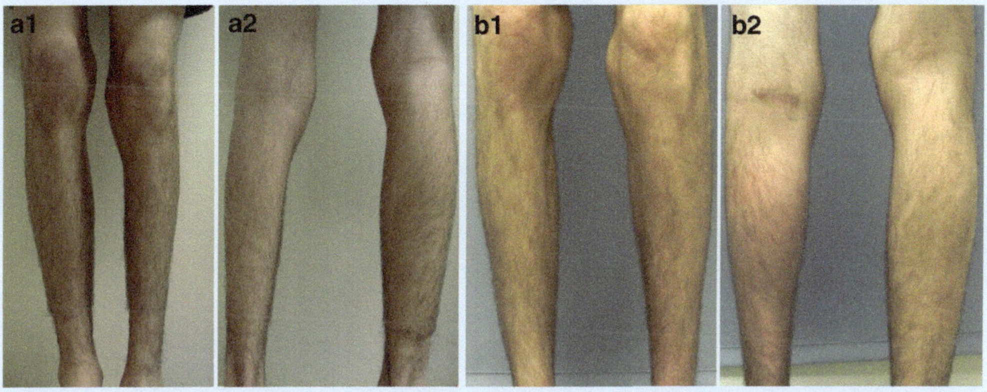

Fig. 8.20 (**a**) Preoperative. (**b**) Postoperative

Case 4 (Fig. 8.21)

A 56-year-old female had back surgery 12 years prior to presenting to the primary author. She had suffered a prolonged recovery with significant disability, leaving her right leg smaller than her left. She presented for augmentation of the affected limb with a style 2, size 1 implant to bring about greater symmetry.

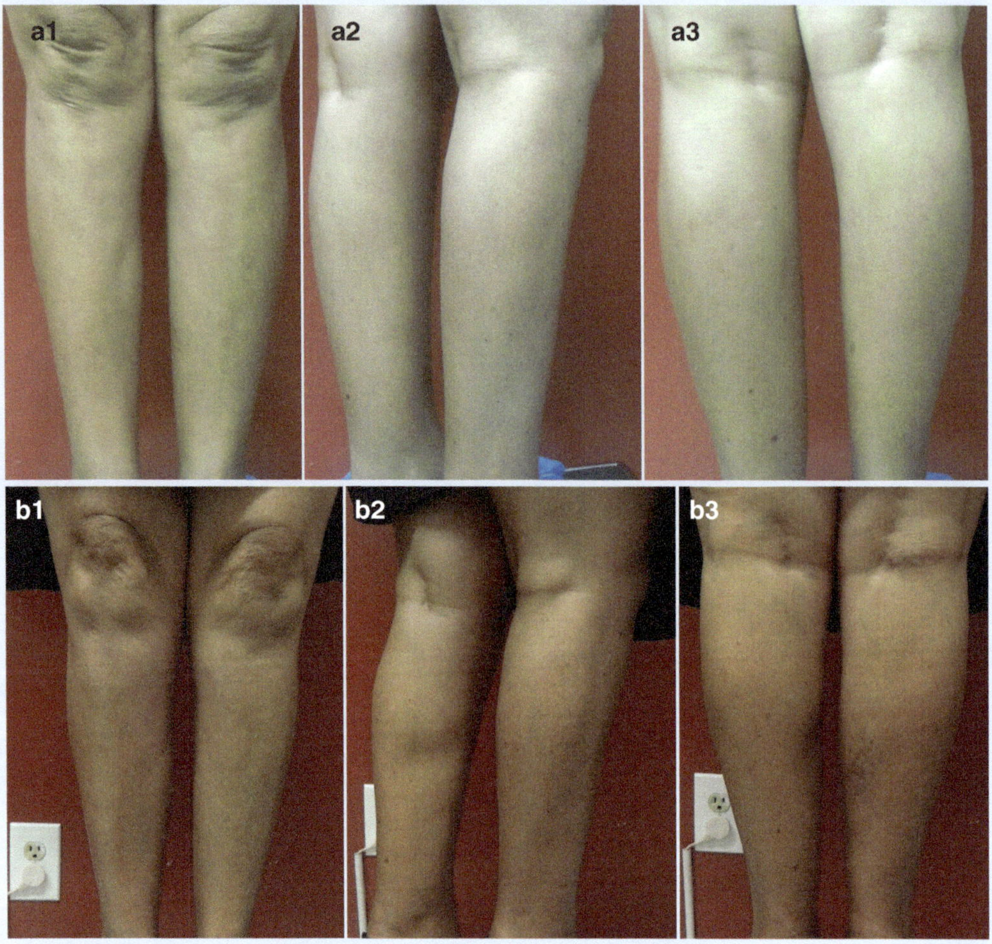

Fig. 8.21 (**a**) Preoperative. (**b**) Postoperative

Case 5 (Fig. 8.22)

A 38-year-old female suffered a trauma to her right leg as a child. She underwent many operations on the affected limb and developed a significant asymmetry. After presenting for consultation, she underwent medial calf augmentation with a style 2, size 1 implant to bring about greater symmetry. She is shown preoperative and 4 months postoperative.

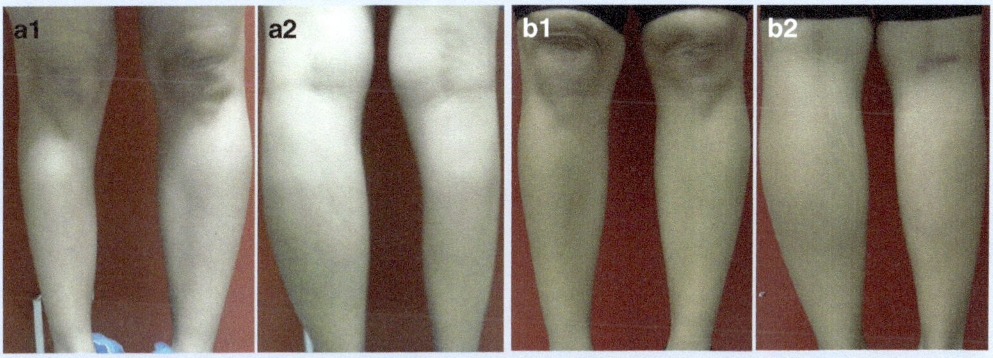

Fig. 8.22 (**a**) Preoperative. (**b**) Four months postoperative

Case 6 (Fig. 8.23)

A 32-year-old female suffered from polio as a child and was bothered by the asymmetry in her legs. She presented for augmentation of her leg and received a style 2, size 1 implant to the left medial calf with improvement in symmetry. She is shown preoperative and 6 months postoperative.

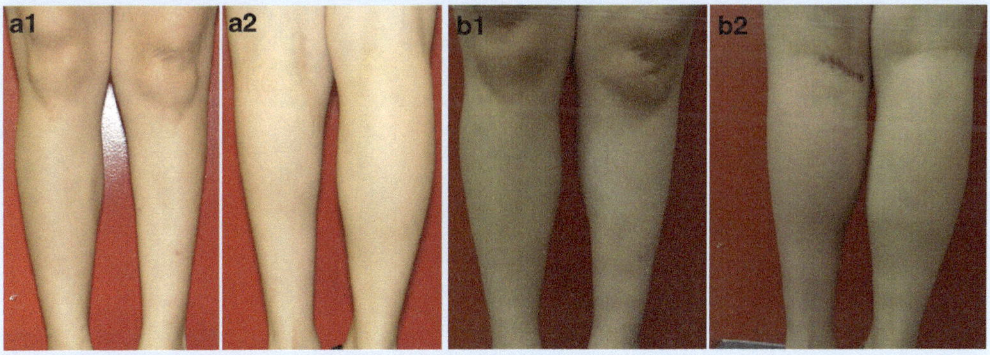

Fig. 8.23 (**a**) Preoperative. (**b**) Six months postoperative

Case 7 (Fig. 8.24)

A 30-year-old male was born with clubfoot deformity of the left leg. He presented for improved symmetry. He agreed to a staged procedure to bring about greater symmetry. First, he underwent augmentation of the medial calf with a style 2, size 2 implant. Eight months later, he underwent lateral calf augmentation with a style 3, size 1 implant. The next step will be either increasing the size of one of the implants or fat grafting to the lower leg, above the ankle.

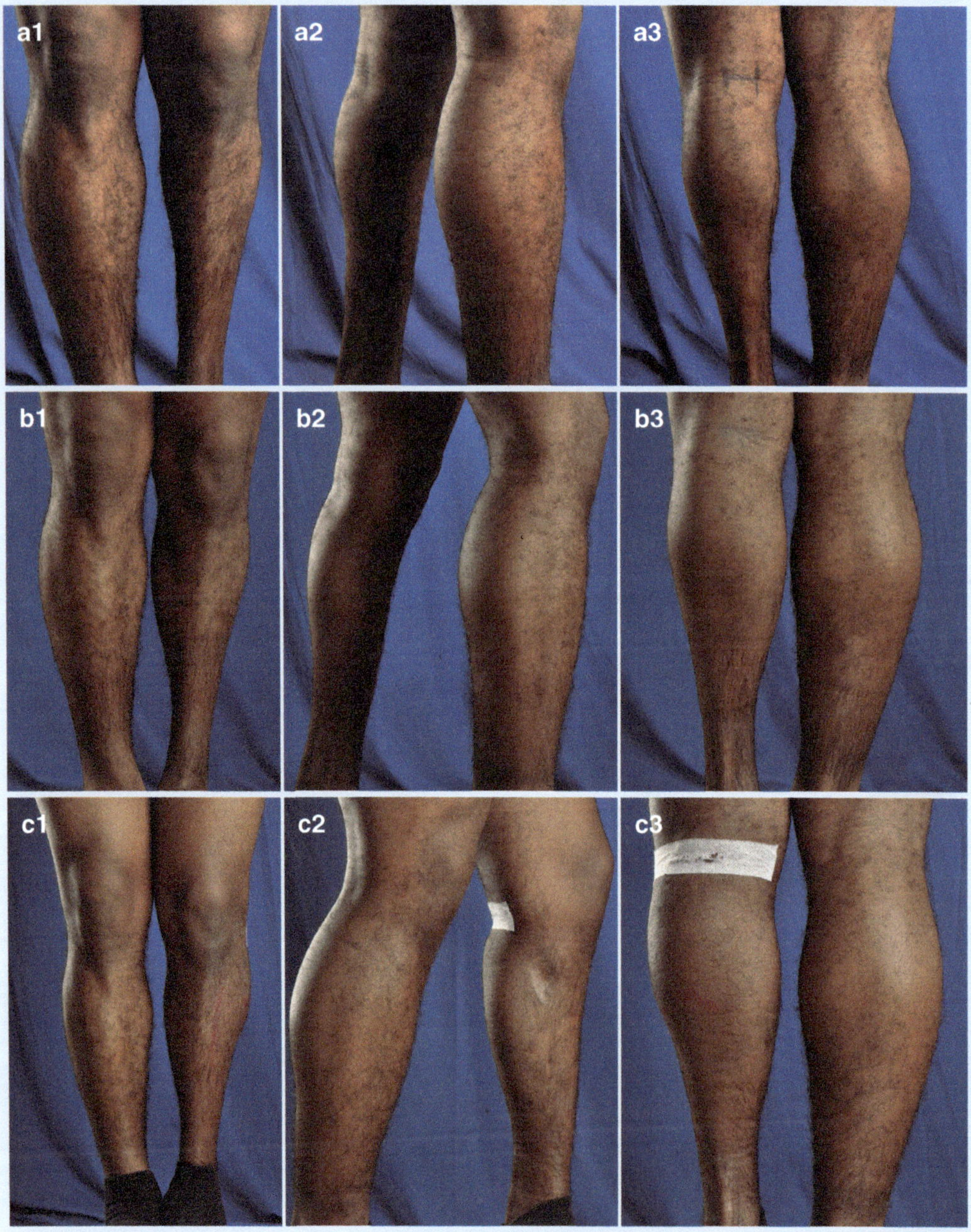

Fig. 8.24 (**a**) Preoperative. (**b**) Eight months postoperative. (**c**) One week after second surgery

Calf Augmentation with Fat Grafting

Over the course of the development of the calf augmentation procedure, some physicians have begun to explore the use of fat grafting to correct hypoplastic calves [1, 19, 20]. The use of fat injection for augmentation was explored to eliminate some of the common complications associated with implants: implant palpability, lack of correction of the ankle region, implant displacement, and the possibility of capsular contracture. Erol et al's [1] study of 2008 looked at 77 patients treated over a 10-year period with autologous fat and tissue cocktail injections, consisting of mini-micrografts of dermis, fascia, and fat. They noted a moderate improvement in 13 % of patients and a good improvement in 87 % of patients. Seventy-five to 200 mL of fat or tissue cocktail was injected into each leg to achieve the results noted in their study. These injections were repeated two to four times at 3-month intervals as was deemed necessary by the investigating physician.

While Eros et al. [1] have used fat grafting for calf augmentation with some success in their patients, the authors' results have been less than impressive. The largest complaint noted in the authors' patients that were augmented with fat is that the overall augmentation is not to their satisfaction or that the augmentation is asymmetric. These complaints are largely due to the variability in fat take and potential for fat cell death. In the hands of many cosmetic surgeons, the average patient can expect a fat take of 50–70 % without the use of stem cells [21–24]. However, this is largely dependent on placement of the fat in a place that has a rich blood supply that can foster the growth of the fat cells. When grafting to the calf, the calf muscles are already largely hypoplastic and so there is a lack of a robust blood supply to support fat cell take, in our opinion. While the authors' results are based solely on fat grafting without the use of tissue cocktail, we do not routinely recommend fat grafting to the calf as the results are inconsistent and there is the potential need for serial injections. On occasion fat grafting was performed to the distal aspect of the leg to produce further symmetry of the legs, particularly in clubfoot patients. But due to the minimal musculature and lack of robust blood supply, the grafting to this area is not reliable. However, the authors continue to look forward to further work in the realm of fat grafting to the calf and will continue to offer it to clubfoot patients in the hope of achieving greater leg symmetry.

Adjunct Procedures

Very commonly patients presenting for calf augmentation will have evidence of lipohypertrophy of the knees and thighs. A liposuction of these areas can often help in producing more shapely legs that are further enhanced by the calf augmentation procedure. These areas should be evaluated in each person presenting for calf augmentation.

Authors' Personal Results [11]

In evaluating the authors' most recent experiences with the technique from 2007 to 2011, it was found that there was an overall satisfaction rate of 92.1 % (186/202) (Table 8.5). Dissatisfaction was primarily due to hypertrophic scarring or an insufficient augmentation.

Table 8.5 Summary data for calf augmentations 2007–2011 [13]

Complication	Number	Percentage ($n=202$)
Infection	4	1.98 %
Seroma	13	6.43 %
Hematoma	1	0.49 %
Asymmetry	20	9.90 %
Hypertrophic/ hyperpigmented scar	30	14.9 %
Capsular contraction	0	0.00 %
Postoperative pain 8–10	19	9.40 %
Dehiscence	0	0.00 %
Satisfied	186	92.1 %
Unsatisfied	16	7.92 %
Compartment syndrome (near)	1	0.49 %
Permanent sensory or motor nerve damage	0	0.00 %

Patient Cases

Case 8 (Fig. 8.25)

A 49-year-old male presented for calf augmentation with style 2, size 2 implants. The patient is shown preoperative and 1 month postoperative.

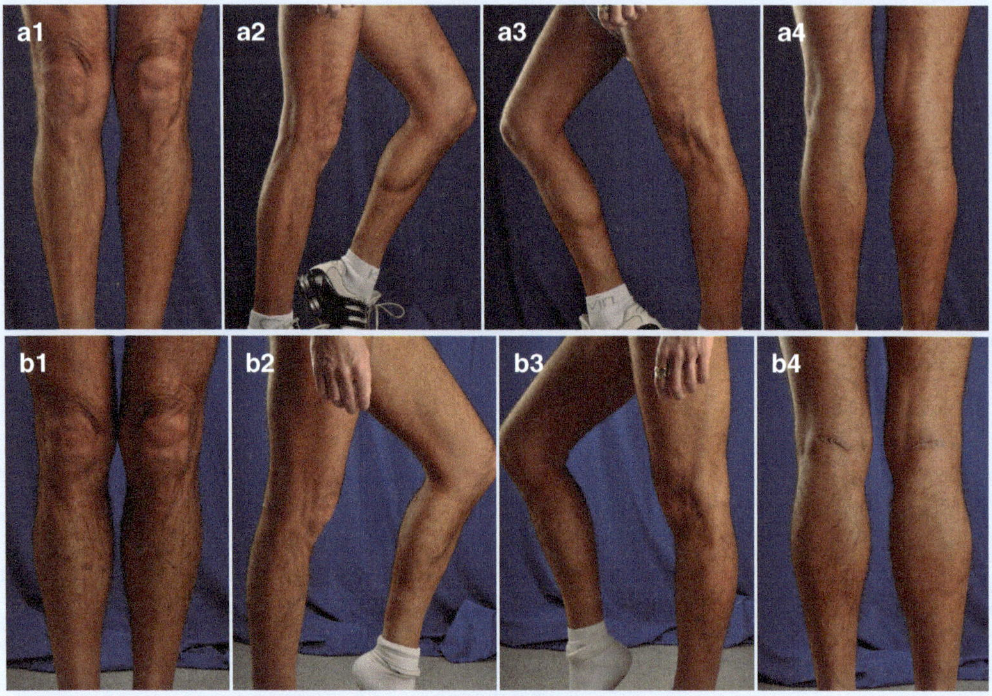

Fig. 8.25 (**a**) Preoperative. (**b**) One month postoperative

Case 9 (Fig. 8.26)

A 44-year-old female underwent augmentation with style 2, size 2 implants and minor liposuction of the right knee to achieve a more aesthetic and symmetric appearance to the legs. She is shown preoperative and 2 months postoperative.

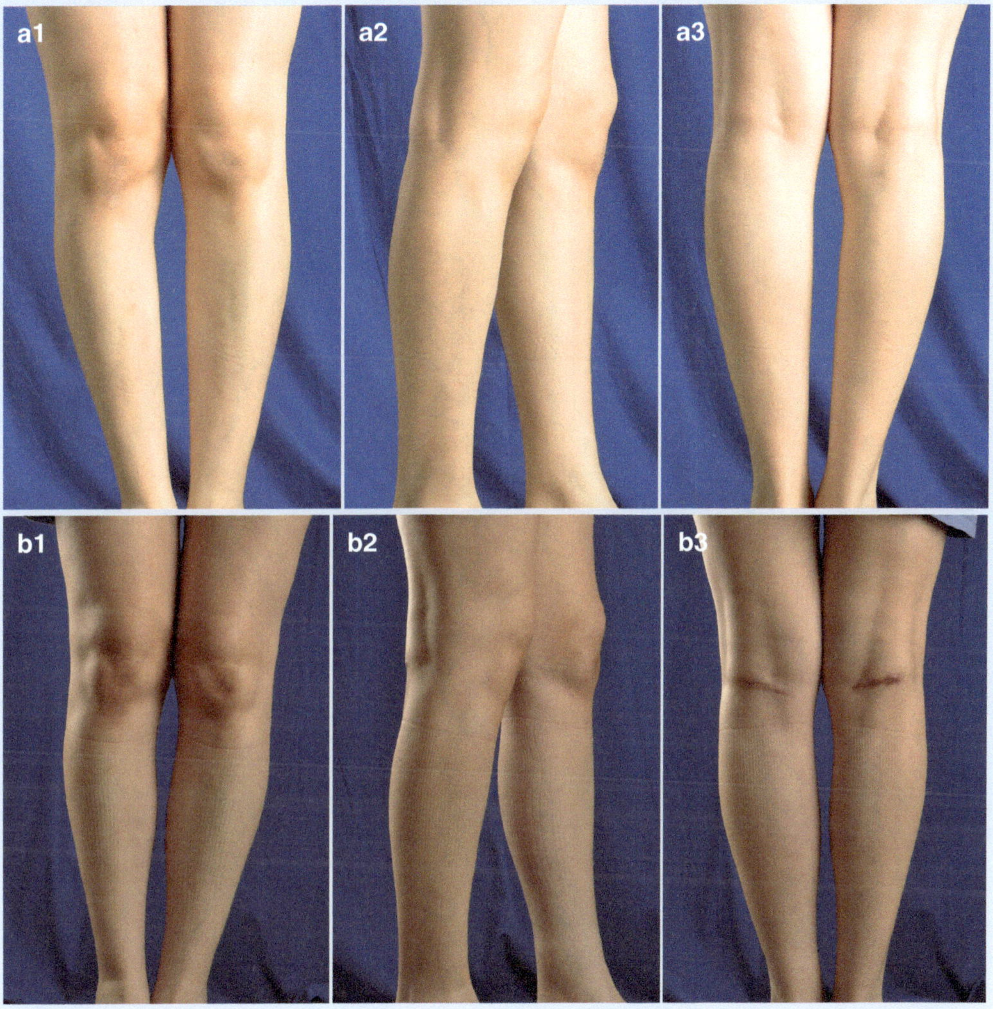

Fig. 8.26 (**a**) Preoperative. (**b**) Two months postoperative

Case 10 (Fig. 8.27)

A 40-year-old female underwent calf augmentation with style 2, size 2 implants. The patient is shown preoperative and 2 months postoperative.

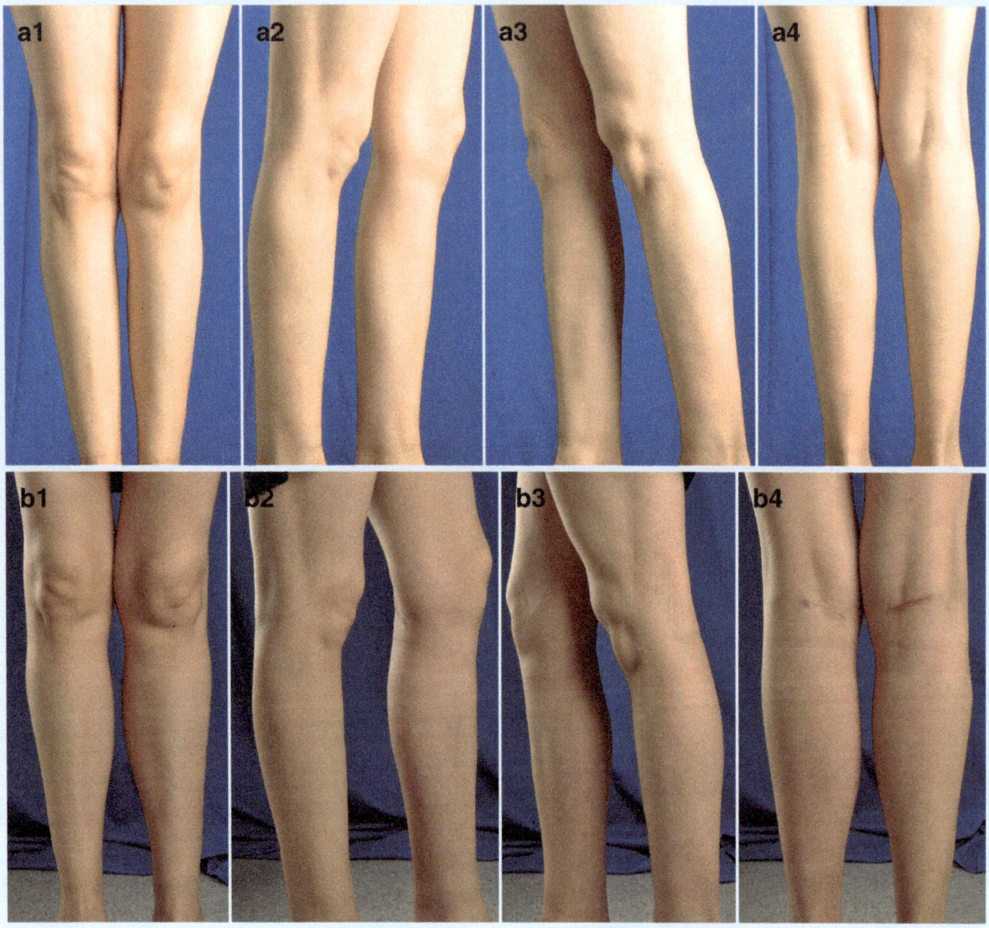

Fig. 8.27 (**a**) Preoperative. (**b**) Two months postoperative

Case 11 (Fig. 8.28)

A 52-year-old female underwent calf augmentation with style 2, size 2 implants. The patient is seen preoperative and 7 months postoperative. Note the hyperpigmented scars which are typical of Latin patients and other higher Fitzpatrick skin types.

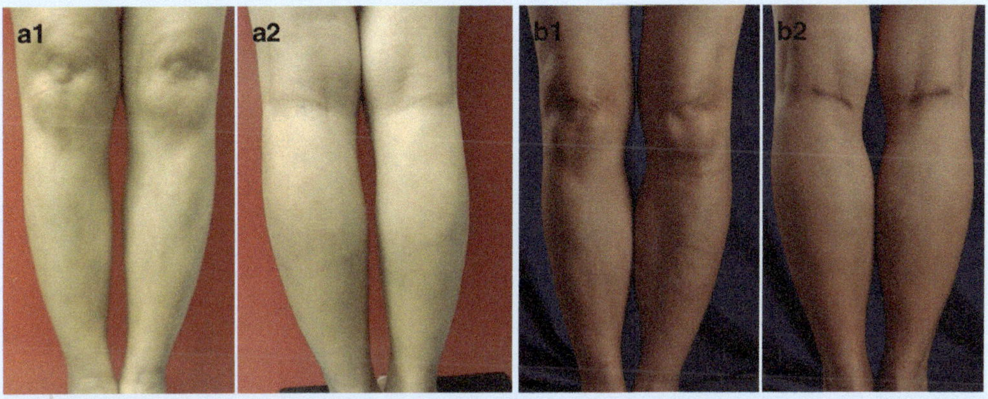

Fig. 8.28 (**a**) Preoperative. (**b**) Seven months postoperative

Case 12 (Fig. 8.29)

A 28-year-old female underwent calf augmentation with style 2, size 2 implants. The patient is shown preoperative and 1 week postoperative. Bruising as noted is very typical for early calf augmentation patients. Swelling extending to the ankles is very common in this early postoperative phase.

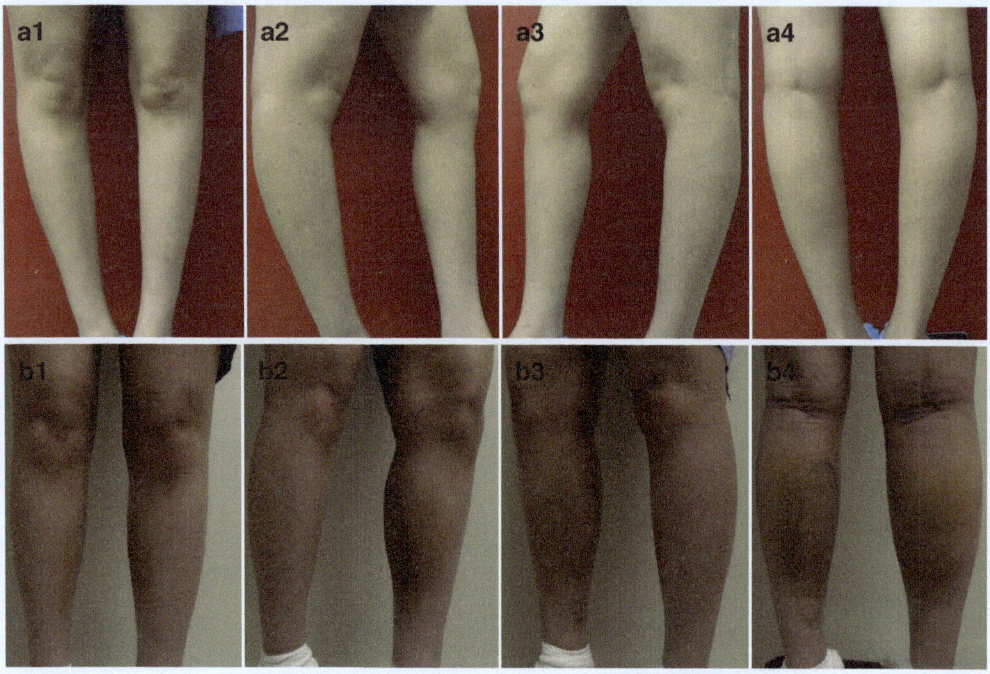

Fig. 8.29 (**a**) Preoperative. (**b**) One week postoperative

Case 13 (Fig. 8.30)

A 29-year-old female underwent calf augmentation with style 2, size 1 implants. The patient is shown preoperative and 6 months postoperative.

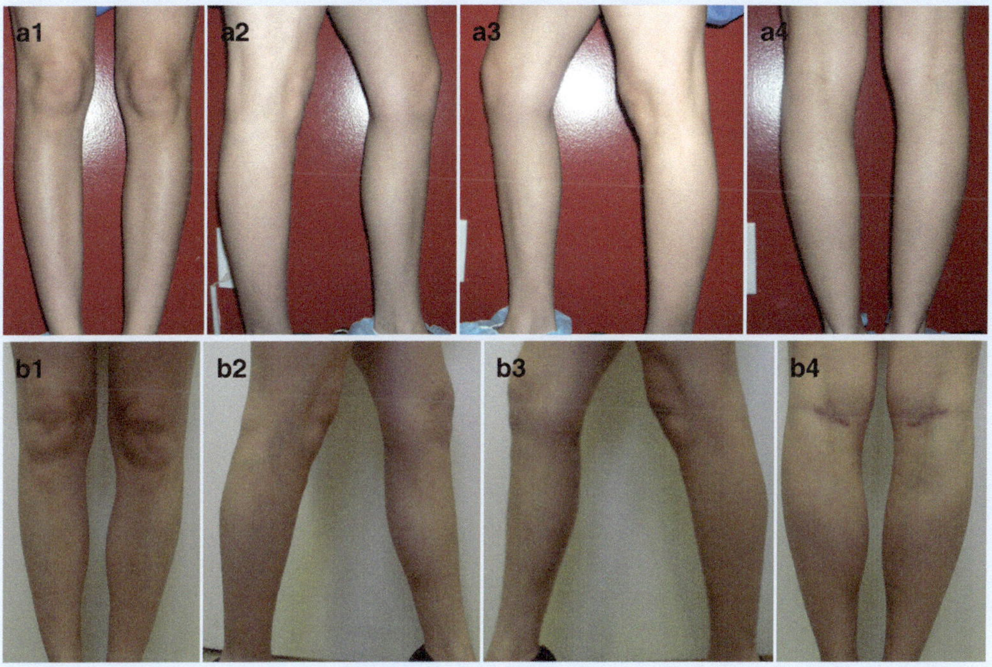

Fig. 8.30 (**a**) Preoperative. (**b**) Six months postoperative

Case 14 (Fig. 8.31)

A 31-year-old male underwent calf augmentation with style 2, size 2 implants. The patient is shown preoperative and 5 months postoperative.

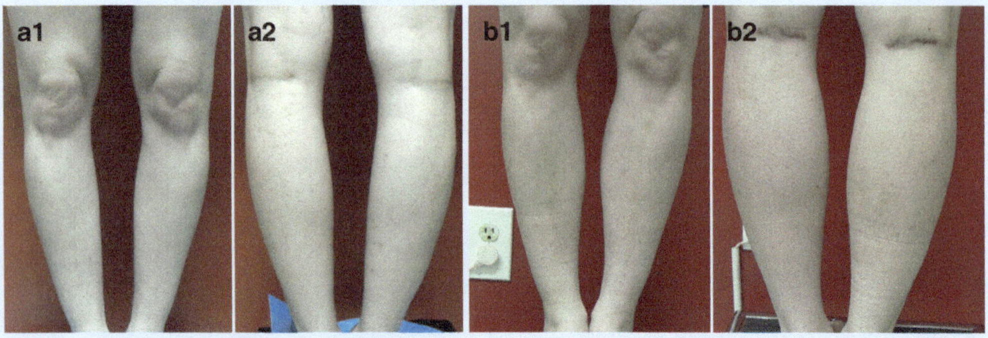

Fig. 8.31 (**a**) Preoperative. (**b**) Five months postoperative

Case 15 (Fig. 8.32)

A 33-year-old male desired to have a more pronounced bulky calf region and underwent augmentation with style 1, size 7 implants. These style 1 implants are well suited for men wanting a more "bulked out" appearance and patients who may be body builders and want an overall enlargement of the entire calf unit. He is shown preoperative and 1 month postoperative.

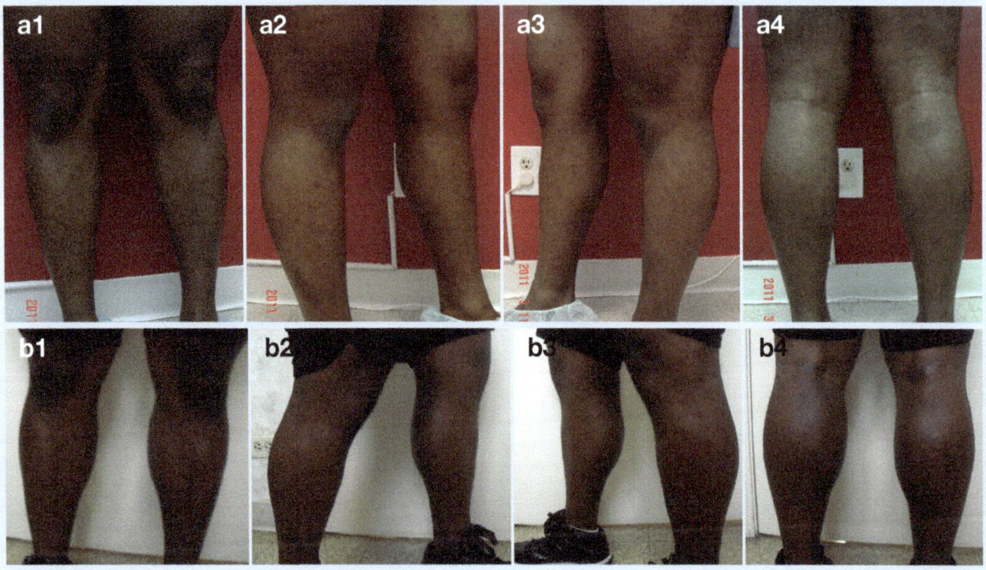

Fig. 8.32 (**a**) Preoperative. (**b**) One month postoperative

Case 16 (Fig. 8.33)
A 46-year-old male suffered from bow legs and felt very self-conscious. He underwent medial calf augmentation with style 2, size 2 implants. He is shown preoperative and 3 months postoperative.

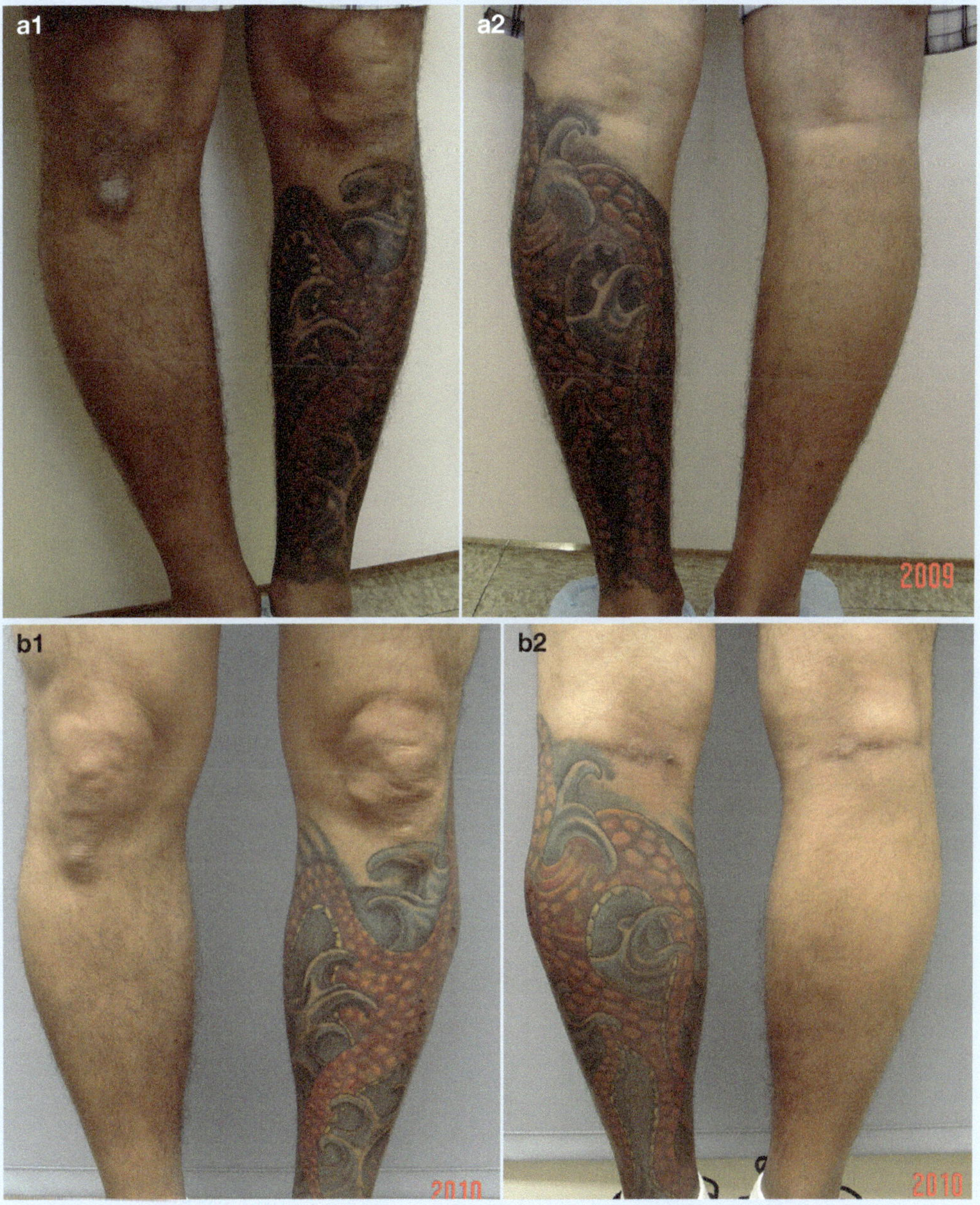

Fig. 8.33 (**a**) Preoperative. (**b**) Three months postoperative

Case 17 (Fig. 8.34)

A 32-year-old female underwent calf augmentation with style 2, size 2 implants. She is shown preoperative and 3 months postoperative.

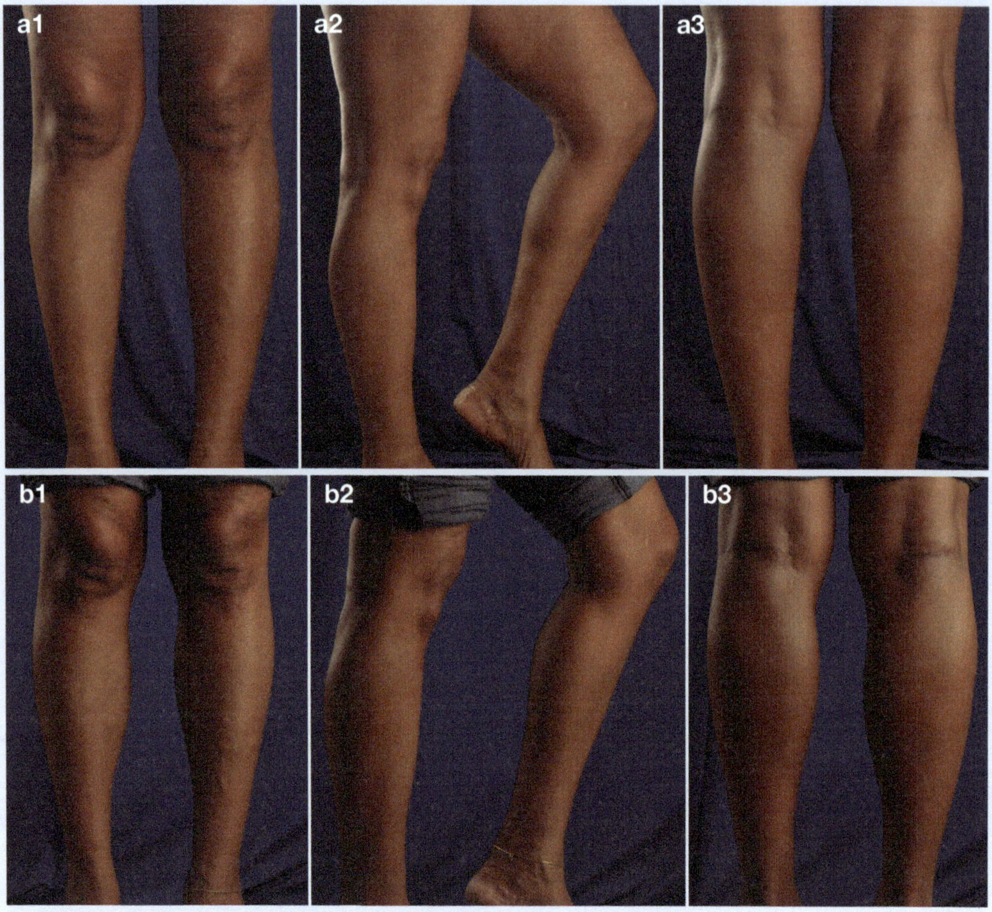

Fig. 8.34 (**a**) Preoperative. (**b**) Three months postoperative

Case 18 (Fig. 8.35)
A 34-year-old male underwent augmentation with style 2, size 2 implants. He is shown preoperative and 4 days postoperative. Bruising seen in the medial calf region is typical for this early phase in healing.

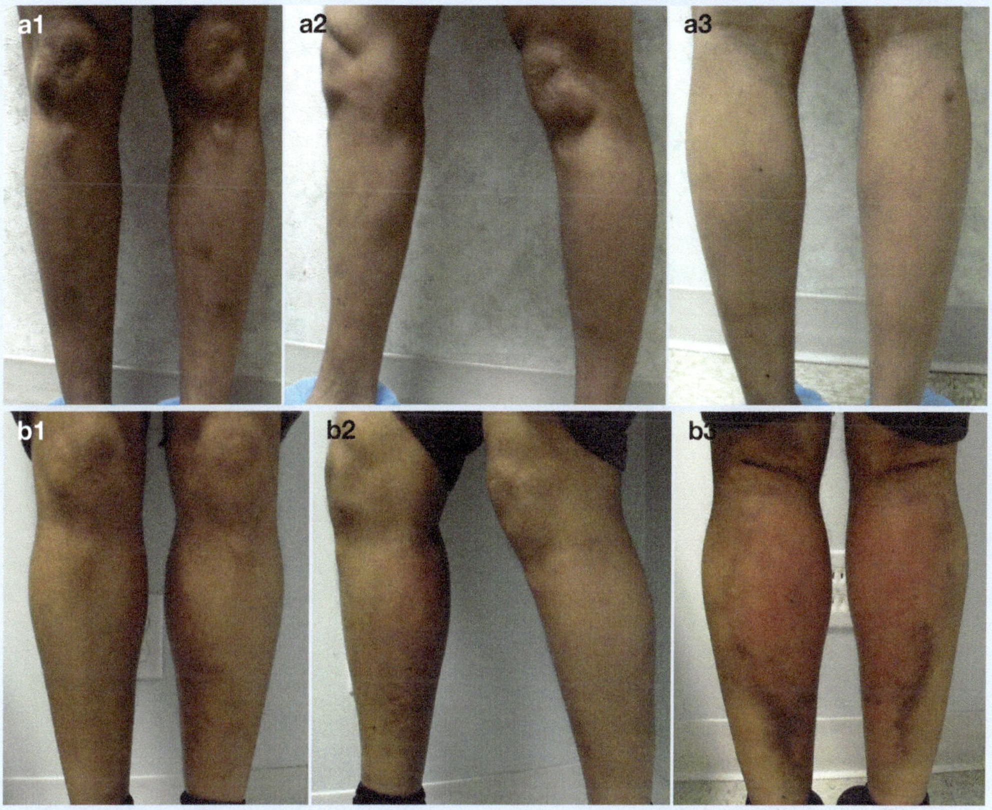

Fig. 8.35 (**a**) Preoperative. (**b**) Four days postoperative

Conclusions

Calf augmentation with silicone implants is a procedure that can nicely enhance the physique in a reliable fashion. The overall satisfaction rate is excellent as long as care is taken to ensure several things: choosing the right implant to meet the patient's expectations, meticulous attention to dissection of the pocket to minimize implant migration, and layered closure to minimize hypertrophic scarring.

References

1. Erol OO, Gürlek A, Agaoglu G. Calf augmentation with autologous tissue injection. Plast Reconstr Surg. 2008;121(6):2127–33.
2. Glitzenstein J. Correction of the amyotrophies of the limbs with silicone prosthesis inclusions. Rev Bras Cir. 1979;69:117–22.
3. Howard PS. Calf augmentation and correction of contour deformities. Clin Plast Surg. 1991;18(3):601–13.
4. Szalay LV. Twelve years' experience of calf augmentation. Aesth Plast Surg. 1995;19(5):473–6.
5. Niechajev I. Calf augmentation and restoration. Plast Reconstr Surg. 2005;116(1):295–305.
6. Aiache AE. Calf implantation. Plast Reconstr Surg. 1989;83(3):488–93.
7. Dini M, Innocenti A, Lorenzetti P. Aesthetic calf augmentation with silicone implants. Aesth Plast Surg. 2002;26(6):490–2.
8. Kalixto MA, Vergara R. Submuscular calf implants. Aesth Plast Surg. 2003;27(2):135–8.
9. Gutstein RA. Augmentation of the lower leg: a new combined calf-tibial implant. Plast Reconstr Surg. 2006;117(3):817–26.
10. Nunes GO, Garcia DP. Calf augmentation with supraperiostic solid prosthesis associated with fasciotomies. Aesth Plast Surg. 2004;28(1):17–9.
11. Chugay P, Chugay N. Calf augmentation: a single institution review of over 200 cases. Am J Cosm Surg. 2013;30(2):64–71.
12. De la Pena-Salcedo JA, Soto-Miranda MA, Lopez-Salguero JF. Calf implants: a 25 year experience and an anatomical review. Aesth Plast Surg. 2012;36(2):261–70.
13. Aiache AE. Calf contour correction with implants. Clin Plast Surg. 1991;18(4):857–62.
14. Carlsen LN. Calf augmentation: a preliminary report. Ann Plast Surg. 1979;2(6):508–10.
15. Vistnes LM. Procedures in plastic and reconstructive surgery: how they do it. Boston: Little Brown & Co; 1991.
16. Carlsen LN. Calf augmentation – a preliminary report. Surg. 1979;2(6):508–10.
17. Cothren CC, Biffl WL, Moore EE. Trauma. In: Brunicardi F, Andersen D, Billiar T, Dunn D, Hunter J, Matthews J, Pollock RE, editors. Schwartz's principles of surgery. New York: McGraw Hill; 2010.
18. Walsh J, Page S. Rhabdomyolysis and compartment syndrome in military trainees. In: DeKoning BL, editor. Recruit medicine. Washington, DC: Walter Reed Army Medical Center Borden Institute; 2006.
19. Veber Jr M, Mojallal A. Calf augmentation with autologous tissue injection. Plast Reconstr Surg. 2010;125(1):423–4.
20. Hendy A. Calf and leg augmentation: autologous fat or silicone implant? J Plast Reconstr Surg. 2010; 34(2):123–6.
21. Coleman SR. Long-term survival of fat transplants: controlled demonstrations. Aesth Plast Surg. 1995; 19(5):421–5.
22. Coleman SR. Structural fat grafts: the ideal filler? Clin Plast Surg. 2001;28(1):111–9.
23. Sterodimas A, de Faria J, Correa WE, Pitanguy I. Tissue engineering in plastic surgery: an up to date review of the current literature. Ann Plast Surg. 2009;62(1):97–103.
24. Sterodimas A, de Faria J, Nicaretta B, Pitanguy I. Tissue engineering with adipose-derive stem cells (ADSCs): current and future applications. J Plast Reconstr Aesthet Surg. 2010;63(11):1886–92.

Deltoid Augmentation

9

Introduction

Trauma, oncologic surgery, and congenital conditions can alter the appearance of the shoulder girdle and produce noticeable asymmetries of the upper extremity. To that end, the author (NVC) designed a prosthesis to help in recontouring the deltoid region and help patients attain greater symmetry between the two arms. In addition, increased publicity given to sculpted physiques has driven many men in search of a more muscular appearance. Despite rigorous workout regimens, some men are not able to gain the volume and definition that they desire in the deltoid region. For that patient, a deltoid implant may help in giving a more muscular appearance.

History of the Procedure

Orthopedic surgeons and plastic surgeons have long dealt with congenital anomalies of the shoulder and injuries to the brachial plexus that produce degeneration of the deltoid muscle and leave asymmetry between the two arms. Silicone prostheses have been used in these cases to help maintain the shape of the arm and achieve greater symmetry between affected and unaffected sides.

Of the known congenital anomalies of the shoulder girdle, Sprengel's disease is the most discussed in the literature, despite its rare occurrence. It results in a congenitally high scapula due to inadequate caudal movement of the scapula during development. Although there is no way to create absolute symmetry between an affected and an unaffected arm, the use of orthopedic procedures such as the Green technique and Woodward technique to reattach the overlying musculature and reposition the bone is the standard of care [1]. Some surgeons have even moved to using artificial silicone grafts to help bridge the gap to a good cosmetic outcome. Saray et al. [2] treated a patient with Sprengel deformity in 2000 using a silicone calf implant, hoping to bring about a more cosmetically appealing result. As noted by Saray, the "orthopedic procedures to correct Sprengel deformity are usually inconsistent and cosmetic results are far from satisfactory." To this end, he and his team set out to correct the patient's "sagging look," which was attributed to trapezius hypoplasia, with a calf implant. A 60 mL calf implant was then placed into a subcutaneous plane via a thyroidectomy-type incision in the neck.

In 2006, Hodgkinson described his work with deltoid reconstruction in patients that had deltoid degeneration following axillary nerve injury [3]. The axillary nerve in trauma victims is typically injured during a significant stretch of the brachial plexus, with disruption of the nerve as it exits the quadrilateral space in the axilla. There have also been cases of iatrogenic axillary nerve injury associated with shoulder operations or fracture reduction [3–6]. The result of these traumatic or iatrogenic injuries is a flattening of the natural convexity of the deltoid region and a weakening of the arm's ability to abduct. Hodgkinson fashioned custom implants for each patient based on

N.V. Chugay et al., *Body Sculpting with Silicone Implants*,
DOI 10.1007/978-3-319-04957-1_9, © Springer International Publishing Switzerland 2014

a moulage preparation of the unaffected deltoid region. This custom-made implant is then placed below the deltoid muscle to help bring symmetry to the two sides.

In 2011, the primary author (NVC) began his work in creating a custom deltoid implant for cosmetic augmentation of the lateral shoulder region. Although the work began on a patient with Sprengel's deformity, subsequent patients merely had hypoplastic deltoid regions and wanted to add volume to achieve a more "bulked up" appearance. Using a technique similar to that employed by Hodgkinson for reconstruction of the deltoid region, the primary author places a custom-made Chugay deltoid implant beneath the deltoid muscle, onto the upper humerus. With this augmentation, patients can expect to see a horizontal increase in volume of approximately 1 in. (2.54 cm) per side.

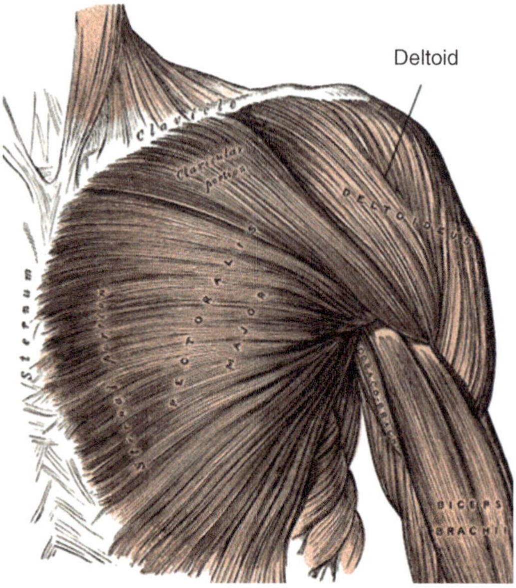

Fig. 9.1 Deltoid muscle overlying shoulder girdle and adjacent muscles

Indications

The primary indication for deltoid augmentation is correction of unilateral defects coming from trauma, oncologic surgery, and congenital anomalies. Congenital abnormalities of the skeleton, such as Sprengel's deformity which results in one shoulder blade sitting higher than the other, can be treated by performing a unilateral deltoid augmentation to bring greater symmetry to the body, particularly in the lateral aspect. Muscular dystrophies and traumatic injuries to the brachial plexus which result in hypotonia to muscles of one arm can similarly be treated with a unilateral deltoid implant to create a more symmetric appearance to the upper extremities. An alternative indication for the procedure may be for augmentation of the deltoid region for purely aesthetic reasons.

Contraindications

A relative contraindication to the procedure is a history of keloid or significant hypertrophic scarring. The deltoid region, along with the pectoral and back regions, is known to have one of the highest occurrences of keloid and hypertrophic scarring [7]. In light of this fact, a person that is already prone to this condition may be a poor candidate for surgery as the risk is already high even without a known predisposition.

Limitations

Augmentation of the shoulder region does not improve function of the muscles of the upper extremity. Patients who present with conditions due to trauma or congenital abnormalities need to understand that the change will be purely cosmetic and will have no improvement in mobility or function of the affected limb.

Relevant Anatomy

The deltoid muscle, or deltoideus, is a triangular-shaped muscle that is responsible for providing the rounded shape to the shoulder region (Fig. 9.1). Rather than being one solid muscle, the deltoid muscle is actually composed of three distinct muscles, as proven in anatomic and

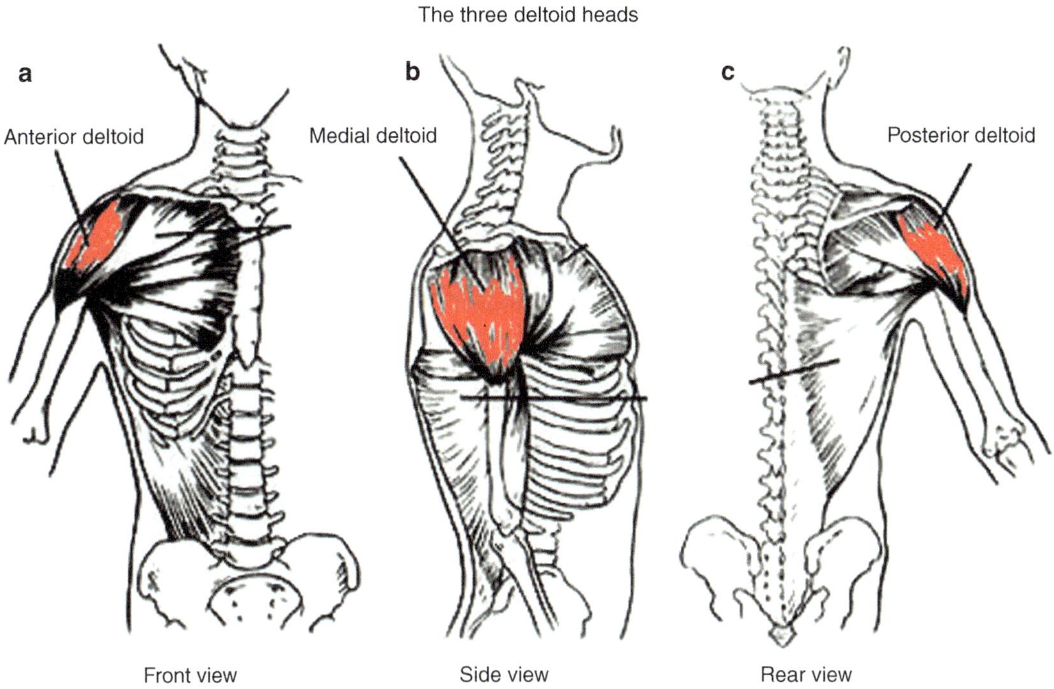

Fig. 9.2 Three heads of deltoid muscle

electromyographic studies (Fig. 9.2) [8]. A study of 30 shoulders revealed an average weight of 191.9 g (range 84–366 g) in humans [9]. The deltoid is made up of three heads: anterior (clavicular), lateral (middle, acromial), and posterior (spinal). The three heads all insert onto the deltoid tuberosity of the humerus. The anterior and lateral heads originate on the clavicle, while the posterior head has its origin on the inferior margin of the spine of the scapula (acromion). While the anterior deltoid often works in synergy with the pectoral muscles in movements of horizontal flexion and medial rotation of the humerus, the lateral deltoid is dedicated to abduction of the humerus at the shoulder joint and the posterior deltoid works in concert with the back muscles such as the teres major and rhomboids to perform horizontal extension and lateral rotation of the humerus. The pectoralis major and the anterior deltoid muscle are closely related and only separated by a small chiasmatic space which allows for the passage of the cephalic vein, preventing the two muscle from being one continuous muscle mass [8]. The deltoid muscle is supplied by the posterior circumflex humeral artery, which arises from the axillary artery. This artery travels posteriorly with the axillary nerve through the quadrangular space of the axilla (Fig. 9.3). The three heads of the deltoid are innervated by the axillary nerve, which arises from the ventral rami of C5 and C6 cervical nerves (Fig. 9.4) [9–11]. Again, this nerve enters from the posterior aspect of the muscle from the axillary region and runs along the medial surface of the muscle. Many orthopedic surgeons recommend that the separation of the deltoid fibers should occur no more than 4 cm from the tip of the acromion as injury to the axillary nerve is a possibility. This has been confirmed in anatomic studies that identify the axillary nerve as being located about 4.6 cm from the tip of the acromion (range 2–6 cm) (Fig. 9.5) [12]. Based on this and other research on the split lateral deltoid approach, it is safe to say that the safe zone for the dissection for placement of a deltoid implant is within 5 cm of the acromion, leaving an area of 5–9 cm below the acromion as a danger zone for potential axillary nerve injury [13].

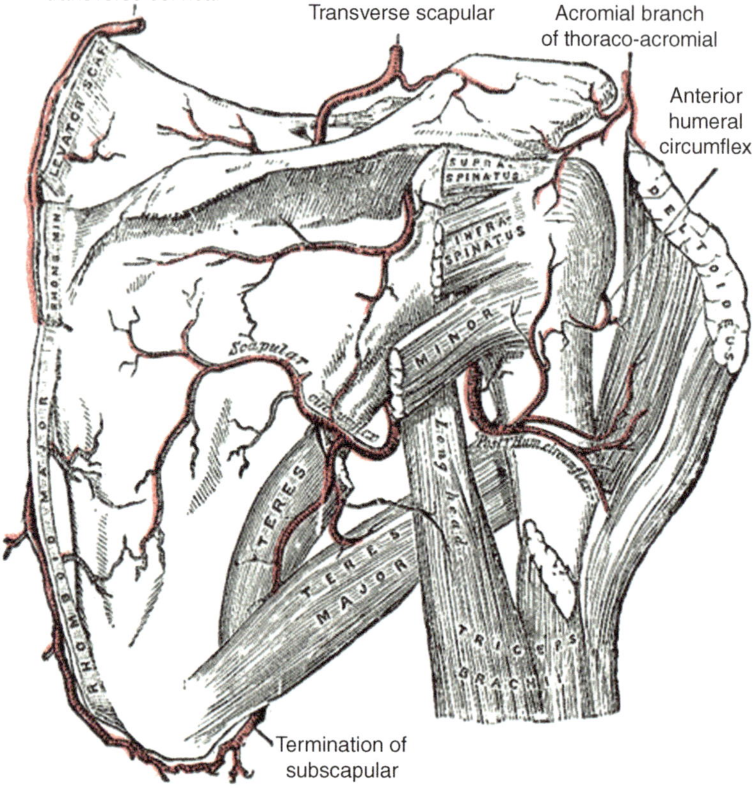

Fig. 9.3 Blood supply to the deltoid

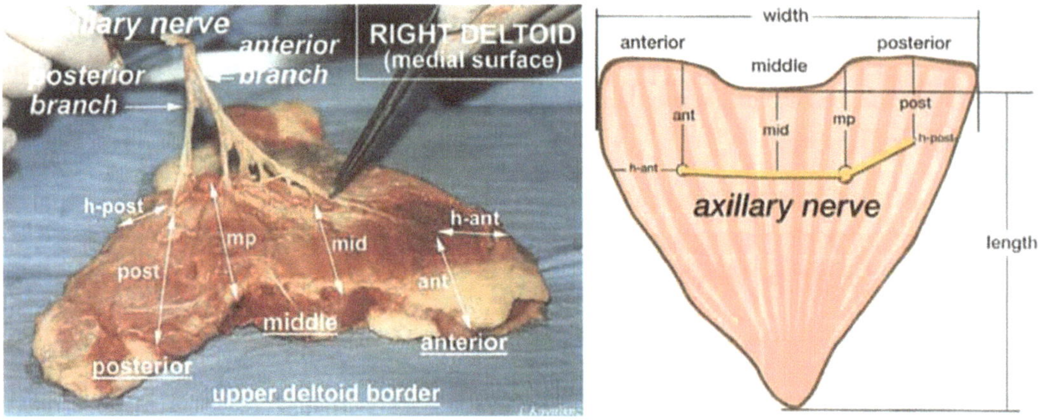

Fig. 9.4 Axillary nerve distribution

Consultation/Implant Selection

A thorough history and physical examination are paramount to preventing complications at the time of deltoid augmentation. During the consultation, patient's expectations are managed and assessment of the patient's mental state is undertaken. It is made clear to the patient the expected augmentation that can be seen with the surgery and limitations of the procedure are also explained (Fig. 9.6). Risks of the procedure, particularly injury to the axillary nerve, are discussed. A person with a notably short deltoid length is at greater danger of damaging the

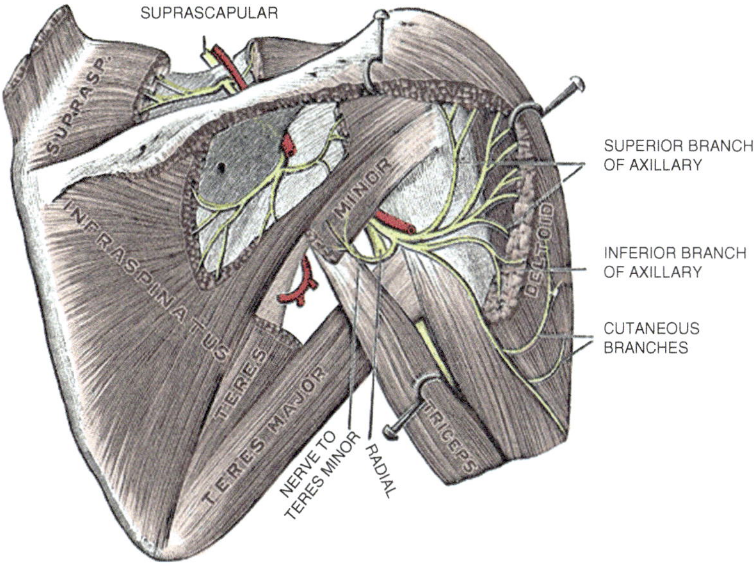

Fig. 9.5 Anatomic dissection of the deltoid muscle and the axillary nerve at its superior border within 5–6 cm of the acromion

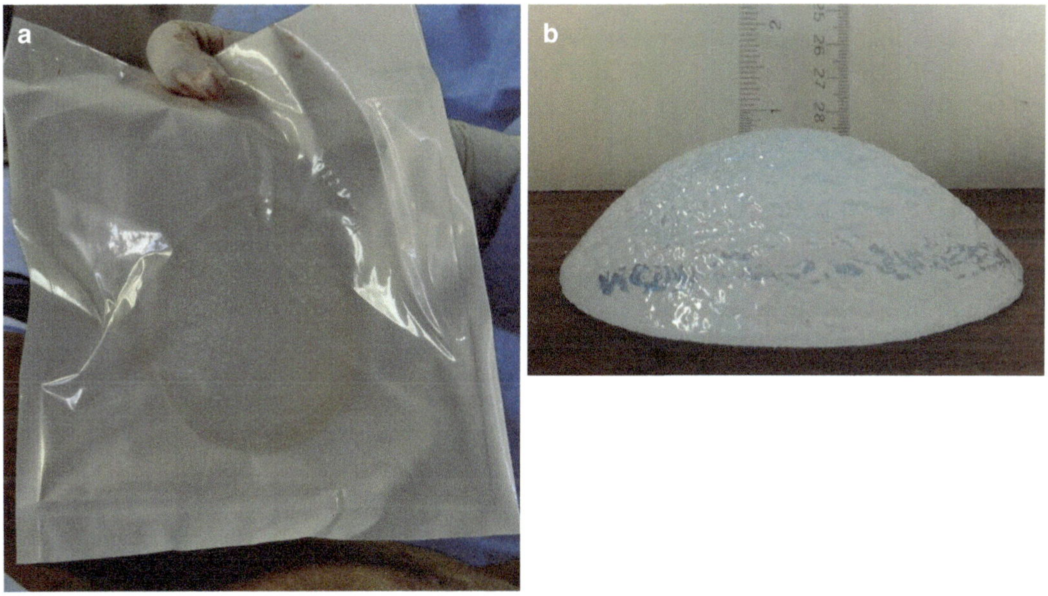

Fig. 9.6 (**a**) The deltoid implant in its packaging prior to implantation. (**b**) Deltoid implant lying flat on the table demonstrating vertical height of approximately 1 inch

axillary nerve at a short distance from the upper border of the muscle [12].

After completion of the history portion of the consultation, an evaluation of the patient's deltoid is made. Any asymmetries or defects are pointed out to the patient. The patient's muscles are then evaluated. The patient is asked to demonstrate a full range of motion of the shoulder girdle and arm to assess for any preexisting nerve injury or palsy. The skin and fat content are similarly assessed at this time as a patient with minimal adipose and thin skin is more at risk for implant palpability. Measurements of the patient's deltoids are then taken: (1) vertical height (length of the muscle) being measured from the level of the acromion to the suspected insertion over the humerus and (2) horizontal expanse of the deltoid (width of the muscle) as noted by palpation of muscle volume.

Table 9.1 Deltoid implants that are available

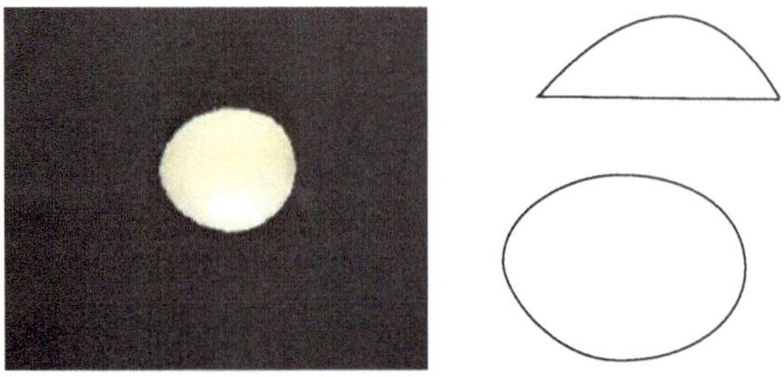

Size	Catalog #	Width	Length	Projection	Volume (cc)
1	1100–01DEL	8.0	10.0	2.0	116
2	1100–01DEL	8.0	10.0	3.0	115
3	1100–01DEL	8.0	10.0	4.0	161

Available Implants (Table 9.1)

Preoperative Planning and Marking

On the day of the surgery, the patient is met in the preoperative holding area. It is here that the patient's consent is verified and again risks, benefits, and alternatives are reviewed with the patient. With the patient in the erect position, the proposed site of incision is marked, measuring approximately 5–7 cm. The site of incision should be in the upper arm, overlying the deltoid muscle and 2 cm below the palpated glenohumeral joint, but being careful to not place the incision too low as axillary nerve injury can be caused with a low lying split of the deltoid muscle (Fig. 9.7). Once the site of the incision is marked, the site of the proposed implant is marked taking into account the patient's anatomy and existing deficit along with the desires of the patient.

Operative Technique

The patient is brought back to the operative suite and placed in the supine position with the arms at the side, with 90 degrees of abduction. If the case is to be done under intravenous (IV) sedation, as is the authors' preference, anesthesia is administered by the anesthesia provider. The patient's arm and chest are prepped sterilely. Twenty milliliters of 1 % lidocaine with epinephrine is injected directly into the substance of the deltoid muscle to achieve adequate analgesia. The site of the incision is identified and incised with a #10 blade scalpel for a length of 5–7 cm. Dissection is carried through the subcutaneous tissues using blunt dissection with a piece of gauze and electrocautery until the fascia overlying the deltoid is reached (Fig. 9.8). Army–Navy retractors are used to expose the fascia (Fig. 9.9). This is then incised with a #15 blade scalpel. Zero Vicryl stay sutures are placed in the fascial edges both superiorly and inferiorly. The deltoid muscle is identified and split in line with its fibers to prevent damage to the substance of the muscle (Fig. 9.10). This splitting of the fibers is performed with a Kelly clamp. Dissection is carried down to the level of the humerus. A submuscular plane is developed for implant placement. This is done with blunt finger dissection and a spatula dissector as needed (Fig. 9.11). Care is taken to create a tight pocket for implant placement as an overly dissected pocket may lead to undesirable implant migration. Hemostasis is attained at this time, as needed, with electrocautery. Once a sufficient pocket has been created, the pocket is irrigated with a solution containing Ancef, gentamicin, Betadine, and normal saline. The irrigant is then aspirated. The pocket is then instilled with 10 mL of 0.5 % Marcaine for postoperative pain control. A custom deltoid implant is then introduced into the pocket (Fig. 9.12). Position is verified and aesthetics are evaluated. Closure is begun by reapproximating the deltoid muscle with 2–3 interrupted 0 Vicryl sutures to minimize the risk of implant extrusion (Fig. 9.13).

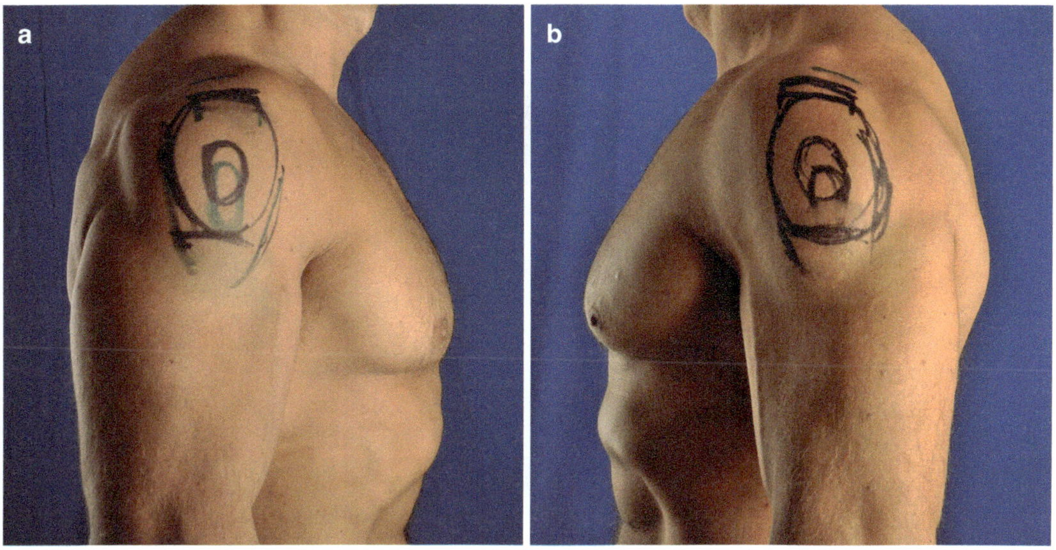

Fig. 9.7 (**a**, **b**) Preoperative markings in patient undergoing bilateral deltoid augmentation

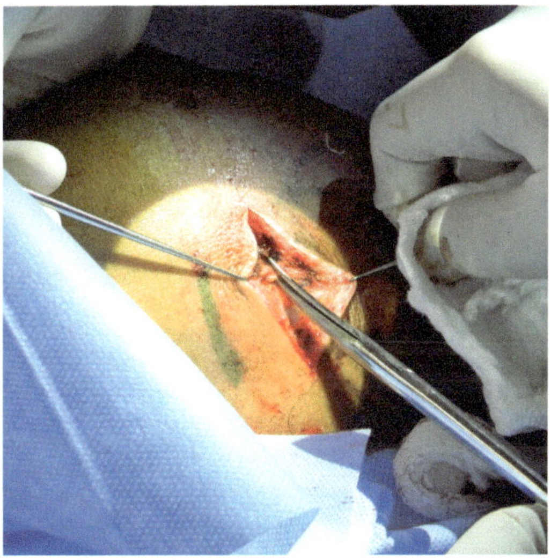

Fig. 9.8 Dissection through subcutaneous tissues using a combination of electrocautery and sharp dissection with scissors

The previously placed stay sutures in the fascia are used as guides to reapproximate the deltoid fascia with 2-0 Vicryl suture. The deep dermis is then reapproximated in buried interrupted fashion with 3-0 Monocryl suture. The skin is closed in subcuticular manner with 3-0 Monoderm Quill suture or with interrupted silk suture (as per surgeon preference). If performing a bilateral deltoid augmentation, the same procedure is mirrored on the contralateral side. After closure is completed, all incisions are dressed with collodion and Robbins tape (Fig. 9.14). The arms are wrapped with Coban to minimize the risk of seroma or hematoma formation. Anesthesia is discontinued and the patient is taken to the postanesthesia care unit (PACU).

Postoperative Care/Instructions

Postoperatively the patient may begin ambulating starting on the evening of the procedure. Patients may experience some difficulty in abducting the operated arm as there is need for accommodation of the implant. This weakness will gradually resolve over the course of the ensuing weeks. Patients may shower the first postoperative day, making sure to keep dressings clean and dry the Robbins tape with a hair dryer on a low-heat setting. Patients are then allowed to begin light activity at week 2 and full unrestricted activity at weeks 4–6. All patients are asked to wear an ACE wrap around the deltoid region for 4 weeks postoperatively to prevent dead space, thereby helping to reduce the risk of seroma formation. If the patient is unable to use an ACE wrap effectively,

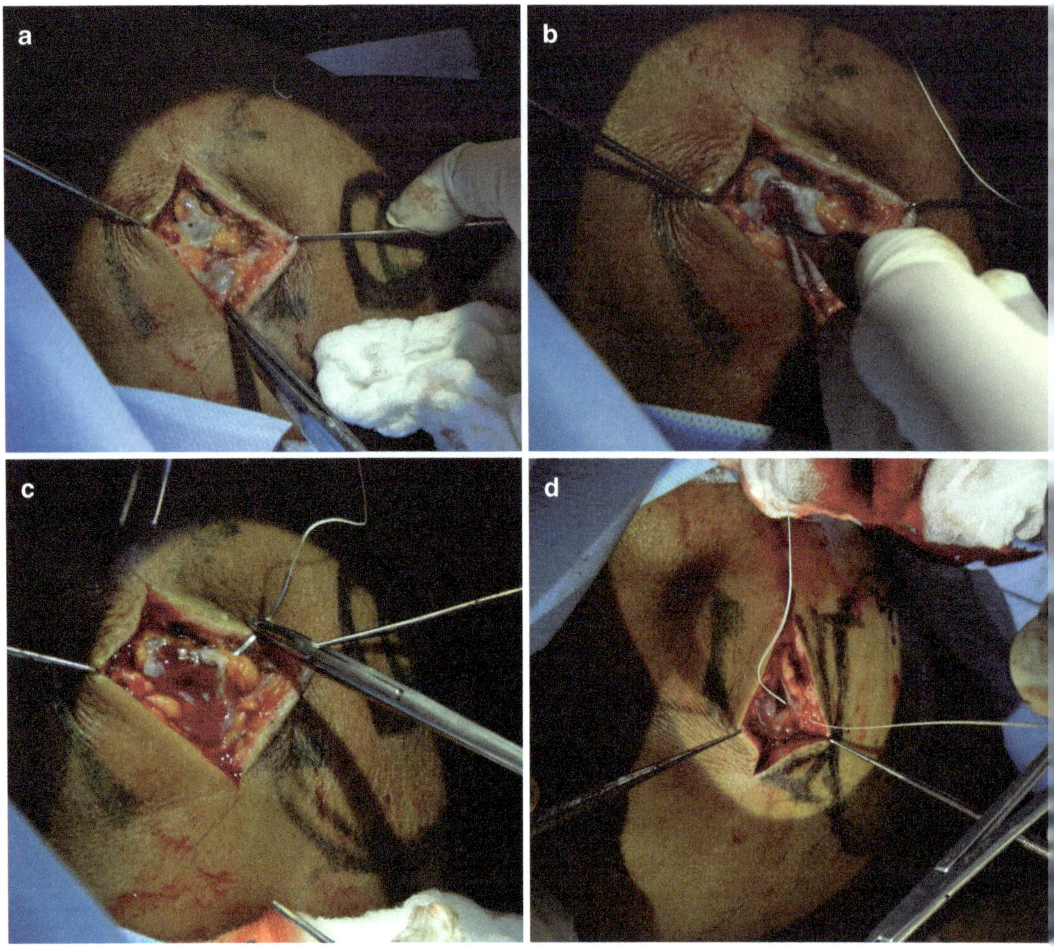

Fig. 9.9 (**a**) Deltoid fascia exposed. (**b**) Incision in deltoid fascia showing deltoid muscle. (**c**) Placement of stay sutures in deltoid fascia. (**d**) Placement of stay sutures in deltoid fascia

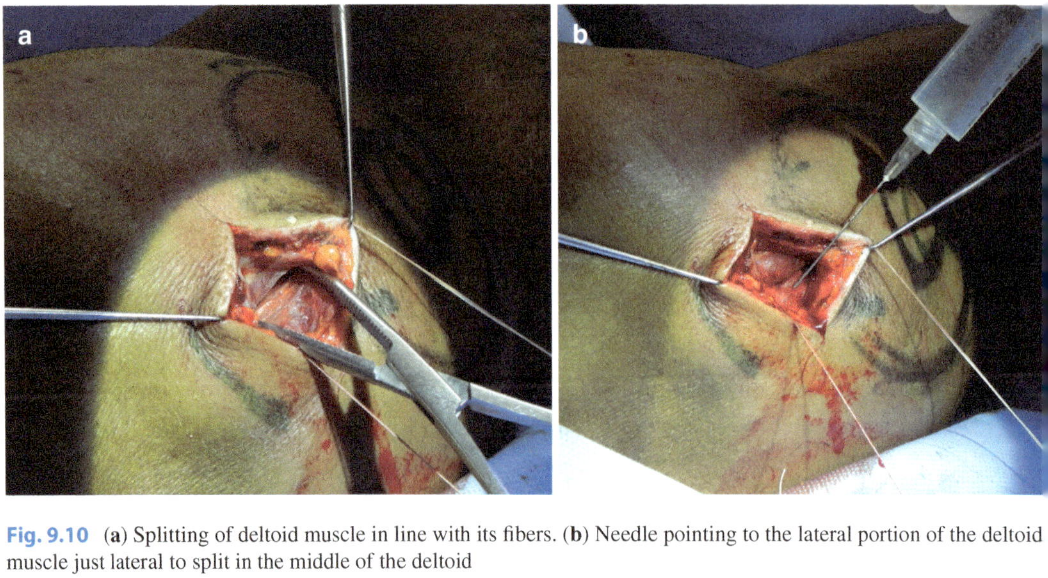

Fig. 9.10 (**a**) Splitting of deltoid muscle in line with its fibers. (**b**) Needle pointing to the lateral portion of the deltoid muscle just lateral to split in the middle of the deltoid

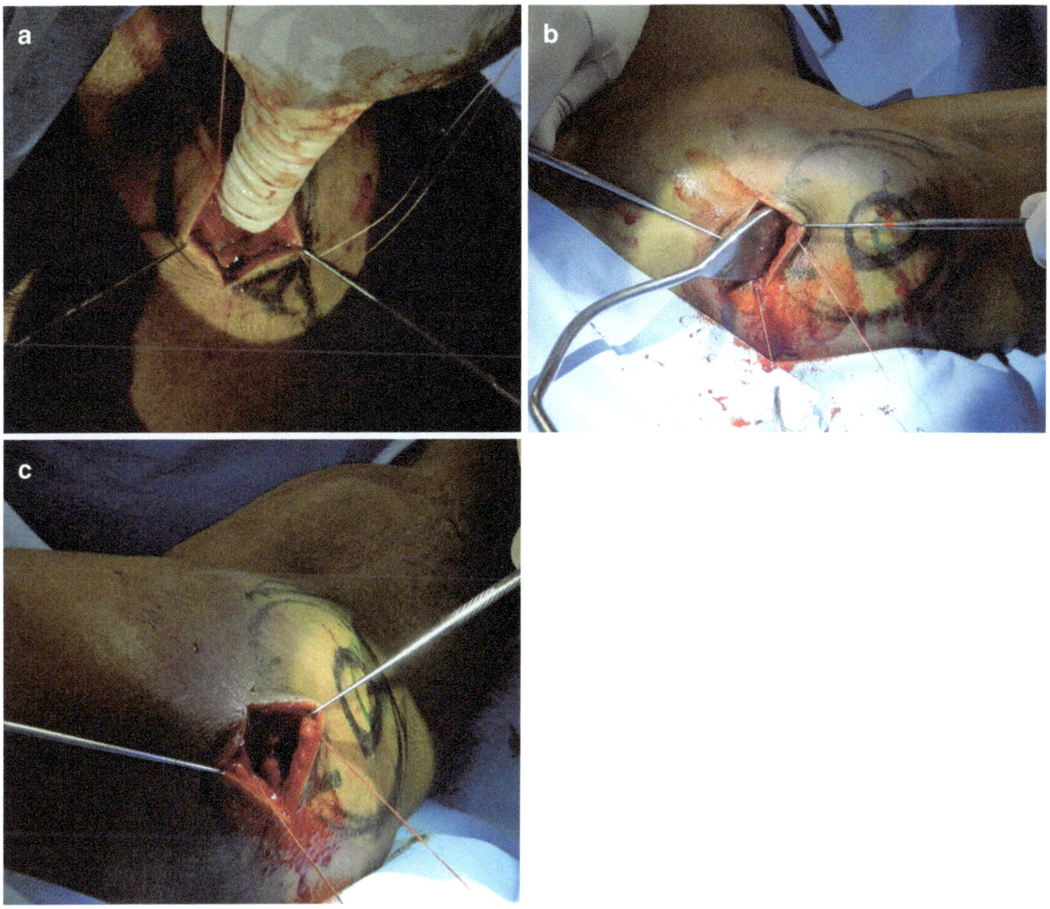

Fig. 9.11 (**a**) Dissection of subdeltoid pocket begun with finger dissection. (**b**) Spatula dissection of submuscular pocket. (**c**) Demonstration of submuscular pocket

a sleeved elastic garment may be used to provide compression to the region. Patients are prescribed both narcotic analgesics along with muscle relaxants (diazepam 5 mg every 8 h as needed for spasm) to assist with postoperative pain and muscle spasms. All patients are prescribed a week-long supply of ciprofloxacin 500 mg bid. If a quinolone allergy exists, the patient is provided amoxicillin with clavulanic acid 500 mg bid for a 7-day period.

Complications

In performing deltoid augmentation, there is a host of complications that can arise (Table 9.2).

Infection

Infection, either superficial or deep, is a possibility in deltoid augmentation surgery. The most likely culprits would be *Staphylococcus aureus* and *Staphylococcus epidermidis*, relatively common skin flora. Prior to making an incision, standard practice should be the administration of 2 g of intravenous (IV) Ancef (or 300 mg IV clindamycin in a penicillin- or cephalosporin-allergic patient). During the procedure, irrigation of the pocket with a standard antibiotic solution containing normal saline, Betadine, Ancef, and gentamicin should be performed. Postoperatively, a 5–10-day regimen of oral antibiotics covering normal skin flora should be administered. If a deep

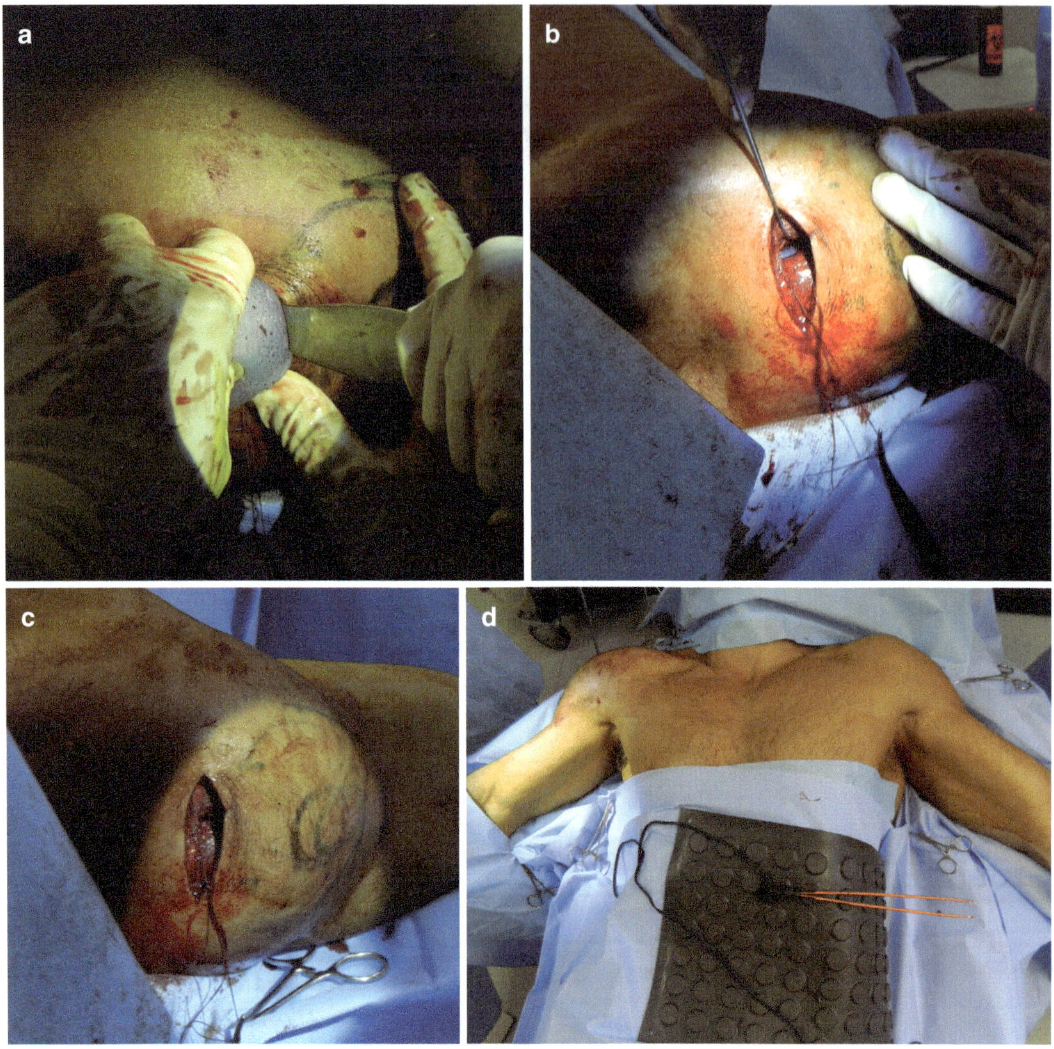

Fig. 9.12 (**a**) Placement of deltoid implant. (**b**) Deltoid implant below muscle noted between fibers of deltoid muscle. (**c**) Deltoid implant in position. (**d**) Right deltoid augmented and left deltoid not augmented

infection occurs, the standard practice is removal of the implant, closure, and possible reimplantation in 3–6 months. There are reports in other forms of implant surgery that conservative management and implant salvage are possible. This should be left at the discretion of the surgeon and performed with careful counseling of the patient.

Seroma

Seromas are statistically the most common complication occurring in implant surgeries. They typically present as new-onset pain, swelling, or asymmetry. The treatment of choice remains percutaneous aspiration. This complication is best prevented with patient compliance with compression garments or the ACE wrap and proper implant placement at the time of surgery, thereby minimizing dead space.

Hematoma

A hematoma is always a possibility in this surgical procedure, where the body of the deltoid

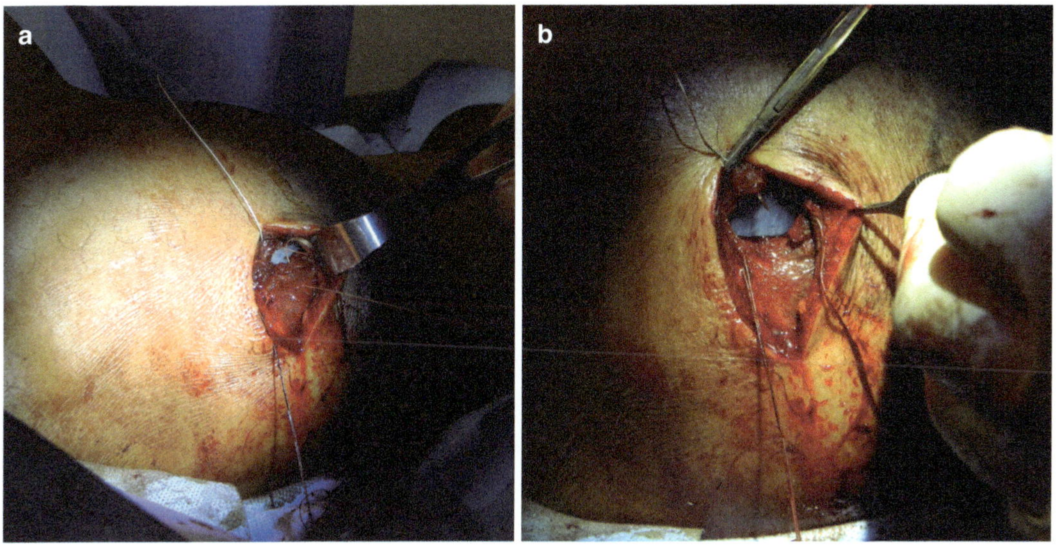

Fig. 9.13 (**a**) Reapproximation of deltoid muscle over implant. (**b**) Reapproximation of deltoid muscle (close-up)

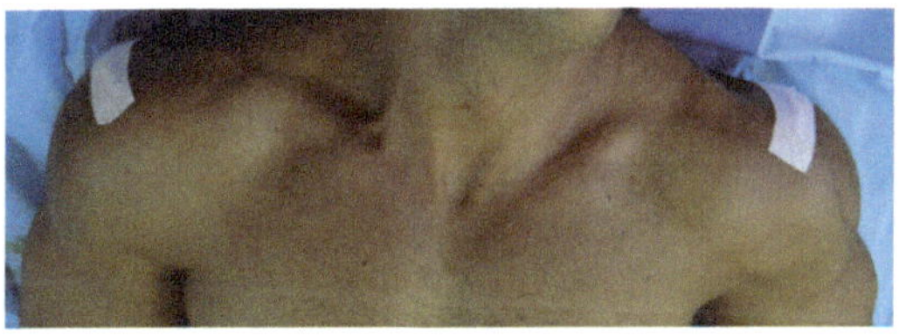

Fig. 9.14 Patient immediately post-bilateral augmentation

Table 9.2 Potential complications of deltoid augmentation

Potential complications of deltoid augmentation surgery
Infection
Seroma
Hematoma
Asymmetry
Implant visibility
Hypertrophic scarring
Hyperpigmentation of the scar
Capsular contracture
Wound dehiscence
Nerve injury (permanent or temporary, motor or sensory)
Compartment syndrome

implant is split in line with its fibers on track to placement of the implant on the humerus. In the event of a hematoma, rapid evacuation, pocket irrigation, and reimplantation are the mainstays of therapy. This complication is best prevented by meticulous hemostasis at the time of surgery and good compression of the deltoid post-op to prevent potential space creation.

Asymmetry

This can occur as a product of preexisting variability in the patient's arms or variability in dissection of the pocket bilaterally. This is best minimized by good preoperative photography and noting any asymmetries preoperatively. To avoid creation of asymmetry, it is important to maintain the same pattern of dissection and pocket creation bilaterally.

Implant Visibility

Due to the submuscular placement of the implant, this is indeed a rare complication. However, those patients that have very thin and atrophic arms to begin with may suffer from implant palpability and visibility. Patients should be counseled on this fact preoperatively if there is a feeling that the patient could be at risk.

Scar Hyperpigmentation and Hypertrophy

The key to reduction of these problems is careful layered closure. Patients with a history of keloid or hypertrophic scar formation may require the use of steroid injected at the site of incision. The deltoid region is well known to have a high risk of hypertrophic and keloid scarring along with the central chest and back regions [7].

Capsular Contracture

This is a possible late sequela of any implant placement, most frequently described in the breast augmentation literature. In the event that a patient presents with signs/symptoms of capsular contracture (e.g., induration of the implant site, tightness in the arm, new-onset pain, new-onset swelling), ultrasound or CT evaluation of the affected extremity is warranted. If a capsule is identified, typically characterized by calcifications, then a partial or complete capsulectomy is warranted. Capsular contracture is best prevented by meticulous hemostasis, good sterile technique, and avoidance of bleeding in the postoperative period. If it is noted early in the postoperative course, our standard therapy is zafirlukast (Accolate) 20 mg daily for a period of 2–3 months. Zafirlukast antagonizes leukotriene D4 and ER receptors. Although primarily used in the treatment of asthma, it has been found useful in the treatment of capsules, particularly in breast augmentation surgery [14–16]. Similarly, the authors find it useful in treating early contractures and have found softening of the affected region after 1–2 months of therapy, thereby avoiding the need for aggressive surgery to excise the capsule. Should the patient have a minimal or incomplete response to zafirlukast, one can consider capsulotomies. A capsulectomy in the area of a deltoid implant would be quite complex and could put major neurovascular structures at risk during the dissection and hence should be approached with caution.

Wound Dehiscence

Wound dehiscence is a product of poor wound closure under too much tension typically. In order to prevent this, meticulous closure in layers is paramount: deltoid muscle (reapproximation of the fibers over the implant), fascia, deep dermis, and skin.

Nerve Injury

In performing a deltoid augmentation, one must always be cognizant of the anatomic location of the axillary nerve. In the field of orthopedic surgery, a split lateral deltoid approach to the shoulder is often used to address proximal humerus fractures and lesions of the rotator cuff. Iatrogenic axillary nerve injury is a well-described complication as the nerve typically lies only 5–6 cm inferior to the tip of the acromion [5, 6]. Much like the technique for split lateral deltoid approach in shoulder surgery, deltoid augmentation seeks to split the deltoid muscle in line with its fibers to gain access the proximal humerus. Care must be taken to anticipate the location of the axillary nerve prior to performing a deltoid augmentation procedure. Bailie [17] noted that the position of the axillary nerve did vary with the position of the arm (neutral vs. 90° abduction vs. 30° extension vs. 45° rotation.). This fact is important to notice as each surgeon may elect to position the patient differently for deltoid augmentation, and this could potentially bring the nerve closer into the surgical field and place the nerve at increased risk of injury. Should the nerve be stretched or severed, an axillary palsy would result. A stretching injury (neuropraxia) will typically resolve within a period of 6–8 weeks. However, a complete transection of the nerve will lead to a reduction in the ability to abduct the affected shoulder.

Compartment Pressure Problems/ Compartment Syndrome

Compartment syndromes, typically seen in trauma, involve an acute increase in pressure inside a closed space, thereby impairing blood flow to the affected space and potentially putting the limb at risk for loss. Clinical signs of compartment syndrome include the 6 Ps: pain, poikilothermia, pallor, paresthesias, paralysis, and pulselessness. In conscious patients, pain out of proportion to examination is the prominent symptom. Pain with passive range of motion is particularly troubling. Compartment syndrome of the deltoid should be considered in the patient who presents with unexplained pain out of proportion to the examination.

Authors' Personal Experience

To date, the authors have performed ten deltoid augmentation procedures for correction of congenital defects, for the correction of defects produced as a result of trauma, and to augment hypoplastic deltoids. No major complications were seen arising from deltoid augmentation. The most frequent complication noted in deltoid augmentation is a hypertrophic scar secondary to the significant amount of motion in the area of the shoulder. 90 % (9/10) of the patients operated on were satisfied with the procedure with only one patient complaining about scarring which was more than he would have expected.

The primary author (NVC) had his beginning with deltoid augmentation when a patient with Sprengel's deformity presented with complaints of asymmetry of the right shoulder particularly in the area overlying the deltoid muscle. To help this patient, the author devised a custom deltoid implant to give greater prominence to the deltoid muscle group. This initial case has since led to the treatment of patients who not only have unilateral deformities due to congenital anomalies and trauma but also to those who simply wish to have a more pronounced deltoid region.

Patient Cases

Case 1 (Fig. 9.15)
A 28-year-old male presented with complaints of asymmetry of his arms secondary to Sprengel's deformity. He wanted to look more symmetric when wearing clothing as none of his shirts fit properly. He underwent right deltoid augmentation with a size 1 deltoid implant. The patient is shown preoperative and 3 months postoperative.

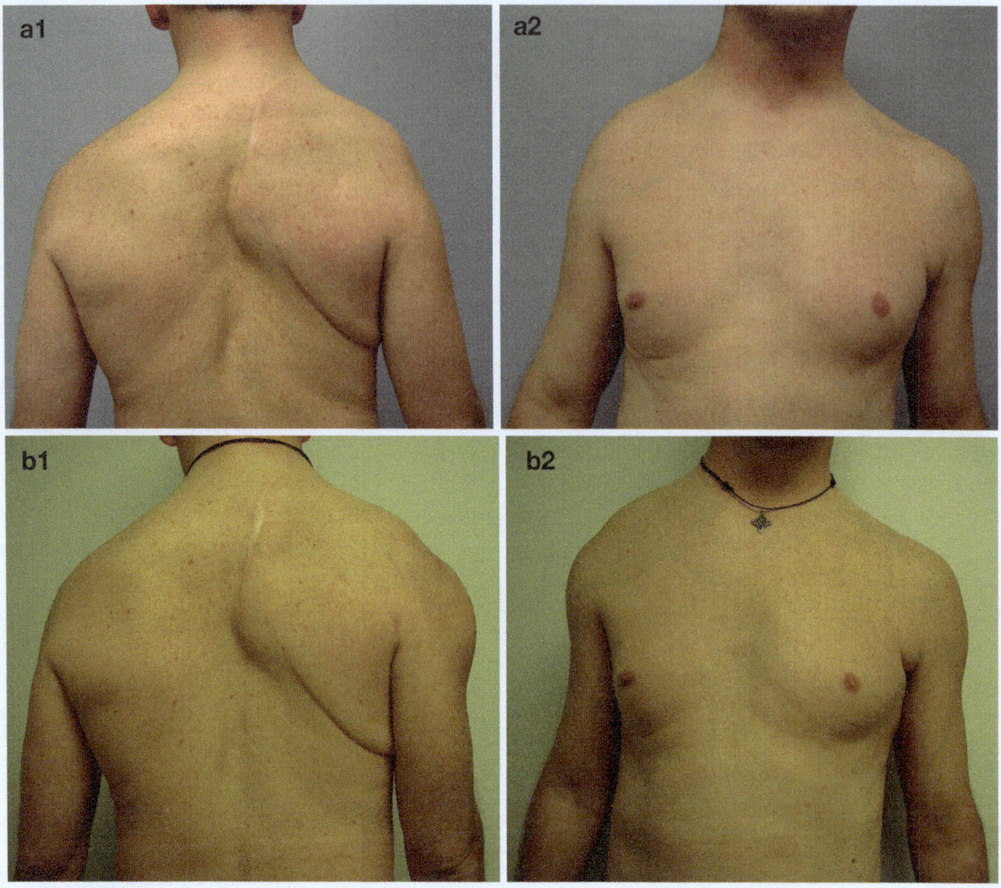

Fig. 9.15 (**a**) Preoperative. (**b**) Postoperative of first patient treated with custom deltoid implant to the right arm

Case 2 (Fig. 9.16)
A 49-year-old male who is an avid participant in physical fitness presented wanting to achieve further definition and size increase in the deltoid region. He underwent deltoid augmentation bilaterally using size 1 deltoid implants. The patient is shown preoperative and 6 months postoperative.

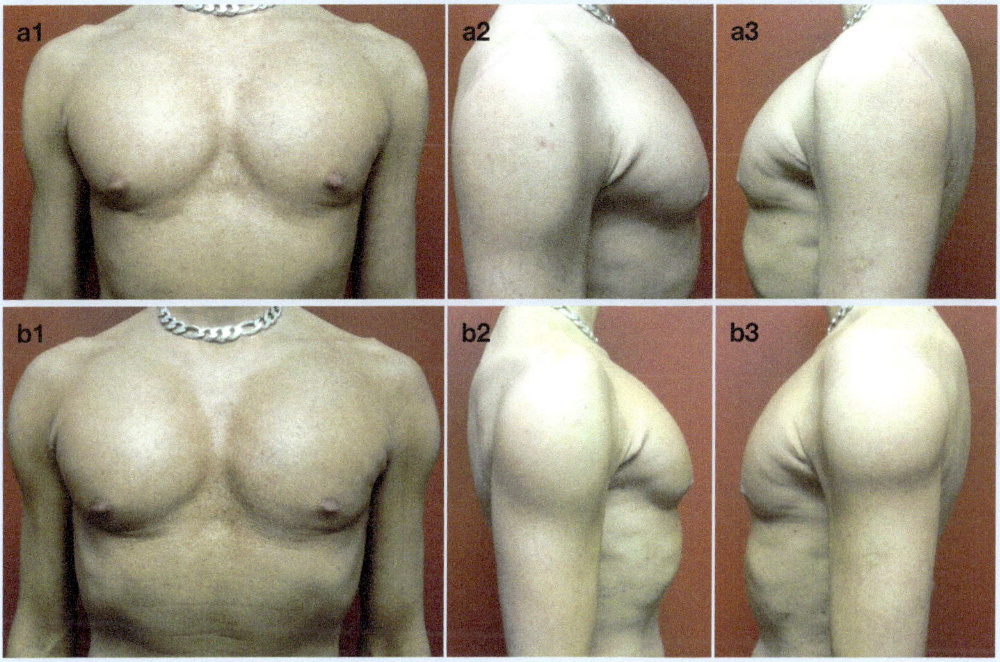

Fig. 9.16 (**a**) Preoperative. (**b**) Postoperative

Case 3 (Fig. 9.17)
A 37-year-old male presented for deltoid augmentation as he was unable to develop sufficient volume in his deltoid region despite an aggressive workout regimen. He underwent deltoid augmentation with size 1 deltoid implants and is shown preoperative and 1 month postoperative.

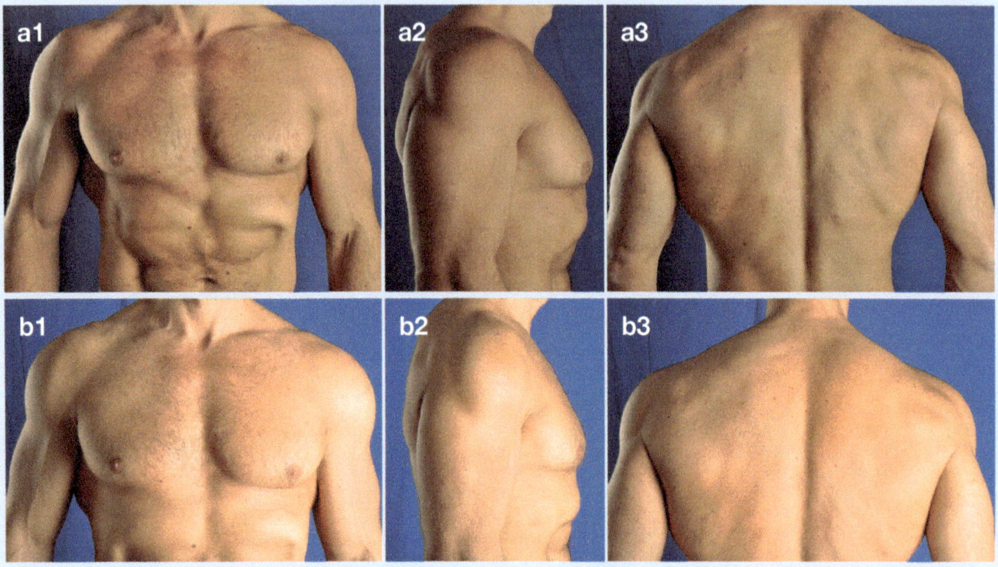

Fig. 9.17 (**a**) Preoperative. (**b**) Postoperative

Conclusions

A semisolid silicone implant can be used as a means of increasing volume to the lateral deltoid region to correct defects left following oncologic procedures, as a result of congenital defects, or following trauma. The implant can also be successfully used to augment a hypoplastic muscle in patients that are not able to achieve the desired results with conventional or even aggressive workout routines.

References

1. Siu KK, Ko JY, Huang CC, Wang FS, Chen JM, Wong T. Woodward procedure improves shoulder function in Sprengel deformity. Chang Gung Med J. 2011;34(4):403–8.
2. Saray A, Eskandari M, Oztuna V. Augmentation of shoulder contour using a calf implant. Aesthetic Plast Surg. 2000;24(5):386–8.
3. Hodgkinson DJ. Contour restoration of the upper limb using solid silicone implants. Aesthetic Plast Surg. 2006;30(1):53–8.
4. Klepps S, Auerbach J, Calhon O, Lin J, Cleeman E, Flatow E. A cadaveric study on the anatomy of the deltoid insertion and its relationship to the deltopectoral approach to the proximal humerus. J Shoulder Elbow Surg. 2004;13(3):322–7.
5. Hoppenfield S, deBoer P. Surgical exposures. In: Hoppenfield S, deBoer P, editors. Surgical exposures in orthopaedics: the anatomic approach. Philadelphia: Lippincott, Williams and Wilkins; 2003. p. 41–60.
6. Perlmutter GS. Axillary nerve injury. Clin Orthop Relat Res. 1999;368:28–36.
7. Lindsey WH, Davis PT. Facial keloids: a fifteen year experience. Arch Otolaryngol Head Neck Surg. 1997;123(4):397–400.
8. Leijnse JNAL, Han SH, Kwon YH. Morphology of deltoid origin and end tendons – a generic model. J Anat. 2008;213(6):733–42.
9. Potau JM, Bardina X, Ciurana N, Camprubí D, Pastor JF, de Paz F, Barbosa M. Quantitative analysis of the deltoid and rotator cuff muscles in humans and great apes. Int J Primatol. 2009;30(5): 697–708.

10. Gray H. Anatomy of the human body. Philadelphia: Lea & Febiger; 1918.
11. Wheeless CR III. Deltoid muscle. In: Wheeless CR III, editor. Wheeless' textbook of orthopaedics. Data Trace Internet Publishing, LLC; 2011. http://www.wheelesson.com/ortho/407. Accessed 20 Sept 2013.
12. Kontakis GM, Steriopoulos K, Damilakis J, Michalodimitrakis E. The position of the axillary nerve in the deltoid muscle: a cadaveric study. Acta Orthop Scand. 1999;70(1):9–11.
13. Cheung S, Fitzpatrick M, Lee TQ. Effects of shoulder position on axillary nerve positions during the split lateral deltoid approach. J Shoulder Elbow Surg. 2009;18(5):748–55.
14. Bastos EM, Neto MS, Alves MT, Garcia EB, Santos RA, Heink T, Pereira JB, Ferreira LM. Histologic analysis of zafirlukast's effect on capsule formation around silicone implants. Aesthetic Plast Surg. 2007;31(5):559–65.
15. Moreira M, Fagundes DJ, de Jesus Simões M, de Oliveira MC, Dos Santos Previdelli IT, Moreira AC. Zafirlukast pocket delivery impairs the capsule healing around textured implants in rats. Aesthetic Plast Surg. 2009;33(1):90–7.
16. Schlesinger SL, Ellenbogen R, Desvigne M, Svehlak S, Heck R. Zafirlukast (Accolate): a new treatment for capsular contracture. Aesthet Surg J. 2002;22(4): 329–36.
17. Bailie DS, Moseley B, Lowe WR. Surgical anatomy of the posterior shoulder: effects of arm position and anterior-inferior capsular shift. J Shoulder Elbow Surg. 1999;8(4):307–13.

10 Quadriceps Augmentation

Introduction

Solid silicone prostheses have been used in multiple areas of the body to give volume to an area that is devoid of substance either due to trauma or post-oncologic procedures and in those who suffer from hypoplasia of a given muscle group due to congenital myodystrophies. In the past decade, it has been the experience in the author's practice that patients are seeking for ways to bulk up further in muscle regions that may be unresponsive to conventional exercise routines. Recently, patients with HIV or on highly active antiretroviral therapy (HAART) have presented to the author's practice seeking bulk in areas that have been ravaged by muscle wasting. It was to that end that a custom silicone implant was devised for a patient to treat muscle wasting in the anterior thigh, which he found particularly vexing.

To further expand the use of a quadriceps implant, one may consider its use in patients that are fit but wish to further enhance the volume in the anterior compartment of the thigh. The quadriceps muscles make up the majority of the volume in the anterior thigh. A person that wishes to increase volume in the anterior thigh has to do more than just cardiovascular work but has to take time and focus in on building up the quadriceps muscles [1]. Many trainers and bodybuilding authors agree that an intensive bodybuilding routine is required to build muscle in the anterior thigh; for some, the intensity of this routine may be prohibitive in getting a "bulked up" quadriceps region.

Indications

Quadriceps augmentation surgery is indicated in patients that have a defect in the anterior thigh region after trauma or post-oncologic procedures. It is also indicated for augmentation of the anterior thigh due to muscle wasting. Finally, there may be a role for quadriceps augmentation in patients who persistently have hypoplasia of the anterior thigh and wish to have an enlarged thigh volume for cosmetic reasons.

Contraindications

Patients with HIV or on immunosuppression therapy are at increased risk of infections. This must be considered in counseling patients for surgery involving muscle implants. Furthermore, an HIV patient with a high viral load is likely not a good candidate as their systemic illness is not well controlled and may put them at risk for increased complications post-op.

Limitations

The current quadriceps implant does not alter the appearance of the vastus lateralis or medialis as it has not been developed to be that large in size and its augmentation scope is limited to the area immediately above the rectus femoris and vastus intermedius.

N.V. Chugay et al., *Body Sculpting with Silicone Implants*,
DOI 10.1007/978-3-319-04957-1_10, © Springer International Publishing Switzerland 2014

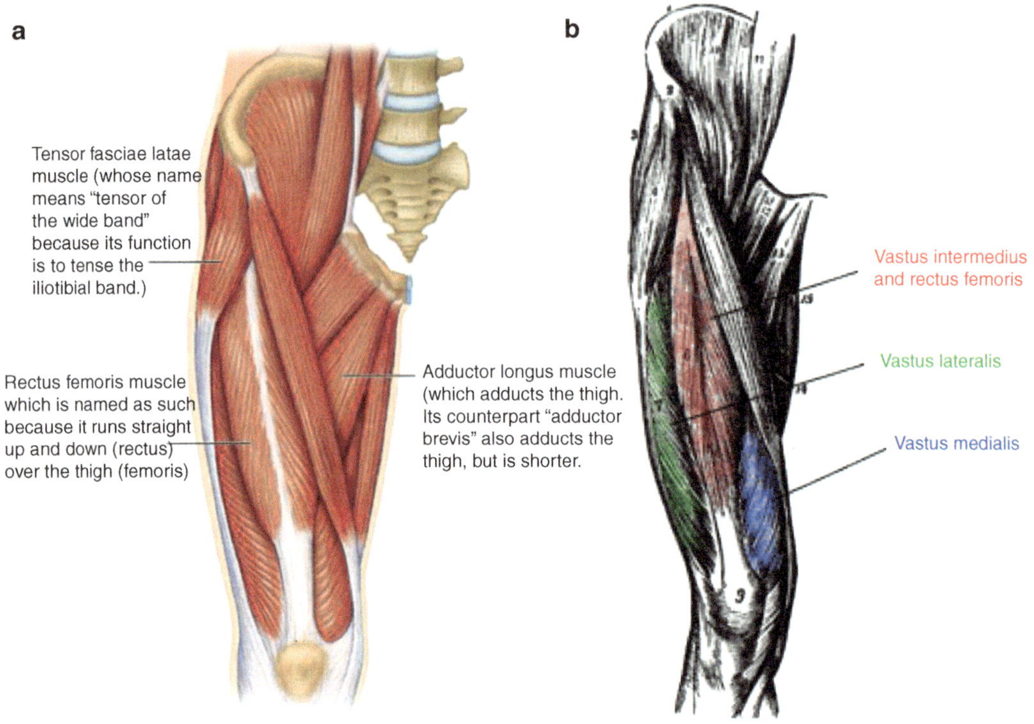

Fig. 10.1 Muscles of the anterior thigh

Relevant Anatomy

The quadriceps femoris (Latin for "four-headed muscle of the femur") is a large muscle group that includes the four prevailing muscles on the front of the thigh: rectus femoris, vastus lateralis, vastus intermedius, and vastus medialis (Fig. 10.1). These muscles act as the primary extensor muscles of the knee and form the volume of the anterior thigh region, overlying the femur. The quadriceps femoris is located in the anterior compartment of the thigh which is bounded by the inguinal ligament superiorly, the capsule of the knee inferiorly, the iliotibial tract laterally, and the femoral neurovascular bundle medially. The fascia overlying the muscles of the anterior compartment is divided into superficial and deep layers. The superficial fascia forms a continuous layer over the whole of the thigh. It consists of loose areolar tissue which is intermingled with fat. Deep to this is the deep investing fascia of the thigh. The deep fascia of the thigh is commonly referred to as the fascia lata. Just like the superficial fascia, it varies in thickness in different parts. It is thicker in the upper and lateral part of the thigh, where it receives a fibrous expansion from the gluteus maximus and where the tensor fasciae latae is inserted between its layers. It is very thin behind and at the upper and medial part of the thigh, where it covers the adductor muscles, and again becomes stronger around the knee. The anterior thigh is relatively free of neurovascular structures, with the majority of structures being deep to the femur or localized to the upper medial thigh (Fig. 10.2). The greater saphenous vein is transmitted through the superficial and deep layers of fascia at the fossa ovalis, located in the upper medial thigh. It is below the deep layer of fascia that the saphenous vein joins the femoral vessels and saphenous nerve (Fig. 10.3) [2]. With the proposed dissection for the anterior quadriceps augmentation, these structures are free from the risk of injury.

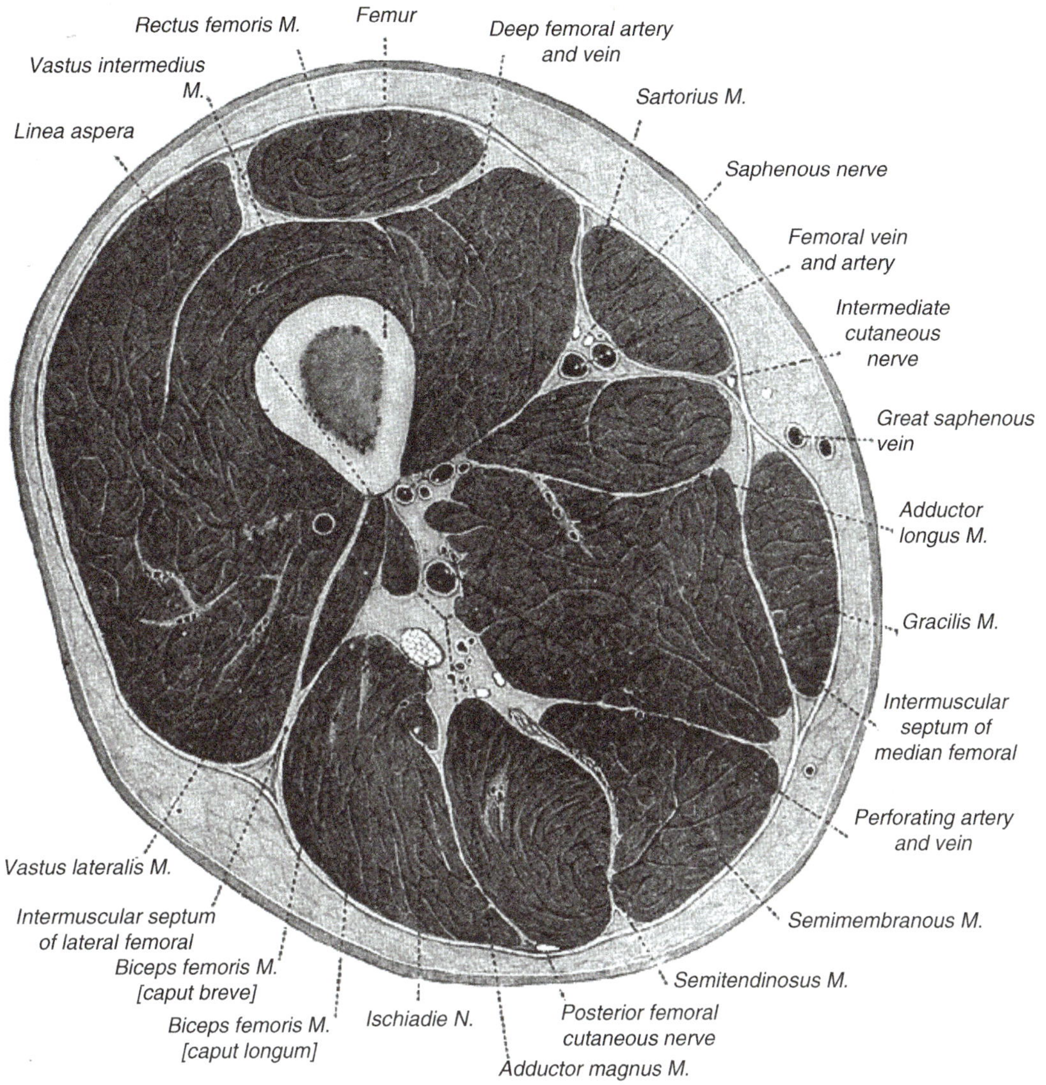

Fig. 10.2 Cross section through mid-thigh. Note the absence of major neurovascular structures in the area of the anterior thigh

Consultation/Implant Selection

A thorough history and physical are paramount to preventing complications at the time of quadriceps augmentation. For patients that do present with HIV or on HAART, further investigation regarding the state of their immunodeficiency should be made. If available, the patient's CD4 count should be requested. An inquiry into any remote or recent infections is made. Questions are posed regarding the patient's reasonable attempts to build the muscle with conventional means. If the patient is suffering from muscle wasting, then there should be an assessment of the reason for the wasting (e.g., muscular dystrophy, muscle wasting of HIV/HAART, inactivity, etc.). During the consultation, patient's expectations are managed and assessment of the patient's mental state is undertaken. It is made clear to the patient the expected augmentation that can be seen with augmentation and limitations of the procedure are also explained.

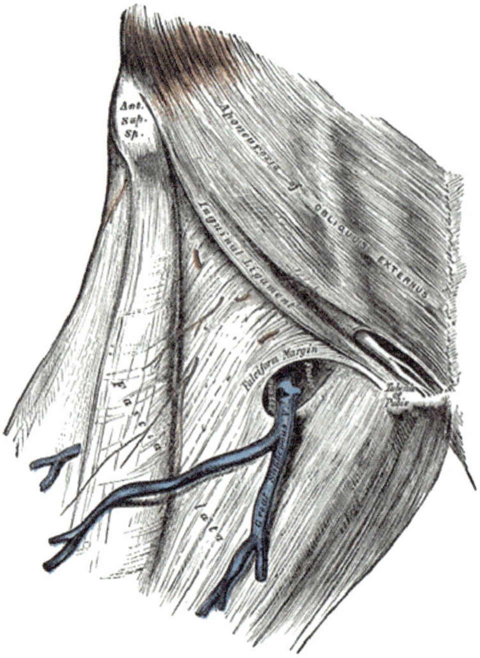

Fig. 10.3 Greater saphenous vein emptying into the femoral vein at the fossa ovalis in the medial thigh

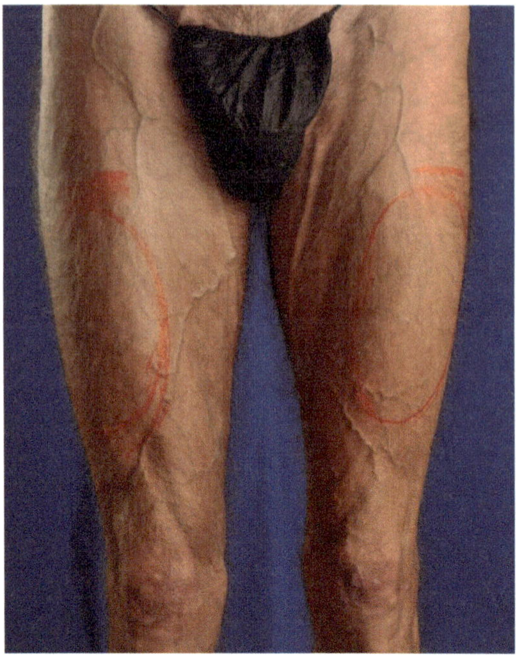

Fig. 10.4 Preoperative marking with location of incision and proposed site of implant

After completion of the history portion of the consultation, an evaluation of the patient's thigh is made. Any asymmetries or defects are pointed out to the patient. The patient's muscles are then evaluated. The skin and fat content are similarly assessed at this time as a patient with minimal adipose and thin skin is more at risk for implant palpability. Measurements of the patient's thighs are then taken: (1) circumference of the thigh at its midpoint and (2) length from the inguinal crease to the patella to ascertain the maximal size of the implant.

Available Implants: Custom-Made for Implantation by Dr. Chugay

The dimensions of the implant used for augmentation are as follows: 10.4 × 15 × 2.5 cm (Fig. 10.4).

Preoperative Planning and Marking

On the day of the surgery, the patient is met in the preoperative holding area. It is here that the patient's consent is verified and again risks, benefits, and alternatives are reviewed with the patient. With the patient in the erect position, the proposed site of incision is marked, measuring approximately 5–7 cm. The site of incision should be in the upper thigh, approximately 8–10 cm below the inguinal crease (Fig. 10.5). Once the site of the incision is marked, the site of the proposed implant is marked taking into account the patient's anatomy and existing deficit along with the desires of the patient.

Operative Technique

The patient is brought to the operative suite and placed in the supine position. Anesthesia is administered. The patient is then prepped and draped in sterile fashion after local infiltration of 25 mL of 1 % lidocaine with epinephrine to each anterior thigh region. Seven centimeter transverse incisions are made in each anterior thigh region in line with preoperative markings. The incisions are made with a 15 blade scalpel. Subsequently, dissection is performed through the subcutaneous tissues using a combination of blunt dissection and a hemostat. Dissection

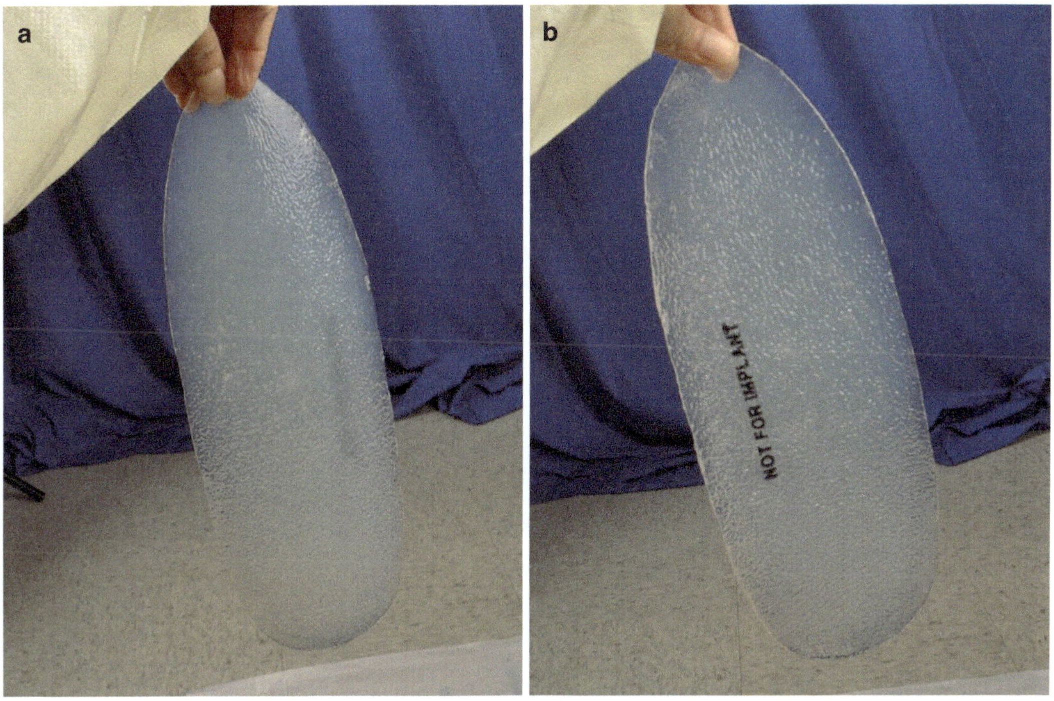

Fig. 10.5 (**a**, **b**) Second generation quadriceps implant for implantation custom-made for Chugay cosmetic. The tapered end (being held) would be placed caudally and the wider portion of the implant cranially, conforming to the normal anatomy of the leg. This implant has not yet been placed but has been created to fill out a larger area of the anterior thigh

is carried to the level of the deep quadriceps fascia. On reaching the fascia, a 15 blade scalpel is used to make a transverse incision (Fig. 10.6). This is then extended with Metzenbaum scissors medially and laterally. At this point 2-0 Vicryl stay sutures are placed in each section of the fascia (Fig. 10.7). A subfascial plane is then dissected over top the rectus femoris muscle using blunt finger dissection and a spatula dissector, ensuring an adequate plane for the implant in the anterior thigh (in line with preoperative markings/patient wishes) (Fig. 10.8). Once a sufficient pocket has been dissected, 15 mL of 0.5 % Marcaine is introduced into the pocket. The pocket is then irrigated with a solution containing normal saline, Betadine, 1 g of Ancef, and 80 mg of Gentamicin. A custom-made silicone implant is then placed into position, making sure to attain symmetry (Fig. 10.9). Once the implants have been placed, symmetry is assessed. At this point closure is begun. The fascia is re-approximated with 2-0 Vicryl suture in interrupted fashion (Fig. 10.10). The deep dermis is re-approximated with 2-0 Vicryl suture in buried fashion. The skin is closed in subcuticular fashion using 3-0 Monocryl Quill Suture. Benzoin and Robbins tape is applied as a dressing. The legs are wrapped with Coban and the patient is taken to postanesthesia care unit (PACU).

Postoperative Care/Instructions

Postoperatively the patient may begin ambulating starting on the evening of the procedure. They may shower on the second postoperative day, making sure to keep dressings clean and dry the Robbins tape with a hair dryer on a low-heat setting. Patients are then allowed to begin light activity at week 2 and full unrestricted activity at weeks 4–6. Patients are asked to wear an ACE wrap around the thigh for 4 weeks postoperatively to prevent dead space, thereby helping to reduce the risk of seroma formation. The legs are to be elevated as much as possible to allow for

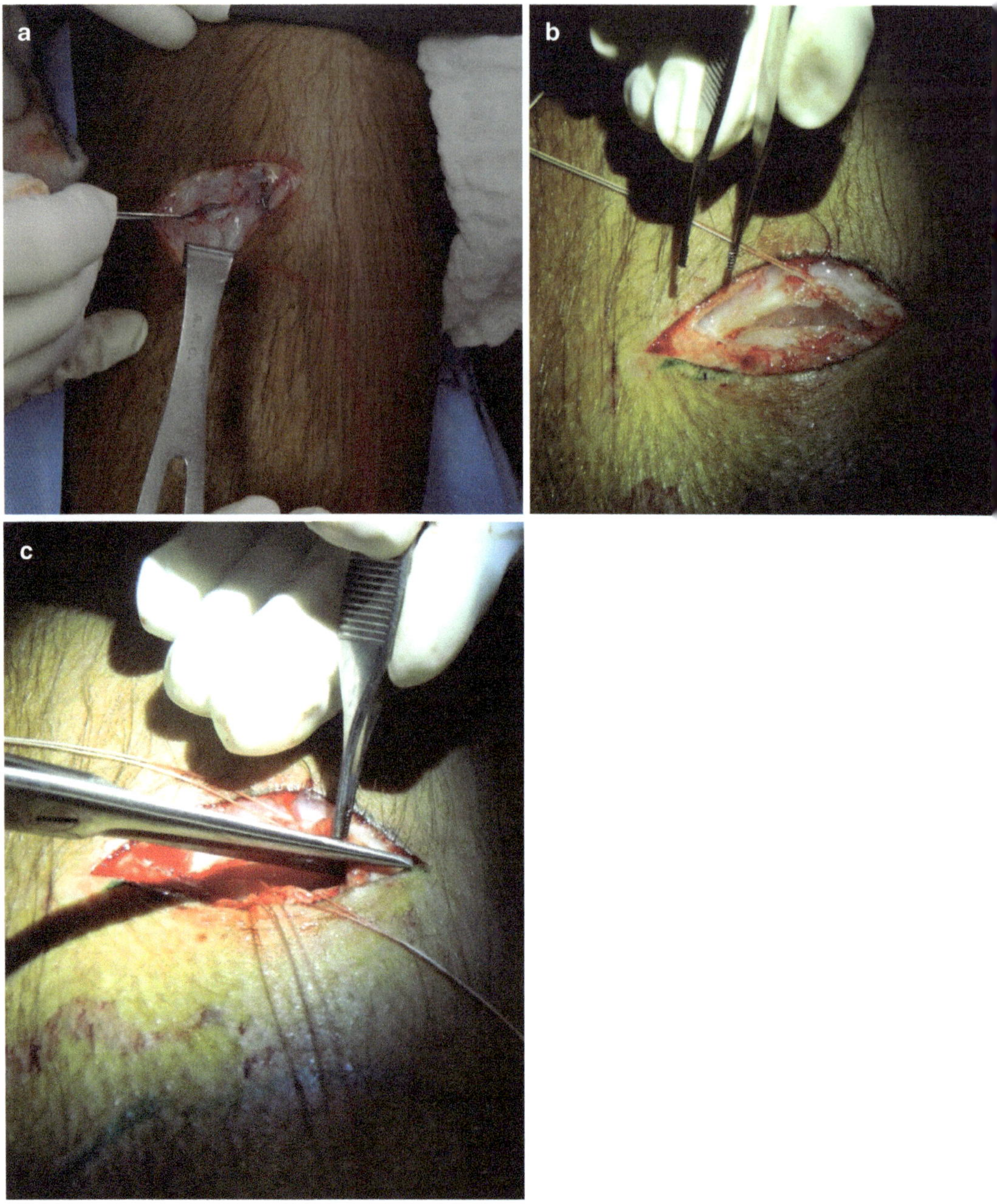

Fig. 10.6 (**a**) Initial incision in the quadriceps fascia. (**b**) Close-up view of incision in quadriceps fascia. (**c**) Extension of incision in quadriceps fascia medially and laterally using Metzenbaum scissors

better lymphatic/venous drainage. Patients are prescribed both narcotic analgesics along with muscle relaxants (diazepam 5 mg every 8 h as needed for spasm) to assist with postoperative pain.

Complications

In performing quadriceps augmentation, there is a host of complications that can arise (Table 10.1).

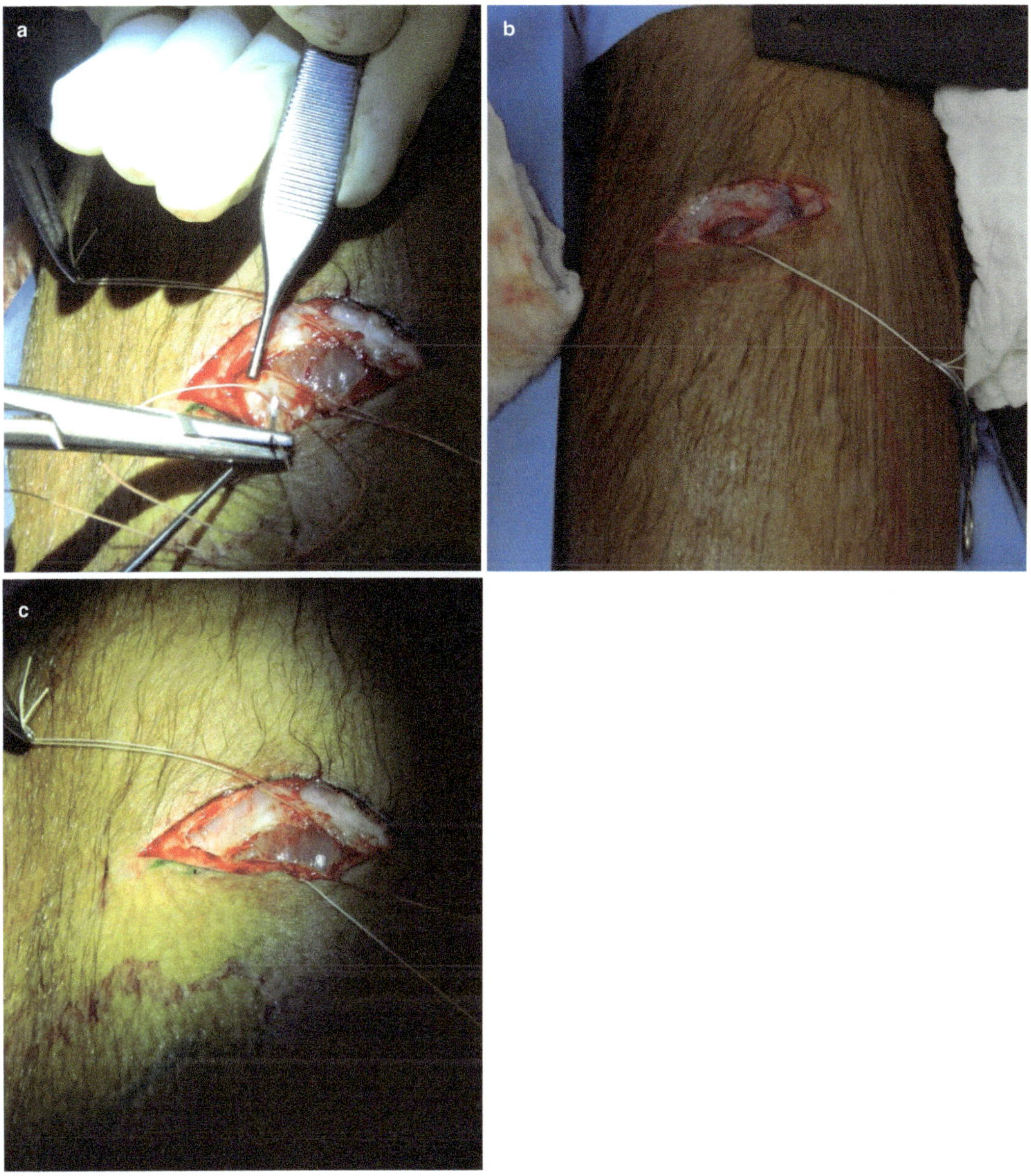

Fig. 10.7 (**a**) Placement of stay sutures in lower portion of quadriceps fascia. (**b**) Stay suture in lower quadriceps fascia (view from a distance). (**c**) Stay sutures in lower portion of quadriceps fascia and upper portion of quadriceps fascia (close). Note two sutures in lower portion of fascia to prevent caudal migration of fascia

Infection

Infection, either superficial or deep, is a possibility in quadriceps augmentation surgery. The most likely culprits would be staphylococcus aureus and streptococcus epidermidis, relatively common skin flora. Prior to making incision, standard practice should be the administration of 2 g of intravenous (IV) Ancef (or 300 mg IV clindamycin in a penicillin – or cephalosporin-allergic patient). During the procedure, irrigation of the pocket with a standard antibiotic solution containing normal saline, Betadine, Ancef, and gentamicin should be performed. Postoperatively, a 5–10-day regimen of oral antibiotics covering normal skin flora should be administered. If a

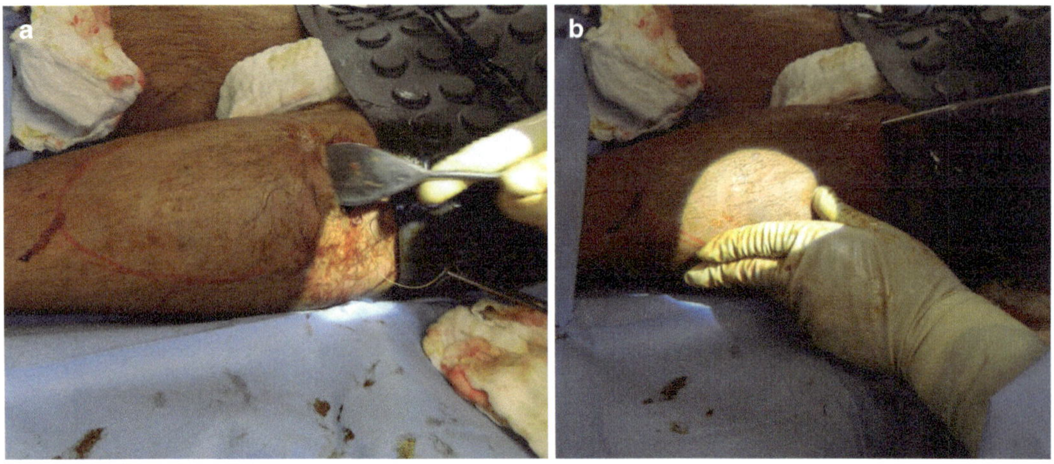

Fig. 10.8 (a) Spatula used for dissection of subfascial pocket in blunt manner. (b) Spatula dissector in position at lateral aspect of pocket, using the external markings as a guide for minimized dissection of the pocket

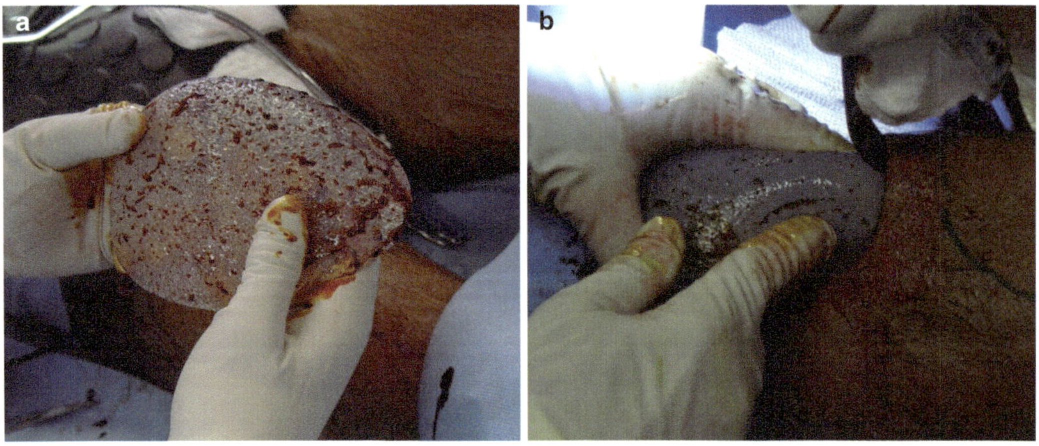

Fig. 10.9 (a) Quadriceps implant covered in Betadine. (b) Implant being placed into left subfascial plane with a folding motion of the implant so as not to require a larger incision at the skin and fascial level

deep infection occurs, the standard of practice is removal of the implant, closure, and possible reimplantation in 3–6 months. There are reports in other forms of implant surgery that conservative management and implant salvage are possible. This should be left at the discretion of the surgeon and performed with careful counseling of the patient. The authors did have a delayed infection that occurred in the one patient. This infection is discussed in further detail below

Seroma

Seromas are statistically the most common complication occurring in implant surgeries. They typically present as new-onset pain, swelling, or asymmetry. The treatment of choice remains percutaneous aspiration. This complication is best prevented with patient compliance with compression stockings and proper implant placement at the time of surgery, thereby minimizing dead space.

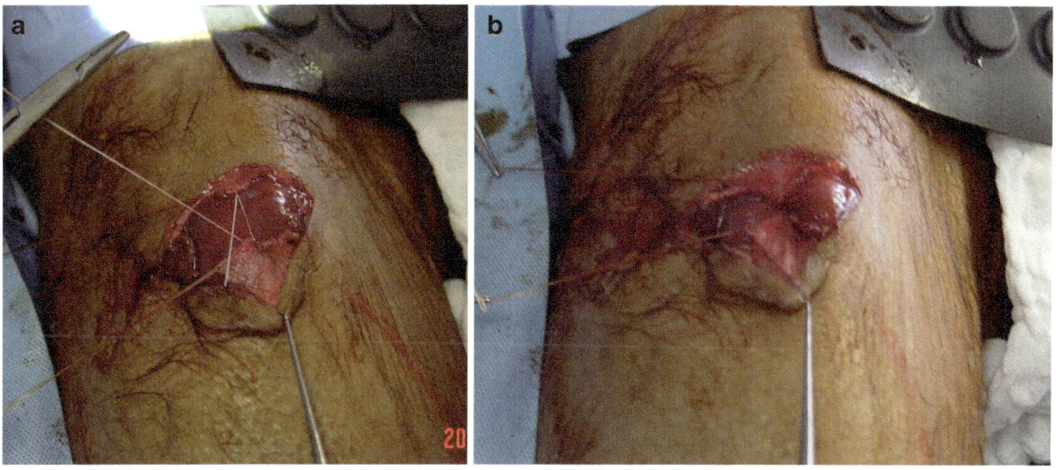

Fig. 10.10 (**a**) 2-0 Vicryl suture being used to approximate quadriceps fascia with rectus femoris visualized (close-up). (**b**) Initial suture approximating quadriceps fascia with further sutures needed medially and laterally to fully approximate fascia

Table 10.1 Potential complications of quadriceps augmentation

Potential complications of quadriceps augmentation surgery
Infection
Seroma
Hematoma
Asymmetry
Implant visibility
Hypertrophic scarring
Hyperpigmentation of the scar
Capsular contracture
Wound dehiscence
Nerve injury (permanent or temporary, motor or sensory)
Compartment syndrome

Hematoma

Although a rare occurrence due to the relatively avascular plane of dissection for the quadriceps augmentation procedure, a hematoma is always a possibility in surgical procedure. In the event of a hematoma, rapid evacuation, pocket irrigation, and reimplantation are the mainstays of therapy. This complication is best prevented by meticulous hemostasis at the time of surgery and good compression of the thigh post-op to prevent potential space creation.

Asymmetry

This can occur as a product of preexisting variability in the patient's legs or variability in dissection of the pocket bilaterally. This is best minimized by good preoperative photography and noting any asymmetries preoperatively. To avoid creation of asymmetry, it is important to maintain the same pattern of dissection and pocket creation bilaterally.

Implant Visibility

Due to the subfascial placement of the implant, this is indeed a rare complication. However, those patients that have very thin and atrophic legs to begin with may suffer from implant palpability and visibility. Patients should be counseled on this fact preoperatively if there is a feeling that the patient could be at risk.

Scar Hyperpigmentation and Hypertrophy

The key to reduction of these problems is careful layered closure. Patients with a history of keloid or hypertrophic scar formation may require the use of steroid injected at the site of incision.

Capsular Contracture

This is a possible late sequela of any implant placement, most frequently described in the breast augmentation literature. In the event that a patient presents with signs/symptoms of capsular contracture (e.g. induration of the implant site, tightness in the leg, new-onset pain, new-onset swelling), ultrasound or CT evaluation of the affected extremity is warranted. If a capsule is identified, typically characterized by calcifications, then a partial or complete capsulectomy is warranted. Capsular contracture is best prevented by meticulous hemostasis, good sterile technique, and avoidance of bleeding in the postoperative period.

Wound Dehiscence

Wound dehiscence is a product of poor wound closure under too much tension typically. In order to prevent this, meticulous closure in three layers is paramount: fascia, deep dermis, and skin.

Nerve Injury

Due to the avascular and relatively structure free dissection performed in the vast majority of cases, permanent nerve injury is rarely a problem. It is quite common for patients to complain of some numbness over the area of the anterior thigh postoperatively; however, this returns within 1–3 months postoperatively.

Compartment Pressure Problems/Compartment Syndrome

Compartment syndromes, typically seen in trauma, involve an acute increase in pressure inside a closed space, thereby impairing blood flow to the affected space and potentially putting the limb at risk for loss. Clinical signs of compartment syndrome include the 6 Ps: pain, poikilothermia, pallor, paresthesias, paralysis, and pulselessness. In conscious patients, pain out of proportion to examination is the prominent symptom. Pain with passive range of motion is particularly troubling. Compartment syndrome of the anterior thigh, while rare, has been reported and should be considered in the patient that presents with unexplained pain out of proportion to the examination [3–5]. In those patients that do present with anterior thigh compartment syndrome, removal of the implant would be recommended. However, there is data to support conservative management in isolated compartment syndrome of the anterior thigh as it is a very large space and difficult to cause significant vascular collapse as the majority of the structures lay deep in the thigh [4].

Discussion

Muscle wasting in HIV-infected individuals is quite common, affecting an estimated 20 % of patients [6, 7]. The Centers for Disease Control and Prevention defines HIV/AIDS wasting syndrome as the involuntary weight loss of greater than 10 % baseline body weight during the previous 12 months or a 5 % loss of weight during the previous 6 months [8]. The wasting in HIV/AIDS is characterized by reductions in lean body mass or fat-free mass, of which skeletal muscle makes up 50–54 % of lean body mass [9]. This wasting syndrome is typically characterized and accompanied by not only the weight loss but also diarrhea, fever, malnutrition, depression, poor appetite, and weakness. Researchers advocate a multimodal approach to treatment of muscle wasting syndrome including a balanced high-protein diet, a regular resistance training workout routine, supplementation of testosterone, supplementation of growth hormone, and possible anabolic steroid use to help maintain and prevent lean muscle mass loss [6, 10]. However, even with these recommended therapies, some patients still cannot achieve the improvement that they would like. Although a quadriceps implant does not solve the underlying problem of HIV wasting, it can improve the mental state of the patient. The patient is given a boost in self-confidence which may improve their quality of life in the long term.

Authors' Personal Experience

To date, the authors have performed one quadriceps augmentation procedure for muscle wasting with aesthetically pleasing results.

Case 1

A 42-year-old with HIV (JM) presented with muscle wasting in the anterior thigh that had become increasingly noticeable since his initial diagnosis and initiation of HAART therapy. Despite a rigorous resistance exercise routine, he was unable to develop or maintain definition in the anterior thigh region to his satisfaction. He suffered from hypertension in addition to HIV. His medications included benazepril and cardizem for hypertension and his antiviral regimen consisting of Prezista, Norvir, Truvada, Retrovir, and Intelence. His laboratory studies were unremarkable beyond the positive HIV test and the mildly elevated triglyceride level of 207 mg/dL (normal range 0–150). A custom implant was created based on measurement of the patient's thigh, resulting in an implant that measured $10.4 \times 15 \times 2.5$ cm. The implant volume was 207 mL. The patient's surgery was uneventful, with successful placement of the implant below the deep quadriceps fascia (Fig. 10.11).

Five months after his augmentation had been completed, the patient presented to the emergency room complaining of redness and tenderness in his right anterior thigh. A CBC was obtained, demonstrating a WBC of 18.2. A CT scan of the leg demonstrated a fluid collection surrounding the implant with dots of air consistent with an abscess. The collection extending from 8 cm above the implant to approximately 1.7 cm below the implant and measured up to 1 cm in maximal thickness. The patient was taken to the operating room for removal of the right quadriceps implant, drainage of a 100 mL collection of purulent fluid, and placement of drains. The fluid was sent for culture and grew streptococcus. The patient was placed on intravenous (IV) antibiotics and had a resolution of his elevated white blood cell count over the course of 3 days. The patient was discharged home on oral Augmentin 875 mg for a course of 10 days.

The patient presented to our office 2 months after drainage of his abscess for re-augmentation of the right quadriceps region as he was so happy with the result of the left quadriceps. The same size custom implant was then placed into the right thigh without incident. At the time of publication of this text, he is one month after his second operation to replace the right thigh implant and has had no complications or sequelae.

After speaking with the patient, it was noted that he had suffered an upper respiratory tract infection 1 week prior to his right implant infection. It is felt that the patient had a seeding of the implant bed with the streptococcus which then produced the remote infection 5 months after his initial surgery. Another contributing factor may be the patient's ongoing battle with HIV and his continued antiretroviral regimen.

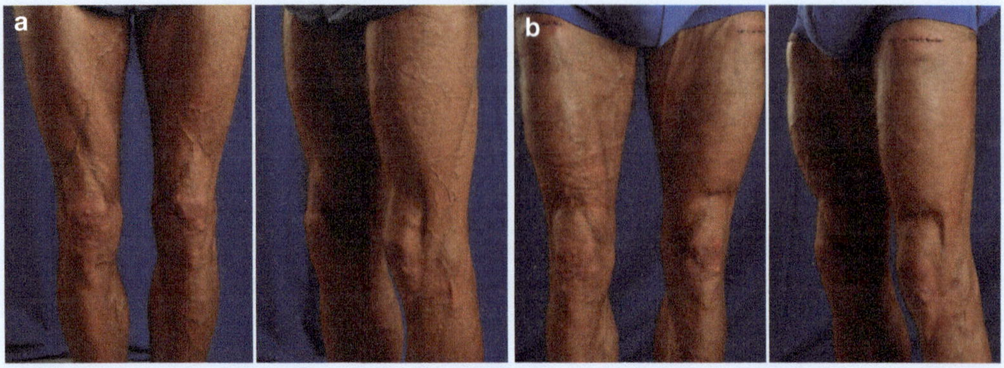

Fig. 10.11 (**a**) Preoperative. (**b**) One week postoperative

Conclusions

A semisolid silicone implant can be used as a means of increasing volume to the anterior thigh in patients with HIV or on HAART and may have a role in purely cosmetic augmentation of the anterior thigh.

References

1. Rivera H. Bodybuilding training principles for creating quadriceps routines: get bigger & defined quads with these bodybuilding quadriceps routines. http://www.bodybuilding.about.com. Accessed 20 Sept 2013.
2. Gray H. Anatomy of the human body. Philadelphia: Lea & Febiger; 1918.
3. Verwiebe EG, Kanlic EM, Saller J, Abdelgawad A. Thigh compartment syndrome, presentation and complications. Bosn J Basic Med Sci. 2009;9 Suppl 1:28–33.
4. Robinson D, On E, Halperin N. Anterior compartment syndrome of the thigh in athletes–indications for conservative treatment. J Trauma. 1992;32(2):183–6.
5. Schwartz Jr JT, Brumback RJ, Lakatos R, Poka A, Bathon GH, Burgess AR. Acute compartment syndrome of the thigh: a spectrum of injury. J Bone Joint Surg Am. 1989;71(3):392–400.
6. Dudgeon WD, Philips KD, Carson JA, Brewer RB, Durstine JL. Counteracting muscle wasting in HIV-infected individuals. HIV Med. 2006;7(5):299–310.
7. Wanke CA, Silva M, Knox TA, Forrester J, Speigelman D, Gorbach SL. Weight loss and wasting remain common complications in individuals infected with human immunodeficiency virus in the era of highly active antiretroviral therapy. Clin Infect Dis. 2000;31(3):803–5.
8. Centers for Disease Control. Revision of the CDC surveillance case definition for acquired immunodeficiency syndrome. MMWR Morb Mortal Wkly Rep. 1987;36(Suppl 1S):1S–15S.
9. Clarys JP, Martin AD, Drinkwater DT. Gross tissue weights in the human body by cadaver dissection. Hum Biol. 1984;56(3):459–73.
10. Kressy J, Wanke C, Gerrior J. Unintentional weight loss/wasting. Tufts University HIV Resources. http://medicine.tufts.edu/Education/Academic-Departments/Clinical-Departments/Public-Health-and-Community-Medicine/Nutrition-and-Infection-Unit/Research/Nutrition-and-Health-Topics/Unintentional-Weight-Loss-Wasting

GPSR Compliance

The European Union's (EU) General Product Safety Regulation (GPSR) is a set of rules that requires consumer products to be safe and our obligations to ensure this.

If you have any concerns about our products, you can contact us on ProductSafety@springernature.com

In case Publisher is established outside the EU, the EU authorized representative is:

Springer Nature Customer Service Center GmbH
Europaplatz 3
69115 Heidelberg, Germany

Batch number: 10732758

Printed by Printforce, the Netherlands